Modern Hip Resurfacing

Edited by

Derek J.W. McMinn, FRCS
McMinn Centre, Birmingham, United Kingdom

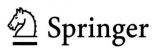 Springer

Derek J.W. McMinn, FRCS
The McMinn Centre, Birmingham, UK

ISBN 978-1-84800-087-2   e-ISBN 978-1-84800-088-9
DOI 10.1007/978-1-84800-088-9

British Library Cataloguing in Publication Data
A catalogue record for this book is available from the British Library

Library of Congress Control Number: 2007943250

Printed on acid-free paper

9 8 7 6 5 4 3 2 1

springer.com

Modern Hip Resurfacing

To the memory of my mother and father,
whose foresight and hard work
allowed me to come from a humble background
and become the first member
of our extended family to
attend university and medical school.

Foreword

When Derek McMinn first told me that he was writing a book about hip resurfacing, I wondered what the book would be entitled, and we discussed this for a short while. My advice was that he should call it: "Hip Resurfacing—How I Made It Work." His immediate reaction was that this title was far too arrogant and would not accurately convey the subject matter of his proposed book. His modesty on this occasion was completely at odds with the mindset required to bulldoze through one of the most controversial devices to be thrust upon the orthopedic market during the past generation. This single-mindedness should have surprised no one—it was precisely this characteristic that he used to ensure a stay of execution for the Royal Orthopaedic Hospital from imminent closure in the early 1990s. His public quip, "The Mr. Blobby School of Accounting," led to the early demise of several promising managerial careers. Freed from the constraints of everyday public practice, he turned his attention toward his pursuit of a lasting solution for the young arthritic hip.

Harboring thoughts after a period of research ironically funded by a Sir John Charnley fellowship at the end of the 1980s, it became abundantly clear to Derek that metal on metal bearing technology had been dismissed far too early and without valid reason. His busy clinical practice as a revision hip surgeon inevitably placed him in close proximity both with failing and successful implants. Fortunately, our predecessors in Birmingham had used a variety of metal on metal prostheses; Derek's insight was to see the wood from the trees—to spot the winning features of an implant whether it be metallurgy, fixation, or geometry. As a result of his clinical observation of many metal on metal bearings enduring over 20 years, Derek was convinced that the metal on metal bearing could offer a solution for the problems of the young adult hip.

At the end of the 1980s apart from the Sulzer group, no one in the world was contemplating a future for the metal on metal bearing, and certainly no one else envisaged a resurgence in hip resurfacing. The notion that a marriage of these two failed concepts would result in a viable option was beyond reasonable comprehension. It was going to take force of personality to convince, first, a manufacturer, and, second, the public to embrace such a procedure. It was in the face of considerable opposition, and with dogged determination not to be deflected from the intended course, that hip resurfacing finally became successful.

Passing acquaintances in bars and fleeting encounters at conferences have all laid claims to the paternity of modern-day hip resurfacing, but the reality is that such claims have only emerged with the benefit of hindsight. The insight that metal on metal bearings may work in a resurfacing scenario clearly was not in itself enough to have a significant impact on the global market; it was only meticulous attention to detail and strength of character that allowed this goal to be achieved.

In the early days, metal on metal and hip resurfacing provoked little reaction apart from faint amusement at the folly of the venture; as the project gathered momentum, however, the establishment and the industry in particular grew increasingly uneasy, cries of "maverick surgeons" and "irresponsibility" were initially muttered, but finally the issue grudgingly found its way on to the agendas of boardrooms around the world.

Gradually, a groundswell of positive opinion driven by the patients themselves emerged. The cat was out of the bag, the public possibly empowered by the Internet were ahead of the game; they *knew* that metal on metal resurfacing worked. Milestones were passed, papers published, and approvals gained, and finally the nightmare of the "trade" was realized. Conglomerates were too unwieldy, too introspective, and too timid to react. One by one over the years, they posed in the friendly guise of acquisition for this technology but predictably they came to spy and copy. Finally, when an honest approach did present itself and was accepted, the ball was no longer ours to run with, the pace of the game no longer ours to dictate—what relief, what disappointment!

Subsequent approval was gained in the U.S. market, and a whole new continent opened up to the technology that McMinn had been involved with, and believed in, for nearly 20 years. The opportunity to launch the product on a grateful and receptive public and professional population without the bad grace and disapproval endured a decade before has perhaps been the most pleasurable reward in this extraordinary journey.

We cannot however be complacent, the future of resurfacing is yet unsure, confounding factors in arthroplasty are always just around the corner. Certainly, the future form of devices will change over the coming years, and vigilance is required for all of our patients both clinically and scientifically. In this book, the priority given to the basic science of the metal on metal bearing and its influence on host tissues is a reflection of the importance attached to it and the recognition that future developments can only come out of a more thorough understanding of past and present practice. We are only just beginning to learn.

In 1993, I presented initial results of metal on metal hip resurfacing at the SICOT meeting in Seoul, South Korea; there were seven delegates in the auditorium! Nowadays, no arthroplasty conference is complete without acknowledging hip resurfacing. Twenty-five years ago, Capello suggested that hip resurfacing merely had to demonstrate *equivalence* to total hip replacement to become the treatment of choice. I suggest that this time is approaching, and the individual responsible for this change of philosophy is the author and editor of this book.

Ronan B.C. Treacy
Birmingham, UK
August 2007

Preface

It was 1987, and the orthopedic world was still coming to terms with a steady stream of long-term failures of metal on polyethylene total hip arthroplasties. Although Hans Georg Willert had published his theory that polyethylene wear–induced osteolysis was the most likely cause of these failures, the debate was still on—many still believed it to be cement disease, intraarticular pressure, or some other unknown cause. Having completed my orthopedic training, I decided to work on a fellowship for a year before taking up a position as an orthopedic consultant. One of the projects I undertook during my fellowship was to review the 10- to 20-year outcomes of Charnley hip replacements that had been performed at the Royal Orthopaedic Hospital in Birmingham since 1966. During my fellowship, I also carried out a large number of revision procedures, and it was clear that revision arthroplasty was going to form a major part of my work over the coming years. During that year, I had the privilege of spending time with Prof. Hans Bucholz and Dr. Eckart Engelbrecht at the Endo-Klinik in Hamburg, with Drs. John Insall and Chit Ranawat at the Hospital for Special Surgery in New York, and with Dr. Bill Harris in Boston learning new techniques in primary and revision arthroplasty.

Toward the end of that year, I was appointed as a consultant to the Royal Orthopaedic Hospital, Birmingham, the oldest orthopedic speciality hospital in the United Kingdom, and wasted no time building up a busy revision joint arthroplasty service. I had to deal not only with in-house referrals but also received a considerable number of difficult cases from colleagues in the West Midlands region covering a population of more than 5 million people. I became adept at techniques such as cementless reconstruction of the deficient acetabulum and reconstruction of the very deficient femur.

Of course, I was also seeing a large number of elderly patients, predominately women, with excellent clinical and radiographic outcomes many years after their Charnley flat back stemmed total hip replacements. However, my revision hip clinics were populated by a completely different group of patients who were in general younger, more active, and predominately men. Furthermore, in this younger population, I was being referred an increasing number of patients for their second, third, or fourth hip revision operations, with each revision operation having failed in a shorter time than did the previous total hip replacement. I started to come to the view that what was a good hip arthroplasty for an elderly, inactive patient would not necessarily be good for a younger, more active patient.

I had been introduced to the concept of hip resurfacing during my orthopedic training, having assisted a number of my senior colleagues with the Wagner hip resurfacing prosthesis. As the new arthroplasty surgeon, I revised many of those patients as well with disappointingly early failures. My own observations from those revision operations and the work of others confirmed that the mode of failure in these resurfacings, where a metal or ceramic head had been articulating on a conventional polyethylene acetabular component, was osteolysis from large volumes of polyethylene debris. It was obvious that Sir John Charnley was spot on when he encouraged joint replacement surgeons to use a small-diameter femoral head on polyethylene total hip replacement in order to reduce the volume of polyethylene debris generated.

Follow-up of another group of patients, however, in my outpatient clinics was particularly revealing with respect to femoral head size. Seven of my senior colleagues at the Royal Orthopaedic Hospital had performed three different varieties of large-headed metal on metal total hip replacements. These patients did not get bearing-related osteolysis at long-term follow-up. It became clear to me that if resurfacing arthroplasty was to be resurrected, then a practical alternative available at the time would be to use a large-headed metal on metal articulation in the resurfacing arthroplasty. Although metal on metal total hip replacements and metal on polyethylene surface replacements had been used at the Royal Orthopaedic Hospital before, both operations had now been abandoned. This was also the situation in most joint replacement centers across the world. Hence, I knew that I had a difficult task; the challenge of combining these two failed systems into what I believed held the clue to a successful arthroplasty procedure and to convince others that we could successfully work toward that goal.

I approached Dr. Ian Brown, managing director of Zimmer Ltd (Swindon, UK), during 1988, and we began discussing how to develop a metal on metal surface replacement for the hip. He had experience of manufacture of metal on metal bearings in the past and was well disposed to the metal on metal resurfacing concept, but after a year, during which time we had an outline of the femoral and the acetabular component design characteristics, Zimmer UK required permission from their parent company in the United States before they could proceed with the project. Zimmer appointed one of their lead surgeon designers from the United States to adjudicate on this matter, and he flatly turned the idea down on the grounds that "surgeons are just not asking for that type of replacement."

I then approached a number of other orthopedic manufacturers who dismissed the idea of a metal on metal surface replacement as insane. Eventually, I was introduced to Mr. Peter Gibson, chairman of Corin Medical Ltd (Cirencester, UK). To my surprise, he had an excellent grasp of the benefits of putting metal on metal and resurfacing arthroplasty concepts together and soon convened a meeting. It was attended by Mr. Mike Tuke, managing director of Finsbury Instruments Ltd (Leatherhead, UK), who had experience in the past of manufacturing the Freeman hip resurfacing; Mr. George Cremore, manufacturing director of Corin Medical Ltd, who had had experience of supervising the manufacture of thousands of metal on metal joint replacements as a young man; Mr. Gibson himself; and me.

At the first meeting, we agreed to proceed with the project, but in order to reduce development cost, they believed that they could start with only one component size. However, I managed to talk them out of that and insisted on having three component sizes available. They wished to use the cobalt chrome castings from the Freeman SLF cup, which they already manufactured, and Mr. Michael Freeman kindly gave permission for his design of cup to be used as the acetabular component for my first resurfacing.

By February 1991, we were ready for the first implantation. Quite unbeknown to me, Prof. Heinz Wagner had been having similar thoughts, and he, too, inserted his first metal on metal hip resurfacing design in February 1991. I had previously visited Heinz Wagner and knew him to be a supreme technical surgeon and from our discussions at meetings respected him as a thoughtful innovator in the field of joint reconstruction. I took great comfort as a young consultant at that time, knowing that there was at least one other surgeon on the same wavelength. I encountered massive opposition from my surgical colleagues both in the United Kingdom and abroad to the idea of a metal on metal resurfacing in subsequent years, and the support from Heinz Wagner kept me going in the teeth of vicious criticism.

This book is an account of my experience with hip resurfacing, starting with the lessons learned from failures of the Wagner polyethylene-containing resurfacings, the challenges we faced solving the issue of fixation of components in the early years, the problems with manufacturing and metallurgy we inadvertently encountered, the solutions to those problems, and finally the development of the Birmingham Hip Resurfacing. My colleagues and I describe herein the Birmingham Hip Resurfacing from concept to 10 years of experience including a major section on surgical technique. This book is an effort to educate orthopedic surgeons on the lessons we learned in an attempt to prevent unnecessary failures for patients in the future.

Derek J.W. McMinn
Birmingham, UK
August 2007

Acknowledgments

It is a pleasure to acknowledge the very considerable help of my wife, Jane McMinn, FRCS, FRCR, at every stage of this hip resurfacing adventure. From the beginning, she allowed me considerable time away from the family pursuing my clinical and research activities and as the resurfacing project took shape supported me in good times and, more usually, in bad times. When the McMinn resurfacing project with Corin went sour, she was a tower of strength. She believed in hip resurfacing and in my ability to turn this into a reliable and durable procedure. The Birmingham Hip Resurfacing (BHR) development could not have happened without Jane's help. For this book, she has turned my scribbles into vaguely presentable English. She has taken on the role of "editor's minder" and has painstakingly proofread and corrected all 31 chapters. She has helped me all these years in her spare time between being director of the Breast Unit at City Hospital (Birmingham, UK) bringing up our three sons, not to mention looking after three dogs, a cat, 500 acres of land, and her prize flock of Dorset Down sheep.

Ronan Treacy joined my team as a registrar and later as a senior registrar and then as fellow. As chairman of the Medical Staff Committee, I led a 2-year campaign to save the Royal Orthopaedic Hospital (Birmingham, UK) from closure. This was ultimately successful, and even at a young age, Ronan had some very good advice to give on tactics. I knew he was a man who could be relied on, and it was a pleasure to join him in the Midland Medical Technologies (MMT) phase of our lives. He has had a huge part to play in this renaissance of the resurfacing procedure. As a young surgeon, he took an enormous risk in our joint development of the BHR. I valued his judgment then and still do when it comes to making tough decisions. In life, one meets people who disappear when the going gets tough; this is when Ronan is perfectly calm and is at his brilliant best. Ronan and I are complete opposites. We have been through some troublesome times, but I can honestly say that we have never had a disagreement over the past 10 years. This is all the more amazing as I seem to have an argument with my shadow most sunny days!

The theatre (operating room) staff at Birmingham Nuffield Hospital have been fantastic over the years. Every surgeon who visits me wants to steal these staff members. They have tolerated droves of visitors over the years, tolerated my obsessional neurotic tendencies, and treated every one of my patients with the respect and care I would want as a patient myself. They have also treated me very well as a patient on 3 occasions. To the current bosses David Stoten and Sue Bliss, I say thank you.

My staff at the McMinn Centre work tirelessly to deliver a good clinical service and produce a good deal of research work. To Pam Charles and her team, well done. This book has tested the strength and resolve of every member of our small team. Joseph Daniel, Hena Ziaee, and Chandra Pradhan have worked very hard over the years to capture the information. Ed Shovelton, Peter Austin, and Claire Doyle in our Media Department have done great work over the past years presenting this information, and hopefully this will be reflected in the quality of the finished book. As I type this piece, all the members of our team are in the office working on the book chapters at 11 PM. To all the members of my team, I promise never to write another book.

The contributors of chapters have been asked because they have valuable work that must be shown to our readers. These people are experts, and I have given them a free hand editorially. They deserve great credit as they all delivered good work against a tight deadline; well done folks.

The biggest thank you must go to my patients. The early patients knew that they were taking a leap in the dark. Their bravery in the absence of hard evidence was humbling. I am so sad for those patients whose procedures did not work out in the early days. To those patients whose resurfacing was a huge success, you have given my team and I the strength to continue the quest for perfection. To the hundreds of patients who happily inconvenienced themselves to be part of the many studies we have carried out; the information from these studies has already changed lives and will continue to do so in the future.

Finally, it is a great privilege to have my book published by Springer, whose name has been synonymous with excellence in medical publishing for many years.

Derek J.W. McMinn
Birmingham, UK
August 2007

Contents

Contributors

Roger W.F. Ashton, BSc(Hons)MechEng
Manufacturing and Product Development Director, Smith & Nephew Orthopaedics Ltd,
Warwick Technology Park, Gallows Hill, Warwick, UK

Tim J. Band, MBA, FIManf, MCQI
Metal on Metal Group Director, Smith & Nephew Orthopaedics Ltd, Warwick Technology Park,
Gallows Hill, Warwick, UK

Joseph Daniel, FRCS, MS(Orth)
Director of Research, The McMinn Centre, Edgbaston, Birmingham, UK

Jonathan W. Freeman, TD, QHS, FRCA
Consultant in Anaesthesia and Intensive Care, Department of Anaesthetics and Intensive Care,
The University Hospital Birmingham NHS Foundation Trust, Edgbaston, Birmingham, UK

Takehito Hananouchi, MD
Fellow, Department of Orthopaedic Surgery, Osaka University Graduate School of Medicine, Osaka, Japan

Anne Hands, MCSP
Senior 1 Physiotherapist, Birmingham Nuffield Hospital, Birmingham, UK

Gabrielle Hawdon, MB BS, B Med Sc, MPH
Clinical Researcher, Department of Surgery, Monash University, Windsor, Australia

Raed Itayem, MD
Consultant Orthopaedic Surgeon, Karolinska Institute
Department of Orthopaedic Surgery, Karolinska University Hospital, Huddinge, Sweden

Amir Kamali, PhD
Research Manager – Implant Testing, Smith & Nephew Orthopaedics Ltd, Warwick Technology Park,
Gallows Hill, Warwick, UK

Dennis R. Kerr, MB BS, FANZCA, Dip ABA
Consultant Anaesthetist, Joint Orthopaedic Centre, Bondi Junction, NSW, Australia

Lawrence Kohan, MB BS, FRACS, FA(Orth)A
Orthopaedic Surgeon, Joint Orthopaedic Centre, Bondi Junction, Australia

Arne Lundberg, MD, PhD
Orthopaedic Surgeon, Associate Professor, Karolinska Institute, Department of Orthopaedic Surgery,
Karolinska University Hospital, Huddinge, Sweden

Henrik Malchau, MD, PhD
Associate Professor, Harvard Medical School, Co-Director, The Harris Orthopaedic Biomechanics,
and Biomaterials Laboratory, Attending Physician, Adult Reconstructive Unit, Orthopaedic Department,
Massachusetts General Hospital, Boston, MA, USA

Callum W. McBryde, MD, MRCS
Specialist Registrar, Birmingham Orthopaedic Training Programme, Research and Teaching Centre,
Royal Orthopaedic Hospital, Birmingham, UK

Stephen McMahon, MB BS, FRACS, FA(Orth)A
Orthopaedic Surgeon, Senior Lecturer Monash University, Melbourne, Malabar Orthopaedic Clinic,
Windsor, Australia

Derek J.W. McMinn, FRCS
Consultant Orthopaedic Surgeon, The McMinn Centre, Edgbaston, Birmingham, UK

Jeff Middleton (deceased)
Previously Head of the Biomechanical Laboratory, Wrightington Hospital, Lancashire, UK; Middleton
Surgical Engineering Research Centre, Upholland, Lancashire, UK

Takashi Nishii, MD
Assistant Professor, Department of Orthopaedic Surgery, Osaka University Graduate School of Medicine,
Osaka, Japan

Martyn Porter, MBChB, FRCS (Ed), FRCS Ed (Orth)
Consultant Orthopaedic Surgeon, Centre for Hip Surgery, Wrightington Hospital, Wigan, UK

Chandra Pradhan, FRCS, MCh(Ortho)
Staff Surgeon, The McMinn Centre, Edgbaston, Birmingham, UK

James W. Pritchett, MD
Seattle, WA, USA

Paul B. Pynsent, PhD
Director, Research and Teaching Centre, Royal Orthopaedic Hospital, Birmingham, UK

James Slover, MD, MS
Assistant Professor, Department of Orthopaedic Surgery, NYU Hospital for Joint Diseases, New York,
NY, USA

Nobuhiko Sugano, MD, PhD
Associate Professor, Department of Orthopaedic Surgery, Osaka University Graduate School
of Medicine, Osaka, Japan

Andrew M.C. Thomas, FRCS
Medical Director, Consultant Orthopaedic Surgeon, Royal Orthopaedic Hospital,
Birmingham, UK

Ronan B.C. Treacy, MB ChB, FRCS, FRCS Orth
Consultant Orthopaedic Surgeon, Royal Orthopaedic Hospital, Birmingham, UK

Erik Wetter, MS
Clinical Systems Development Manager, RSA Biomedical AB, Uminova Science Park, AMEÅ, Sweden

Hena Ziaee, BSc(Hons)
Biomedical Scientist, The McMinn Centre, Edgbaston, Birmingham, UK

1
Development Perspectives

Derek J.W. McMinn

Hip arthritis in its early stages involves the loss of a few millimeters of articular cartilage on the femoral head and acetabulum. From the pioneering hip resurfacing work of Charnley using double cups of Teflon (more correctly, polytetrafluoroethylene) in the 1950s right through to the end of the 1980s, surgeons were attracted to the resurfacing concept with replacement only of the worn-out parts. Over these 40 years, however, the major problem was excessive wear of the resurfacing materials, and the hip resurfacing operation fell into disrepute. I was able to witness the problem of wear of the bearing parts in my revision practice when large numbers of Wagner resurfacings had to be converted to total hip replacements (Figs. 1.1–1.3).

The particular problems with the Wagner were loosening of components and collapse of the femoral head. These extremely disappointing results in the hands of many surgeons encouraged the view that the concept of hip resurfacing arthroplasty was flawed. However, closer examination of the failure patterns show that this was a failure of materials rather than a failure of concept.

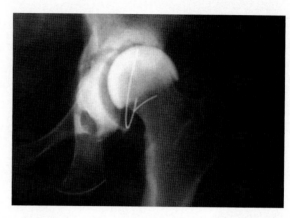

FIG. 1.2. Common form of failure in ceramic on polyethylene resurfacing. Linear osteolysis has loosened the acetabular component, which migrated into a vertical alignment. Severe wear of the acetabular component edge occurred with fracture of the peripheral metal cup marker.

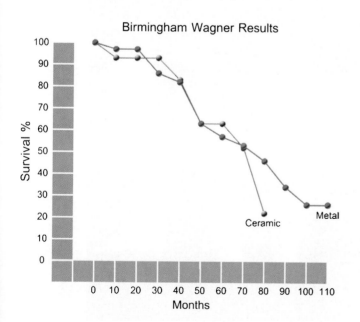

FIG. 1.1. Poor results on survivorship analysis with the ceramic on polyethylene and metal on polyethylene resurfacings performed in Birmingham.

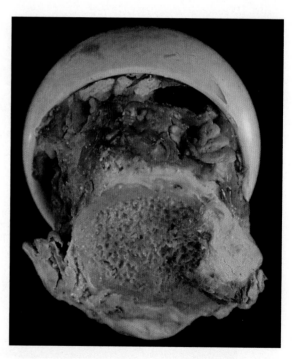

FIG. 1.3. Femoral head and neck removed at revision surgery with solidly fixed ceramic femoral component. Loose acetabular cup and acetabular osteolysis necessitated revision 9 years after implantation.

In this soundly fixed ceramic femoral component, the bone quality in the base of the femoral head looks excellent (Fig. 1.4). Although there are trabeculae streaming down from the tips of cement keyplugs, the concern is that large cavities are present in the polar aspect of this femoral head. Do these cavities represent avascular necrosis of the femoral head, stress shielding of the polar aspect of the femoral head, or osteolysis? The presence of a head-neck junction cavity starts to look like osteolysis (Fig. 1.5). Histology on the bone of this femoral head confirmed that the cavities were due to osteolysis from polyethylene debris (Figs. 1.6–1.8). Presumably, the intermittent high pressure in the hip joint cavity drove the polyethylene debris through the entry point at the femoral head-neck junction into the substance of the femoral head bone.

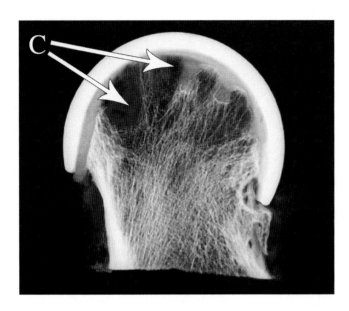

Fig. 1.4. Microradiograph of coronal slice of ceramic femoral component on femoral head and neck. Cavities (*C*) are present in femoral head.

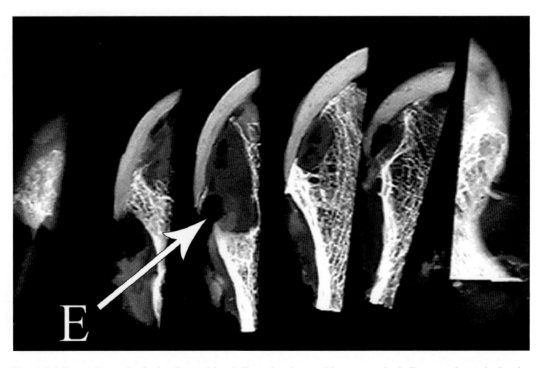

Fig. 1.5. Microradiograph of other femoral head slices showing cavities present including a cavity at the head-neck junction and what appears to be an entry point (*E*).

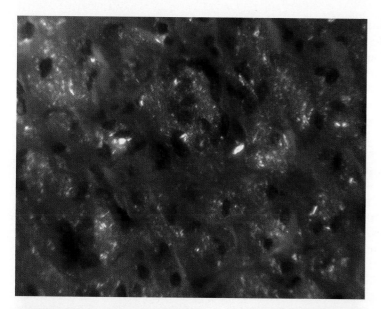

FIG. 1.6. Macrophages laden with polyethylene particles present in one section of the femoral head. This appearance was seen on every slice of the femoral head.

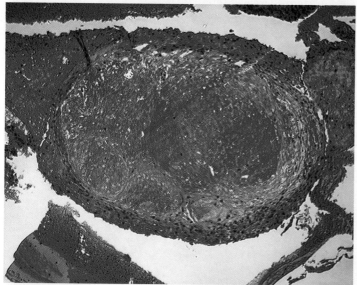

FIG. 1.7. Two-millimeter-diameter granuloma present on one section of femoral head. Granulomata were present on every slice of the femoral head.

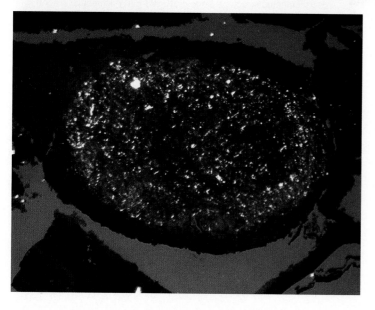

FIG. 1.8. Polarized light microscopy shows granuloma full of polyethylene debris.

With cemented polyethylene-containing hip resurfacing components, polyethylene particles gained access to the acetabular bone-cement interface, giving a predominately linear pattern of osteolysis and resulting in cup loosening. As can be seen from the above figures, even with cemented femoral resurfacing components, polyethylene debris gained access to the femoral head bone, and if acetabular loosening in these early resurfacings did not occur, then the system failed by femoral head collapse when femoral head destruction by osteolysis became severe enough. With cementless porous-ingrowth, acetabular components loosening was much less of a problem, but severe acetabular osteolysis occurred, often giving major problems at revision surgery (Figs. 1.9 and 1.10).

It was clear that polyethylene could not be used as the bearing material in hip resurfacing. First, the combined thickness of the polyethylene cup together with the thickness of the required acetabular cement mantle or cementless metal shell, plus the thickness of the femoral component and femoral cement mantle, led to a bulky implant that required excessive bone removal for implantation. The necessary use of a large femoral head size in the resurfacing arthroplasty led to excess polyethylene debris, osteolysis, loosening, and collapse of femoral heads. A bearing material had to be found that would be durable for use in young, active patients and would be durable when used with a large-diameter articulation. In addition, the bearing material had to be capable of manufacture as a thin component to avoid excessive resection of valuable bone stock in young patients. Ironically, such material had in fact been in successful clinical use for more than 30 years but had not been used in resurfacing arthroplasty in any significantly large study, or so we thought.

Maurice Muller performed 18 metal on metal hip resurfacings in the 1960s. He gave up using this implant when Sir John Charnley convinced him of the benefits of the metal on polyethylene articulation. Muller told me later that he very much regretted having given up metal on metal articulations either for resurfacing or total hip replacement. Gerard also performed a small series.

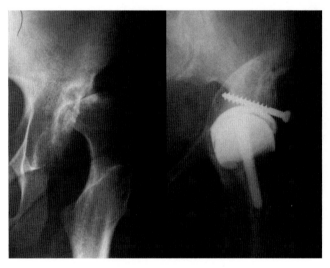

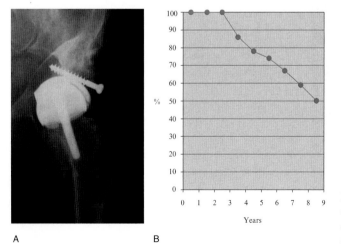

FIG. 1.9. (A) Severe DDH treated with cementless Buechel-Pappas resurfacing and structural bone graft. (B) Early acetabular osteolysis 4 years postoperatively.

FIG. 1.10. (A) Severe acetabular osteolysis 5 years postoperatively. (B) Buechel-Pappas survivorship analysis in Oswestry. This implant employed ethylene oxide–sterilized polyethylene in the bearing (Images courtesy Prof. James Richardson, MD, FRCS).

Metal on Metal Total Hip Replacement

Over the past 20 years, I have had the opportunity of following up patients who have had three different varieties of large-headed metal on metal total hip replacement (THR) performed by seven of my predecessors (Fig. 1.11). Most of these patients were seen for another problem and were surprised that I was interested in their well-functioning old metal on metal THRs. It is quite remarkable that most of these patients are clinically and radiographically excellent.

The biggest number of metal on metal THRs performed in Birmingham, United Kingdom, were of the Ring uncemented type. The surgeon who performed these (the late Robert Duke, FRCS) was allergic to bone cement (even wearing three pairs of gloves) and the uncemented Ring (Fig. 1.12) was his only THR. The acetabular component came in one size only and had an external surface of smooth cobalt chrome. The femoral component had three sizes, and again the stem surface was smooth cobalt chrome. Not surprisingly, in almost all instances, long-term x-rays show a radiolucent line at the implant-bone interface on both the acetabular and femoral sides. Despite interface access, I have never seen osteolysis associated with this implant.

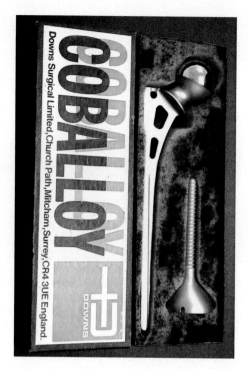

FIG. 1.12. Ring THR stem and cup in original, now rather faded, box.

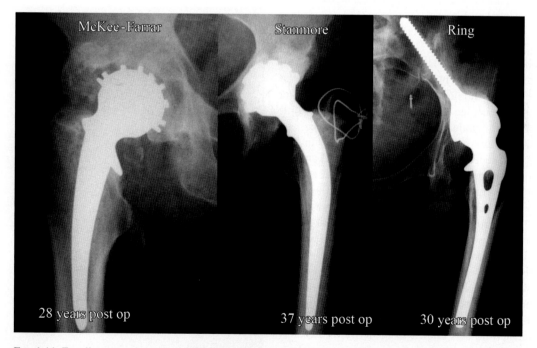

FIG. 1.11. Excellent outcomes after McKee-Farrar at 28 years follow-up, Stanmore at 37 years follow-up, and Ring at 30 years follow-up. No osteolysis. Note radiolucent cement has been used on McKee-Farrar.

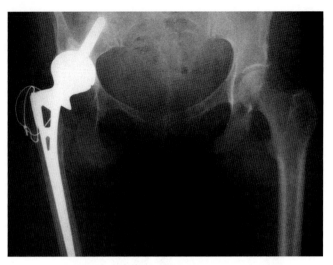

FIG. 1.13. A 56-year-old woman with pain after Ring THR 23.5 years before.

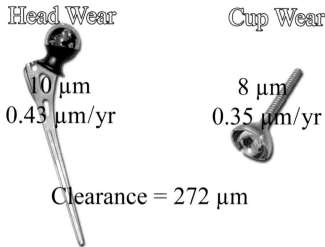

FIG. 1.14. Wear and clearance measurements of the components removed from the patient of Fig. 1.13.

It is remarkable how well patients performed clinically with this Ring THR. With good-quality radiographs, it could be seen that most patients developed an implant-bone radiolucent line, yet the vast majority of patients had no pain associated with this. However, I have had the opportunity of revising a small number of patients with Ring THR implants where loosening was associated with pain.

This woman had a Ring THR performed by Peter Ring at the age of 32 years (Fig. 1.13). Her diagnosis was developmental dysplasia of the hip (DDH), and the cup was inserted with a high hip center. She always had a degree of discomfort after surgery, but this did not stop her being active. After her THR, she had children, led an active life, and had a full-time occupation. Her pain gradually increased over the years, and approximately 5 years before the radiograph taken in Fig. 1.13, Peter Ring's successor made an attempt at revising her THR through a trochanteric osteotomy approach. Her components could not be removed, the greater trochanter was wired in position, and she continued to have discomfort on walking. She eventually tracked down Peter Ring who had retired, and he advised her to consult with me regarding revision surgery. At surgery, the acetabular component was loose with a thin film of soft tissue between the implant and bone. The femoral component was removed after division of the bone bridges growing through the upper femoral component fenestrations. There was no metallosis or osteolysis.

In this patient, who was known to be active, remarkably little wear of the bearing parts has occurred with only 10-μm wear on the femoral head and 8-μm wear on the acetabular component. This represents 0.43 μm per year wear on the femoral head component and 0.35 μm per year wear on the acetabular component (Fig. 1.14). The diametral clearance on this bearing was 272 μm, and with the current state of knowledge this would be regarded as a large clearance. The lack

of osteolysis around the acetabular component in this patient with proven acetabular component loosening gives support to the view that normal low wear from these metal on metal bearings does not cause osteolysis (Fig. 1.15).

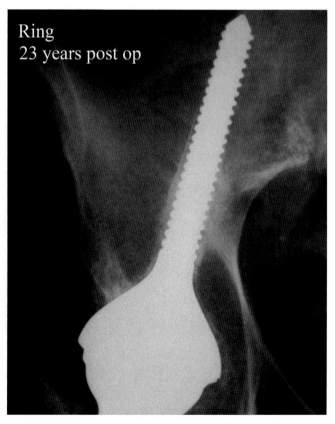

FIG. 1.15. Radiolucent line around smooth Ring cup. Another patient with interface access but no osteolysis.

I have some examples where I have had to revise a cemented metal on metal THR for osteolysis. In the revision of the patient below, the bearing looked pristine and bone cement was firmly adherent to the McKee-Farrar cup (Fig. 1.16). However, loosening at the cement-bone interface had abraded large volumes of cement debris. The femoral component was solidly fixed, and there was no metallosis (Fig. 1.17). In order to minimize the size of the operation in this elderly patient, the acetabulum was bone grafted, metal reinforcement was used, and the original McKee-Farrar cup was recemented with a good outcome.

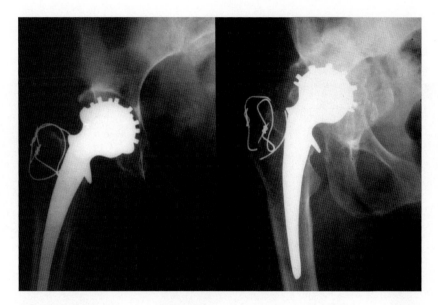

FIG. 1.16. McKee-Farrar postoperatively and after 20 years with severe pelvic osteolysis. At revision, no metallosis but massive production of cement debris.

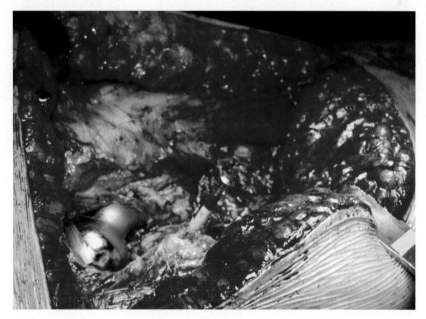

FIG. 1.17. Intraoperative photograph of patient of Fig. 1.16 during revision. Note absence of metallosis.

I also have some patients with less severe osteolysis after loosening of their cemented metal on metal THRs. For example, the following patient had acetabular cup loosening and moderate osteolysis 28 years after a McKee-Farrar THR that had been cemented with radiolucent cement (Fig. 1.18).

Before her THR, she had undergone a femoral osteotomy with a poor outcome. At operation, the femoral component was solidly fixed, the bearing showed no visible wear, and there was no metallosis. The patient was a frail 79-year-old and in order to minimize the extent of revision surgery, the femoral component was left *in situ*, the acetabular floor was bone grafted, and the cup was recemented with a good outcome.

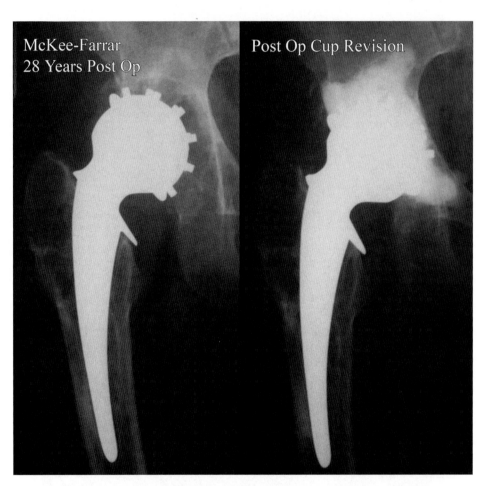

FIG. 1.18. Cup loosening and acetabular osteolysis 28 years after a McKee-Farrar THR. Acetabulum bone grafted and cup recemented. Note radiolucent cement used at original operation.

I also have some examples of osteolysis of the femur with loosening of the cemented femoral component of metal on metal THRs. The loosening and micromovement was usually at the implant-cement interface with osteolysis produced at an area of defective cement mantle (Fig. 1.19).

We had good evidence that metal on metal bearings exhibited low wear and in the absence of other debris did not cause osteolysis. The metal on metal bearings could be manufactured in different sizes and the components could be kept thin without reducing implant strength and risking fracture. Metal on metal bearings therefore seemed ideal to resurrect hip resurfacing.

There remained only the problem of convincing other surgeons and an implant manufacturer that combining two unattractive ideas would make an attractive implant (Fig. 1.20)!

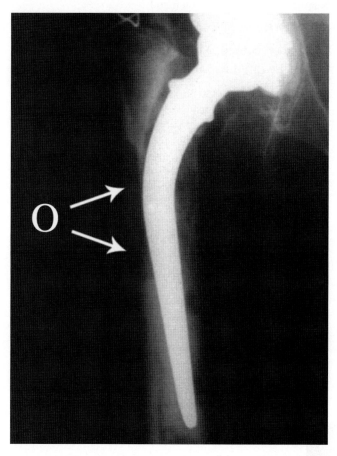

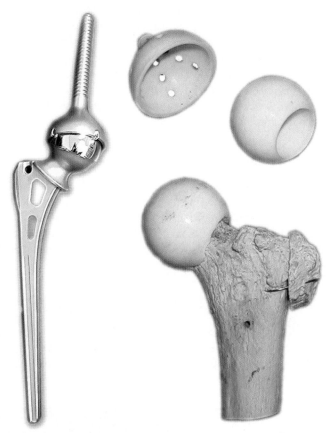

FIG. 1.19. Severe femoral focal osteolysis (O) in a patient with loose femoral component of Stanmore metal on metal THR with micromotion and cement generation at stem-cement interface 23 years postoperatively.

FIG. 1.20. Combining metal on metal bearings with Charnley's hip resurfacing concept proved a hard sell.

Why Were Metal on Metal Prostheses Abandoned?

Why, when the metal on metal implants were behaving well, were they abandoned in favor of metal on polyethylene articulations?

Difficulty with Manufacture of Cobalt Chrome

Cast cobalt chrome is very hard and difficult to manufacture. To give surgeons an idea how hard this material is to cut, one needs to attempt to saw through the material with a hacksaw from a hardware store. Certainly an impression can be made on the metal, but the teeth soon start to wear off the saw.

In implant manufacture, the teeth of cutting tools are much harder than those of a hacksaw, but wear of tools is a major issue and presents difficulty maintaining accuracy as wear of the cutting tools occurs. This difficulty translates into long machining times, frequent sharpening, replacement of tools, and increased man hours and cost. It was recognized at the time that a high degree of sphericity and a defined clearance with a polar bearing articulation were important for success, and with relatively unsophisticated machines available at the time, increased reliance was placed on the skill of the machinist again adding cost to the implant.

Ease of Manufacture of Polyethylene

By comparison with as-cast cobalt chrome, polyethylene was easy to manufacture. Charnley manufactured polyethylene cups himself in his workshop in 1962, and in 1963 a machine was built at Wrightington that could manufacture polyethylene cups in 4 or 5 minutes. The cost advantage over a metal on metal bearing is obvious.

Good Initial Results of Metal on Polyethylene Prostheses

The early results achieved by Charnley with polyethylene cups were outstanding. Neither Charnley nor Thackrays patented polyethylene as part of the bearing couple of joint replace-

ments, and indeed Charnley encouraged other innovators like Bucholz and Muller to use the same bearing material.

This meant that a number of different manufacturers were able to make their own joint replacements without having to have the same expertise or production costs required in the manufacture of metal on metal couples. This opened up a whole new era of surgeons and engineers designing their own joint replacements with an increasingly large number of manufacturers eager to oblige to their own and the designer's financial advantage. Disappointingly, the greatest innovator of them all, Sir John Charnley, did not benefit financially in the same way as did a mass of lesser lights who followed.

In the midst of this bonanza for designers and corporations, there was no appetite to return to an expensive and difficult bearing couple like metal on metal.

Michael Freeman, MD, FRCS: His Part in the Downfall of Metal on Metal

For the three orthopedic surgeons in the world who do not know him, Mike Freeman is one of the brightest and most articulate investigators one will ever meet. He has been a formidable debater at international conferences over the years, usually destroying the case of his opponent. Like a top-quality defense attorney, his use of words and clarity of thought could get his client away with blatant murder. He is, however, not shy about criticizing his own efforts. I helped organize a conference a few years ago, and we had invited Freeman to speak about ankle replacement. He started: "Gentlemen, my ankle replacement is the worst thing that ever hit the human frame. I shall now proceed to discuss salvage of the failed ankle replacement." If Freeman's ankle replacement was the worst thing to hit the human frame, then his Imperial College London hip (ICLH) hip resurfacing was the second worst thing. When he persuaded Peter Ring to abandon metal on metal articulations, the new Ring press-fit uncemented polyethylene cup was equipped with the Freeman osseous peg; this implant was a disaster and probably the third worst thing to hit the human frame (Fig. 1.21).

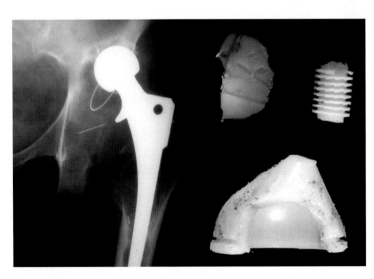

Fig. 1.21. Gross acetabular and femoral osteolysis with failed Ring metal on polyethylene THR. On the right is a disintegrated Ring, uncemented, polyethylene cup.

For metal on metal bearings, it was regrettable that Freeman was leading the case for the opposition. It is more helpful to have the Johnnie Cochran types on your side. Freeman clearly disliked cobalt chrome on cobalt chrome bearings and produced several pieces of work that were extremely damaging. Together with his colleagues Swanson and Heath [1], Freeman designed a joint simulator machine and reported the testing of several joint types including the McKee and Charnley hips.

For the Charnley hip, they ran the simulator to 4 million cycles and reported that *no* wear particles had been produced during the test, which they estimated to represent 4 years of use in the normal human. This needs to be viewed against a backdrop statement by Wilson and Scales in 1970 [2] (designers of the Stanmore metal on metal THR) "… if the wear products of polyethylene do not produce an undesirable tissue response; neither adjacent nor in tissues remote from the implant, then metal on metal bearings will be discarded." We now know, but it was not known in 1970, that polyethylene debris–associated osteolysis turned out to be the major problem with hip arthroplasty. No polyethylene wear particles on Freeman's simulator; this was just the encouragement that the new wave of Charnley surgeons wanted to hear and was another nail in the coffin of the decreasing band of metal on metal users. This proved to be the first of a string of totally misleading results from hip simulator machines, as we shall see later. In contrast, the McKee metal on metal prostheses produced "visible quantities" of metal debris on the simulator machine—hardly encouraging news for the followers of McKee.

Freeman produced two pieces of work relating to the frictional torque of metal on metal bearings compared with metal on polyethylene bearings [1,3]. Together with his colleagues, Anderson and Swanson, Freeman reported that the frictional torques of metal on metal bearings were higher than those of metal on polyethylene articulations. However, the maximum torques from the metal on metal articulations were 4 to 20 times lower than the torque required to loosen cups cemented into the acetabulum. Not deterred by this finding, Freeman still recommended metal on polyethylene on the grounds that the heat produced by curing bone cement might cause thermal damage to bone thus weakening the fixation and arguing that the lower torque of the metal on polyethylene bearings might allow the acetabular fixation to survive. As we will see later, the friction factor with a "run-in" Birmingham Hip Resurfacing (BHR) is as low as a 28-mm metal on polyethylene articulation. However, that is recent information, and the frictional torque issue in the 1970s was a concern for surgeons who wished to continue with metal on metal bearings.

Freeman produced two pieces of work relating to malignancy from metal wear particles [1,4]. In his 1973 *Journal of Bone and Joint Surgery* paper, Freeman and colleagues showed that injection of "massive doses" of cobalt chrome particles into the muscle of rats produced a variety of malignant tumors.

Local and distant site tumor potential weighed heavily on the minds of metal on metal surgeons. Freeman, many years later, is reported to have said, "I now know that even a nylon suture can cause tumors in rats—so I was wrong!" Happily, he does seem to have been wrong, at least in relation to local site tumors adjacent to metal on metal implants.

Perhaps the most devastating piece of work from Freeman was in relation to metal sensitivity and metal on metal joints [5]. Evans, Freeman et al. performed skin sensitivity tests on 14 patients with failed metal implants. Nine patients had positive tests; the suggested hypothesis was that these patients had a delayed hypersensitivity reaction to the released metal ions that caused vascular occlusion, bone necrosis, and implant loosening. Completely contrary and better evidence came later from the Hospital for Special Surgery, New York [6], unfortunately too late to save metal on metal implants. The paper of Evans, Freeman et al. was accompanied in the same issue of the *Journal of Bone and Joint Surgery* by an editorial [7] that gave no comfort to potential users of metal on metal joints. To a variable degree, concern around this issue still persists today. Metal hypersensitivity in a large population of BHR patients out to 10 years follow-up is discussed later. Happily, it seems to represent a very small clinical problem. As we shall see later in this book, cobalt, chromium, and molybdenum are the main constituents of the alloy used for metal on metal joints, and they are all essential elements. These three elements are all present in the diet, are in body tissues, and are essential for life. It is hard to see how a patient could be allergic to one of these elements and still survive. Surely that would be just as serious as a patient developing an allergy to oxygen. As we will see later, there are many trace elements also present in the cobalt chrome alloy, and the potential exists for allergy to some of these nonessential trace elements.

It is ironic that after so much work to help kill off the historic era of metal on metal joints, when the BHR was developed by Midland Medical Technologies (MMT), Finsbury Instruments was engaged to carry out a major part of the manufacturing, and Mike Freeman was a shareholder in that company. Mike Freeman has been nothing but helpful to me personally. The comments above should not be seen in any way as detracting from the contribution of one of the greatest innovators in the field of joint replacement alive today.

Sir John Charnley's Influence

During the late 1960s and early 1970s, surgeons across the world experienced initial success with all varieties of THR and attention then focused on which type of THR would prove more durable. Charnley concentrated on the issue of frictional torque. He built a pendulum comparator to demonstrate the superiority of the 22-mm metal on polyethylene Charnley joint over all other varieties of bearing couple (Fig. 1.22). Thanks to the generosity of Prof. Mike Wroblewski, I have had the opportunity to visit the Wrightington museum and to use and videotape the Charnley pendulum comparator. My senior colleagues had warned me that they believed the McKee joint was run on Charnley's pendulum without lubrication, so I went to Wrightington armed with a small bottle of fresh human synovial fluid. I liberally bathed the McKee-Farrar articulation in human synovial fluid before inserting the ball into the cup. The maximum load that the technician would allow me to apply to the apparatus was 80 lb (36 kg). When the pendulum bobs were released, the metal on metal couple came to a juddering halt after 3 half swings and made a screeching noise.

The Charnley joint kept on swinging smoothly for 10 half swings. I thought there might be some grit or other foreign body in the articulation. The metal on metal couple was duly carefully cleaned and the experiment repeated several times with an equally dismal result (Fig. 1.23).

With the 36 kg of air pressure applied to the stationary metal on metal articulation, I tried to move the pendulum arm back and forth, and although movement could be obtained, the resistance to such movement was very high. Video footage of the Charnley pendulum comparator in action can be seen on the DVD accompanying this book. I understood clearly at that time why so many thousands of orthopedic surgeons who had visited Wrightington in the years before myself were completely convinced of the superiority of the metal on polyethylene articulation, and I could easily understand why none of them would ever insert a metal on metal articulation again. I found myself unconsciously looking toward the heavens in order to get a reply from Charnley on how he had managed to set up this awful rig that showed metal on metal in such an appalling light. No reply was forthcoming, and I left Wrightington that day devastated.

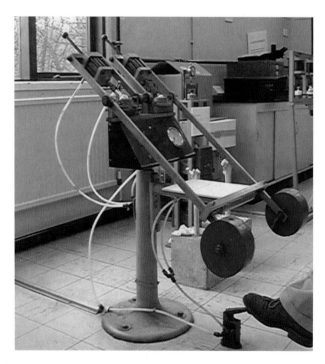

FIG. 1.22. Charnley pendulum comparator.

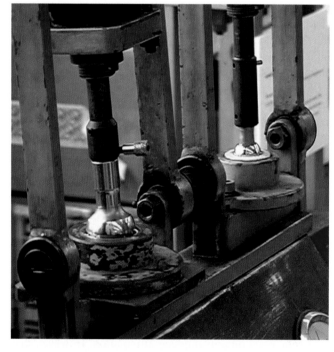

FIG. 1.23. The McKee-Farrar metal on metal couple (nearest) came to a juddering halt despite the application of human synovial fluid, and the Charnley metal on polyethylene couple (farthest) kept on swinging.

I have no definite answers on why the Charnley pendulum comparator is so awful for a metal on metal articulation. The first terrible thought was that as the metal on metal bearing behaved so badly at 36 kg, surely at loads up to 500 kg experienced in the hip of a sportsman the metal on metal bearing would be completely jammed. Charnley wrote an interesting section in his book [8] on this very subject. He described the situation whereby a patient could still function normally with bilateral intermittently jamming McKee-Farrar hips. I have seen many patients with excellent outcomes after 20 years of use of a metal on metal articulation, and I found it very hard to accept that their joints could intermittently jam each time the joint was loaded without loosening the components over those 20 years. The design of a metal on metal joint is critical to its performance, and in particular it is known that equatorial bearings perform worst when loaded, acting as a clutch mechanism. The best design for a metal on metal joint is a polar bearing. The McKee-Farrar joint that Charnley used, he claimed, was an annular bearing, which is suboptimal. An annular bearing is halfway between a polar bearing and an equatorial bearing. Like equatorial bearings, annular bearings have high frictional torque under load.

The design of the pendulum comparator is complex, and it does require that the center of articulation of the bearing couple under test is lined up with the center of rotation of the two outer roller bearings. The direction of load on this pendulum comparator is distinctly odd and quite different to the loading in the normal hip as Charnley's own work showed. In the pendulum comparator, the load is directed through the femoral component with the head-cup contact area moving in an arc described by the amplitude of the pendulum. This would give a multidirectional cup wear pattern, and Charnley knew that this did not occur in the human hip.

In a high-wearing polymer, such as the Teflon cup used by Charnley from 1958–1961, the direction of loading and wear can easily be appreciated (Fig. 1.24). The loading is in one direction, unlike Charnley's pendulum comparator where the loading is multidirectional. This may have implications for the lubrication and performance of metal on metal bearings.

We built a small pendulum that performed much better with metal on metal joints than did Charnley's apparatus. However, I could not rest until I had a pendulum apparatus constructed that loaded the hip joint in a more satisfactory fashion than did Charnley's pendulum comparator and also did not have the hazards of Charnley's two roller bearings incorporated in the apparatus. The pendulum furthermore had to load the hip joint to 500 kg, and the metal on metal articulation under test would have to be manufactured to modern standards (Fig. 1.25).

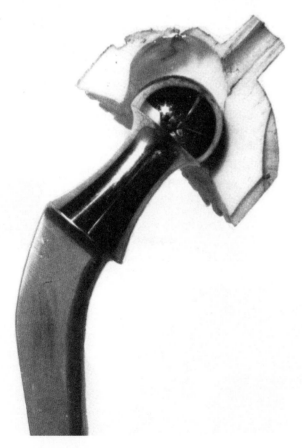

FIG. 1.24. Total wear-through of a Charnley Teflon cup after 3 years showing vertical direction of wear track. (Reproduced with permission from Springer).

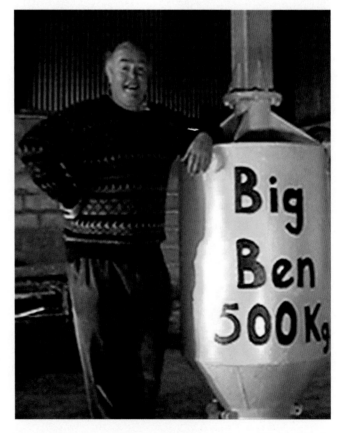

FIG. 1.25. Author standing beside 500-kg concrete-filled steel bob. This weight was necessary to give realistic high loading on prosthetic hip joints.

Under the guidance of structural engineers, a large building was steel reinforced in order to prevent collapse of the building by a swinging half-tonne pendulum. When testing a bearing with this apparatus, the pendulum is started at a fixed point, and the number of swings taken for the pendulum to come to a standstill is recorded. A number of runs are then performed on each bearing. It is appreciated that peak loads in the hip of an active person can reach six to nine times body weight, which means that a sportsman engaged in high-level sport will generate a load across the hip joint in the region of 500 kg and above.

Until we started building this pendulum, I had not fully appreciated what a massive load 500 kg is. In addition, observing this monster pendulum swinging makes one appreciate how clever the normal hip joint design is to cope with these huge loads (Figs. 1.26–1.28).

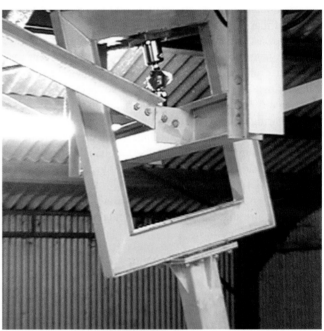

FIG. 1.27. Loading area for test hip joint prostheses high in roof space. When stationary, a hydraulic ram is attached to distract the apparatus and load a new joint for testing.

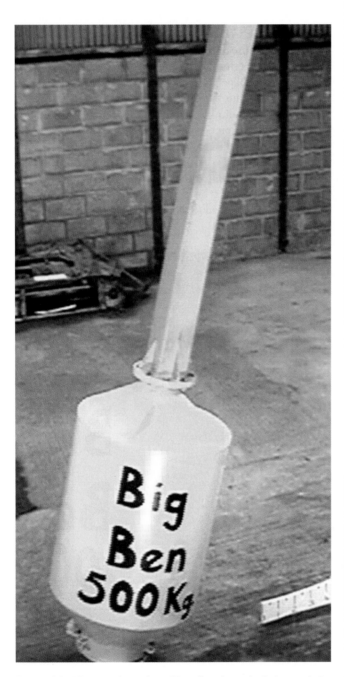

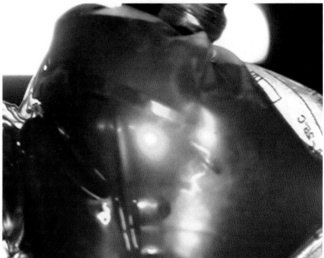

FIG. 1.26. Big Ben in action. Happily, the calculations of the structural engineers were correct, and the pendulum did not cause collapse of the building.

FIG. 1.28. This shows metal on metal couple with the acetabular component on top. Outside the prosthesis is a membrane containing serum and hyaluronic acid.

Results Obtained Using 500-kg Pendulum

When the metal on polyethylene bearings are considered, it can be seen that the 22-, 28-, and 32-mm bearings decrease the number of swings per run and then come to a plateau. The different-sized metal on metal bearings have been tested in serum and hyaluronic acid (HUA) (substitute for synovial fluid) and blood. Of course, these metal on metal bearings in patients are initially bathed in blood and later in synovial fluid.

Unlike the results from Sir John Charnley's pendulum comparator, it can clearly be seen that the frictional torque of these different-head-sized metal on metal bearings are not very different from a range of metal on polyethylene bearings in common clinical use (Fig. 1.29). It can be concluded, therefore, that frictional torque with these metal on metal bearings is not the issue that Sir John Charnley thought it would be. This relatively low frictional torque from the metal on metal bearings is entirely consistent with the clinical experience of historic metal on metal joints having lasted 30 years or more.

We made some other interesting observations using this apparatus. I tried running both the metal on polyethylene and metal on metal articulations dry and in lubrication fluid. With the metal on polyethylene joints, the number of swings to a standstill when run dry was slightly greater than when run in lubricating fluid, so all further tests with metal on polyethylene were run dry. The situation was completely different with the metal on metal articulations. When these were run dry, there was a loud screeching noise, and the bearings were destroyed after one run. The metal on metal bearings performed much better with a lubricant, and I tried calf serum, serum and hyaluronic acid, blood, and finally engine oil. The serum with added hyaluronic acid was marginally better than serum alone, but with both lubricants the metal on metal bearings emitted a low-grade grinding noise on movement. In addition, occasional squeaks could be heard. With blood as the lubricant, all noise ceased, and the number of swings to a standstill with each bearing size was improved compared with the same bearing with serum and hyaluronic acid as the lubricant. It should be noted that in the early weeks after implantation of a metal on metal bearing, these joints are bathed in blood. I also ran some metal on metal joints with engine oil as the lubricant. Interestingly, blood was just as efficient a lubricant as engine oil.

I was interested in attempting to investigate the effect of diametral clearance between the head and cup on the frictional torque. An electrical circuit was set up to detect when the head and cup were no longer in electrical contact. For this experiment, serum with added hyaluronic acid was used as the lubricant. In these newly manufactured metal on metal joints, no effect of reducing clearance was seen until the diametral clearance was reduced to 25 µm at which time electrical contact between the head and cup was broken. The relevance of all this will be seen in later parts of this book, suffice to say now that metal on metal joints exhibit the phenomenon of "run-in" with increasing usage. The surface profile of a newly manufactured metal on metal joint is distinctly inferior to the surface profile of a run-in joint, and as we shall see, this has implications for the lubrication of newly manufactured and run-in metal on metal joints.

Another interesting observation related to the metal on metal couples when subjected to 500 kg of static load. In Sir John Charnley's pendulum comparator with 36 kg of static load, the metal on metal articulation was virtually locked. In my pendulum with 500 kg of static load, the cup and the whole pendulum apparatus can be easily rotated on the prosthetic head using only little finger pressure. See Big Ben in action on the DVD that accompanies this book.

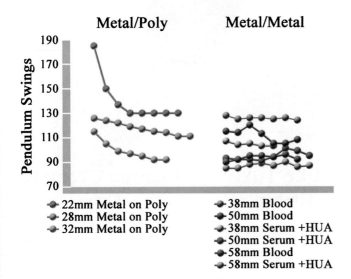

FIG. 1.29. With the 22-mm metal on polyethylene articulation, it can be seen that the number of swings to a standstill on each run decreased down to a plateau. Across the range of sizes, the metal on polyethylene frictional torque is broadly similar to the metal on metal frictional torque.

Development of My Metal on Metal Hip Resurfacing

I made good progress during 1988 with Ian Brown and his team at Zimmer UK, Swindon. We had agreed on the design for the femoral and acetabular components. I had used the Harris-Galante I acetabular cup and eventually ended up performing more than 1000 implants. I have not had cause to revise a single case for loosening but like many others have had my fair share of problems such as dislocation, infection, a handful of tine fractures with liner breakout, and rather too many cases of late pelvic osteolysis.

Fixation, however, has never been a problem with this implant. One of my patients developed recurrent dislocation and ended up being revised elsewhere by a surgeon who believed that uncemented fixation was not very powerful. An attempt was made to remove the cup shell without first breaking down the implant-bone interface. The surgeon extracted the cup but also removed the rest of the acetabulum, which he discovered was very powerfully attached (Fig. 1.30).

I wanted fibermesh on the acetabular resurfacing cup that we were designing, but we could not decide whether to go with commercially pure titanium or cobalt chrome fibermesh. Titanium fibermesh, of course, was used on the H-G1 cup, but we worried about dissimilar metals when diffusion-bonding it to cobalt chrome with the potential for galvanic corrosion. Cobalt chrome fibermesh was a possibility, but some of the Zimmer team worried that it might not be as friendly for bone ingrowth as titanium. Zimmer US had an extensive experience developing fibermesh, and I hoped to get some guidance from the United States. However, Jorge Galante turned the idea of a metal on metal resurfacing down flat. Sadly, the hip resurfacing project with Zimmer ended.

The Corin Years

Peter Gibson, Corin, and Mike Tuke, Finsbury, were instrumental in getting the metal on metal hip resurfacing project started. However, it was George Cremore, with his metal on metal manufacturing know-how, who was the key player once the decision had been made to proceed with the project (Fig. 1.31). I supplied George with new and used McKee-Farrar and Ring implants in the expectation that he would reproduce the excellent bearing characteristics of these implants.

We eventually agreed that there would be three component sizes. Corin wanted to use the Freeman superolateral fins (SLF) cup castings as these were readily available to them, leaving just three new femoral castings to be manufactured. Michael Freeman agreed to his cup design being used. I brought up the subject of porous coating on the acetabular cup, but this was rejected. I was very taken with a statement from Michael Freeman that he used to justify his design of nonporous coated acetabular cup: "To get bone ingrowth into a porous surface you need stability, but if you have stability who needs porous ingrowth."

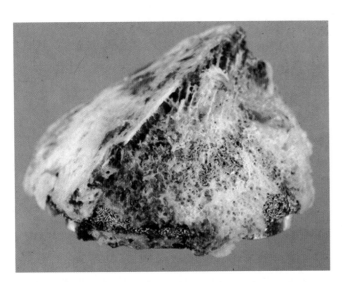

FIG. 1.30. Harris-Galante I cup shell together with osseointegrated acetabulum removed at revision surgery.

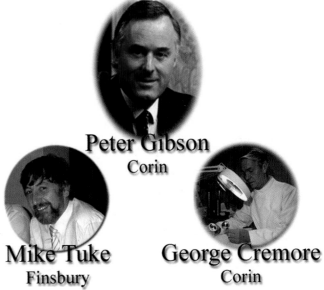

FIG. 1.31. Three key players.

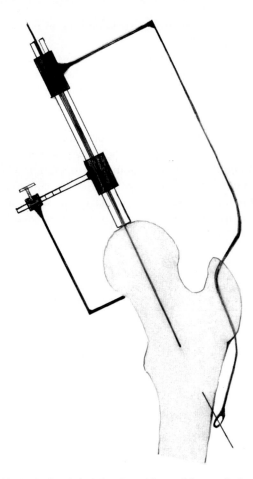

Fig. 1.32. Author's original drawing of femoral jig supplied to Corin.

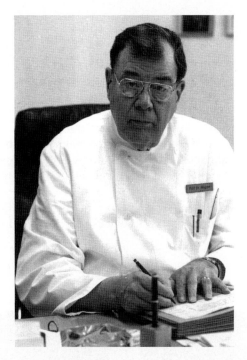

Fig. 1.33. Prof. Heinz Wagner (1929–2001).

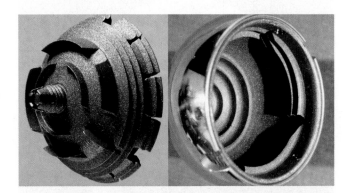

Fig. 1.34. Initial variety of cementless metal on metal resurfacing. Cup and head had porous titanium ingrowth surfaces with cobalt chrome articular surfaces. Femoral component was of a "screw-on" type.

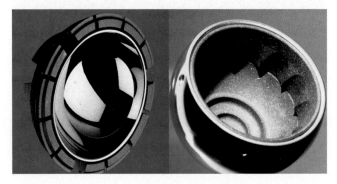

Fig. 1.35. Second variety of cementless implant with femoral component changed to impacted press-fit type. (Images courtesy Prof. Michael Wagner, MD, PhD.).

This sounded like a logical argument to me at the time, and we applied this also to the femoral component, aiming for a design that would achieve stability as a press fit without worrying about a porous ingrowth surface. I set about designing a set of instruments; most of these were obvious adaptations of what had gone before, but the jig to place the femoral guide wire was new and turned out to be very useful (Fig. 1.32).

By February 1991, we were ready to insert the first metal on metal resurfacing. Unknown to me, Prof. Heinz Wagner had also been developing his metal on metal resurfacing, and he too inserted his first model in February 1991 (Fig. 1.33).

Heinz and Michael Wagner inserted two varieties of metal on metal resurfacing and reported their results in 1996 [9] (Figs. 1.34 and 1.35). Heinz and Michael Wagner eventually abandoned hip resurfacing due to fixation problems.

Pilot Series

Seventy implants of my press-fit design were inserted between February 1991 and February 1992 (Fig. 1.36).

In our publication in 1996 [10], we reported an 8.6% aseptic revision rate at 44 to 54 months follow-up. At revision of these loose press-fit components, both components were confirmed to be loose at reoperation. There was no macroscopic metallosis, and the femoral heads were viable on visual inspection and on histology. There was no osteolysis, but a thin soft tissue membrane was present at the interface in all cases.

The survivorship graph shows the disappointing outcome with these press-fit devices (Fig. 1.37). However, a number of these patients still continue to perform well (Fig. 1.38).

At the end of 1 year, I was not happy. I had a meeting with Michael Freeman and told him about the troubles I was having with the press-fit implant. I reminded him about his advice related to stability and porous ingrowth, and quick as a flash he told me that the SLF press-fit cups with a metal on polythylene total hip replacement were fine and my problems must be due to the metal on metal bearing. I said I could not carry on doing this operation with such a high failure rate, but to my surprise he said something along the lines of "now that you have started you have got to perfect it," and his concluding words were "slap a bit of cement on my son."

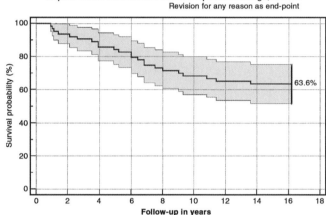

FIG. 1.37. Poor results with press-fit resurfacing.

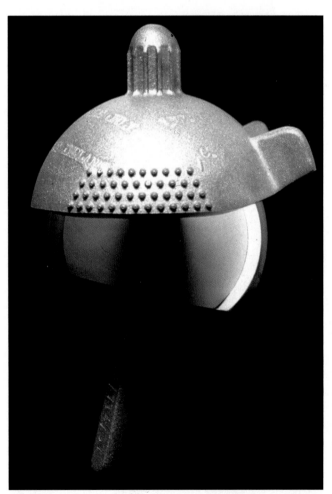

FIG. 1.36. Nonporous, non–HA-coated, uncemented, press-fit components. Note superolateral fins (SLF) Freeman cup design.

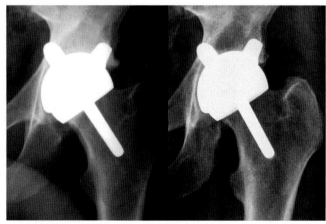

FIG. 1.38. Satisfactory clinical and radiologic outcome 1 year and 16 years after press-fit resurfacing.

I had similar advice from Prof. Mike Wroblewski who told me that I needed to get a large team around me and "make this device work." I decided to alter the implant and go with cemented fixation on both the acetabular and femoral components, but in the mean time we had a number of patients who were agitating to have their hips resurfaced. As a stopgap measure, we decided to have the acetabular and femoral components HA-coated (Fig. 1.39).

The early results with the HA-coated implants were excellent. A survivorship curve on this tiny number of patients (six) is hardly very meaningful, but two patients have had to be revised for femoral loosening (Fig. 1.40).

I was nervous about carrying out cementless fixation of femoral components, and I restricted myself to patients with good-quality bone in the main.

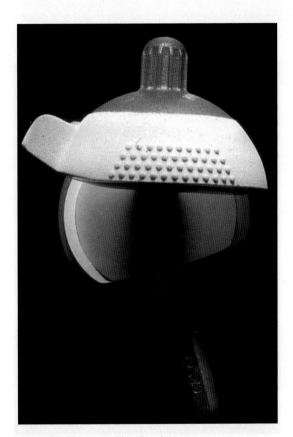

FIG. 1.39. HA-coated head and cup.

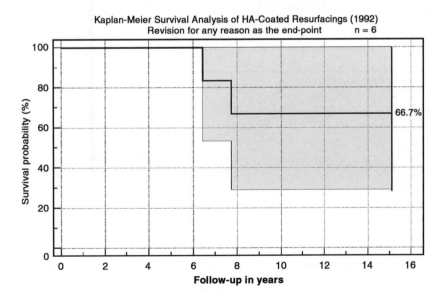

FIG. 1.40. Poor results with HA-coated components due to femoral loosening.

The implant was modified for cemented fixation, and I carried out 43 procedures between March 1992 and December 1993 (Fig. 1.41).

Cemented femoral components solved the femoral loosening problem, and I have not had a femoral loosening since I started the cemented femoral series in March 1992. However, the cemented acetabular cup fixation was terrible. At the time when we reported our early results in 1996, one patient had undergone revision surgery for infection and three patients had undergone revision for cup breakout from the cement mantle. These three patients with early breakout had been revised to an HA-coated acetabular component with a good outcome. The radiology of the cemented acetabular components was poor; at 1 year, 11% had a complete three-zone radiolucent line at the cement bone interface.

At 2 years, 22% had a complete radiolucent line, and at 3 years 67% had a complete radiolucent line. Not surprisingly, these progressive radiolucent lines turned into later cup loosening requiring revision surgery. The survivorship curve shows that this was the worst hip implant I have ever personally performed (Fig. 1.42).

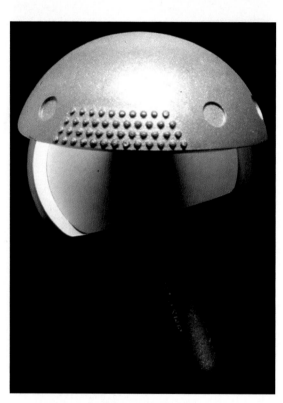

FIG. 1.41. Cemented cup and femoral components. Recesses in cup for cement fixation.

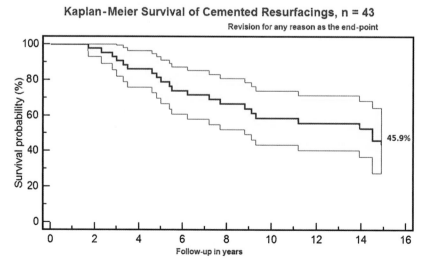

FIG. 1.42. Very poor results with cemented cup, cemented head resurfacings due to acetabular failure.

In some patients, cemented cup resurfacing lasted a good number of years. However, I have come to realize that this cemented cup resurfacing design was so bad that the patients would have been better off if their implant had failed sooner. When late de-bonding occurred between the implant and cement, a tremendous amount of cement debris was generated, and this caused osteolysis (Fig. 1.43). X-ray gives an overoptimistic picture. At revision, one is faced with a mess from massive amounts of cement debris (see the DVD that accompanies this book).

With loosening at the cement-bone interface (Fig. 1.44), cement debris production and osteolysis was not as severe. Revision of these failed cemented cup resurfacings to THR gave us the opportunity of examining femoral head viability in these femoral heads with securely fixed femoral components. Histologic examination of these femoral heads showed normal hemopoietic marrow (Fig. 1.45).

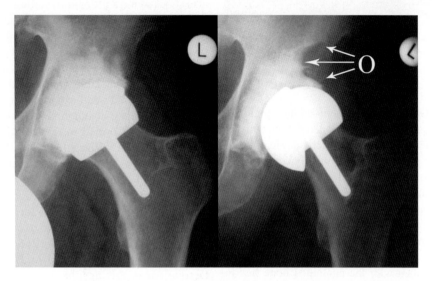

Fig. 1.43. Satisfactory appearances of cemented cup resurfacing at 1 year. Severe osteolysis (*O*) in pelvis at 13 years caused by cement generation at de-bonded implant-cement interface.

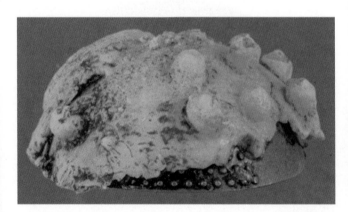

Fig. 1.44. Cemented cup removed for loosening.

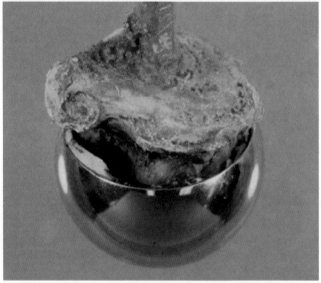

Fig. 1.45. Solidly fixed femoral component revised for cemented cup loosening.

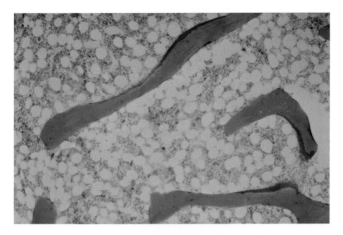

FIG. 1.46. Viable femoral head after resurfacing using a posterior surgical approach.

I had a number of femoral heads examined histologically by Prof. Archie Malcolm, and he considered that none of them showed any evidence of avascular necrosis. He did suggest, however, that we could go further and give the patients tetracycline 2 weeks before their revision surgery. Because we had a number of patients needing revision for their failed cemented cup resurfacing, we were able to do this (Fig. 1.46, Fig. 1.47).

These cemented femoral components were soundly fixed to the underlying bone. In order to obtain histology of the femoral heads, the implant with the contained bone had to be sectioned. Mr. Brian Mawhinney performed a number of these sections for me, and all of the samples we had exam-

ined by Prof. Malcolm showed viable femoral heads. Brian Mawhinney and Archie Malcolm left Newcastle, and I have not had further femoral head histology since then, as most histology labs seem incapable of sectioning through the femoral component.

I was becoming increasingly nervous about the cemented cup fixation in view of the progressive radiolucent lines, but two surgeons from abroad showed interest in using this device. Harlan Amstutz from Los Angeles was one of these. I told him about my early cup breakouts and the progressive radiolucent lines, and he believed that further features on the back of the acetabular cup would prevent breakouts. He also shocked me a little bit by telling me that the radiolucent lines were due to my poor acetabular cement technique! I did point out to him that I had carried out a lot of cemented polyethylene cups in the past without any of these problems, but he was undeterred. Corin made deeper grooves in the acetabular cup back and supplied him with the implant (Fig. 1.48). Harlan continued carrying out this cemented cup for 2 years after I had abandoned it. No doubt all the measurements being performed were useful in developing his own resurfacing, the Conserve Plus. Don Howie from Adelaide, unlike Harlan Amstutz, did come and see me performing these cemented cup resurfacings. I also told him that I had already decided to give this fixation method up and would move to an HA cup as soon as this became available. The day that Don Howie came to visit me, I did one resurfacing, and my senior registrar at the time, Eric Isbister, carried out two or three other cases. Don Howie watched them all. Despite our misgivings, he decided to start implanting the cemented cup and cemented femoral component device, and again Corin supplied this to him. I enquired of both of these surgeons a few years ago about their results, and I was interested to learn that their cemented cup results appeared to be at least as bad as my own.

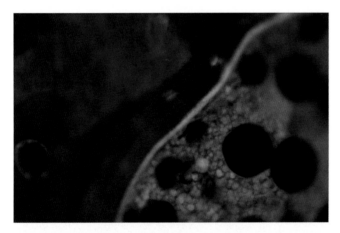

FIG. 1.47. Femoral head bone in a patient with a previous cemented femoral component that was solidly fixed. The resurfacing operation had been performed through a posterior surgical approach. Reason for revision: cup loosening. Under ultraviolet light, uptake of fluorescent tetracycline can be seen on a trabecula.

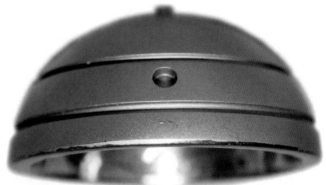

FIG. 1.48. Deeper fixation features for cemented cup provided for Dr. Amstutz.

About 14 years after the event, I was giving a talk abroad, and Michael Freeman was in the audience; I described the excellent results I had achieved with the cemented femoral component but the terrible carnage I had caused with the cemented acetabular component that had behaved worse than any cemented polyethylene cup I had ever inserted. The only polyethylene cup that I had experience revising that came close to being as bad as this implant was the cemented Exeter metal-backed cup. In that device, we also saw cup breakout from the cement mantle (Fig. 1.49) and accelerated cup loosening (Fig. 1.50).

I was amazed at the end of my talk when Michael Freeman stood up and asserted that he only meant me to cement the femoral component and not the acetabular component! Afterwards, I tried to think how I could possibly have known that, when I was seeing loosening with the press-fit acetabular component and his advice was "slap a bit of cement on my son." Perhaps Michael was worried about being associated also with the fourth worst implant to hit the human frame!

I had often wondered why my cemented resurfacing acetabular cup was so much worse than the cemented McKee-Farrar cup. I now think that the answer lies in the spikes on the outer surface of the McKee-Farrar cup (Fig. 1.51).

In my cemented resurfacing cups, the patients with thin cement mantles seemed to develop cup loosening. The patients with thick cement mantles seemed to be less prone to bone-cement interface loosening, but they developed late cup-cement de-bonding. The McKee-Farrar cup spikes guaranteed a thick cement mantle around the cup. I speculate that this reduced relative movement between the cement and bone. In addition, the spikes guaranteed that the cup could not break out from the cement mantle, either early or late.

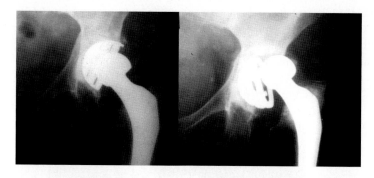

FIG. 1.49. Postoperative x-ray of Exeter metal-backed cemented cup and cup de-bonded from cement mantle.

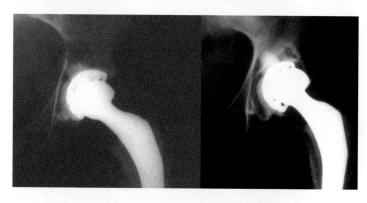

FIG. 1.50. Postoperative x-ray of Exeter metal-backed cemented cup and accelerated loosening at cement-bone interface.

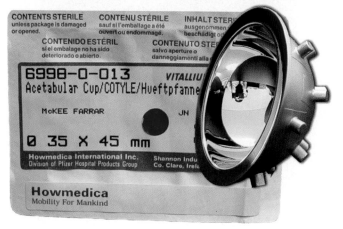

FIG. 1.51. Spikes on the back of McKee-Farrar cup with its original box.

The Hybrid Series

The best acetabular fixation I had seen with my resurfacings, even though the numbers were only tiny, was in the HA-coated cup device. I did not want to return to this device because I had been used to the Harris Galante cup filling the acetabular cavity; Michael Freeman's SLF cup was a cut-away device that just did not fill the acetabulum, at least it did not fill the arthritic acetabulum after it was reamed. It seemed to me that a device that took maximum surface area contact would do better with respect to fixation and impingement of the anterior and posterior acetabular walls, which regularly protruded and required trimming with the Freeman SLF cup. A new cup was designed for cementless HA-coated fixation that had a 180-degree outer sector angle to obtain maximum bony contact and support. The cup was made eccentric in thickness, and the inner sector angle was kept exactly the same as the SLF articular surface.

There was no cup introducer for the early SLF resurfacing cup design, and we just used a block of plastic to impact the cup. The new cup would have an introducer and antirotation flanges. In addition, I had modeling done. We decided that a peripherally expanded acetabular cup would be better than a hemispherical cup at getting a good initial press fit. I designed-in four sets of antirotation fins and eventually this was manufactured. We started inserting this device in March 1994. The first problem related to the antirotation fins. These were to be arranged so that one set bit into the pubis and another set into the ischium. However, the anterosuperior set of antirotation fins regularly hit against sclerotic bone in the anterosuperior acetabulum, and instead of biting into this bone, a common occurrence was that the fins caused the acetabular cup to stand away from the acetabulum in that region.

The posterosuperior set of fins created another problem. This region of the acetabulum is, of course, unsupported and relatively thin, and a regular occurrence on impacting the cup was that these posterosuperior fins split the acetabulum in a radial direction (Fig. 1.52). This problem was solved by removing the superior two sets of fins leaving only fins to bite into the soft bone of the pubis and ischium (Fig. 1.53). The peripherally expanded acetabular component caused me much trouble with insertion, and failure to fully bottom-out the cup was a common occurrence in my practice.

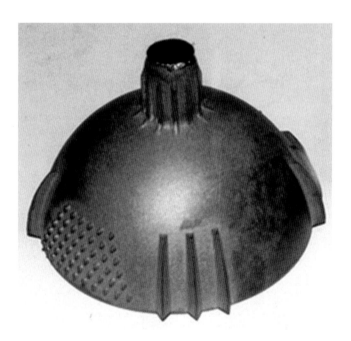

FIG. 1.52. New variety of cup before HA coating. Three of the four sets of antirotation fins can be seen.

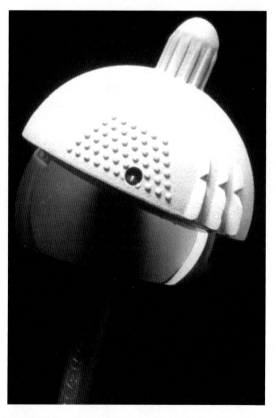

FIG. 1.53. McMinn Hybrid Resurfacing used from March 1994 to December 1996.

When others started using this device, there was much trouble with this design feature. I knew this had to go, but Peter Gibson and the Corin company had been very obliging in modifying the design of the resurfacing to try and get it to work for me. I could not bring myself to ask them to change it again after such a short time in use, so we worked around this problem basically by overreaming the acetabulum. A review of my cases by Dr. Christian de Cock showed that the early results with this device were very good but also showed that failure to seat the acetabular component was a common occurrence (Fig. 1.54). This did not, however, create any clinical problems and, unlike the press-fit, uncoated devices, patients made a rapid and excellent recovery after this hybrid fixed device.

On my postoperative radiographs, only 13 of the first 100 cases had no radiolucent lines in any zone (98 of the 100 were alive at 3 years for comparison). However, on the 3-year-plus radiographs, most of the radiolucent lines had gone with new bone filling the gaps. Seventy-four hips of the 98 had no radiolucent line in any zone at the 3-year-plus time period (Table 1.1).

Eighty hips were classified as Charnley category A or B. These patients had no built-in restraint from other conditions to their activity level. These patients had very good function from their hips (Table 1.2).

At last, I had a hip resurfacing design that gave a good early outcome in patients and, despite the difficulty with cup insertion and poor seating, the radiology at the interfaces improved with time. I started developing more confidence in the device and allowed my numbers to gradually increase. I was grateful to many colleagues in the United Kingdom for referring me young patients who they thought would be suitable for hip resurfacing. Most of these early hybrid designs continue to work well in patients (Fig. 1.55).

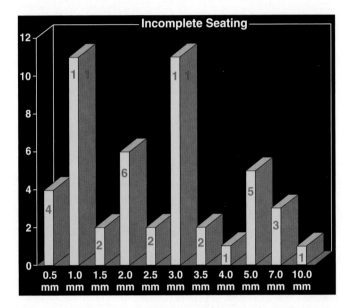

FIG. 1.54. Forty-eight of the first 100 cups were not fully seated. Incomplete seating varied from 0.5 mm to 10 mm.

TABLE 1.1. Cup radiolucent lines

Post-op		3+ years	
One Zone	13	One Zone	15
Two Zone	47	Two Zone	7
Three Zone	25	Three Zone	2
No Radiolucency	13	No Radiolucency	74

TABLE 1.2. Merle-D'Aubigné scores in charnley A + B categories

80 Hips		
Pain	➤	5.99
Walking	➤	5.95
Movement	➤	5.96

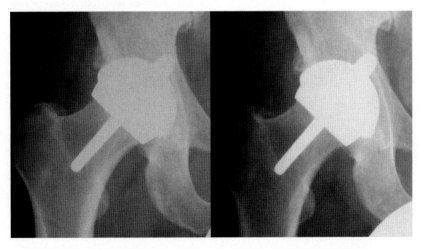

FIG. 1.55. Perfect radiographic outcome 2 years and 12.7 years after McMinn Hybrid Resurfacing performed in 1994. The patient is a keen golfer with a 6 handicap.

Although things were going well on the clinical front, changes occurred at Corin that were unsettling. Peter Gibson sold a large chunk of his shares in Corin, and the new investors brought in their own managing director. From that day I saw the culture of the company change with the dollar becoming the new God. Cost-cutting and increased profits seemed the overriding target. The animals were in charge of the zoo.

I spent my time training new surgeons who wished to take up the resurfacing method in several different countries. I was increasingly being invited to give talks at various meetings on hip resurfacing. It was an interesting fact that when my resurfacings were distinctly suboptimal in the pilot study years, I only had a modest amount of grief from surgeons around the world who objected to hip resurfacing. The opposition started to intensify when the hybrid devices were obviously working well. I had to endure sequential arguments with time, along the lines of:

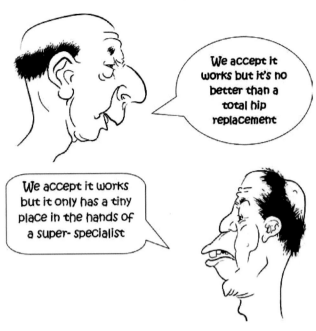

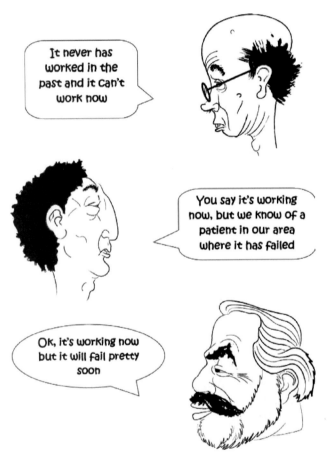

Dealing with all these sceptics was no problem because when I came back from conferences, I was able to listen to patients who were absolutely delighted, and my wine cellar was looking distinctly healthy from the many gifts I had received. Everything was going well until the end of 1996 when a few of my patients started to report a screeching noise from their

hips in the immediate postoperative period. Other surgeons from around the world reported the same problem, and we think there were about 20 patients from different centers who reported this early noise from their hips.

It is relevant for me now to describe all the noises that a metal on metal hip resurfacing can make at different time periods. In the early postoperative period, it is common for patients to report a knocking or tapping noise. We have investigated this with standing and leg dangling x-rays of the hip and have observed 2 mm of distraction of the hip with dangling in patients who report a knocking noise. We think this is caused by a hip capsule full of blood, and pain inhibition of various muscles around the hip in the early postoperative period allowing the head to displace slightly out of the cup. When the leg is loaded, a relocation noise occurs. This noise is generally reported on the ward, and when the patient returns for their 2- to 3-month postoperative review, the noise has gone. Unlike the common early postoperative tapping noise, a screeching noise is very rare and to my knowledge has occurred in about 1 per 1000 cases in my series. I have of course had the same noise reported by other surgeons around the world. This noise occurs typically at around the 6-month postoperative stage. My patients who have developed this have been very careful in the early postoperative period and then around the 6-month stage they have gone mountain climbing. I have had a patient on top of a mountain telephone me, and holding their mobile phone beside their hip, I could hear a loud screeching noise with each hip movement. I believe that if we could magically place a hip resurfacing into a patient's hip without producing any bleeding, then I think every patient would get noise from their hip in the early postoperative period. It is the blood after surgery that bathes the hip joint and acts as an excellent lubricant that allows the hip to "run in" without any noise. We know from retrievals that a small patch on the acetabular cup and a larger patch on the femoral head are run in. I speculate that the timid and careful patient runs in a smaller patch and at the 6-month stage when they go mountain climbing, a different and larger patch is required, particularly on the head, to accommodate walking with a flexed hip. The problem now is that they are "running in" a new patch without blood and instead have synovial fluid lubricating the hip joint and a noise is produced. I advised patients who had this noise to engage in intensive swimming, trying to reproduce the noise by various movements and running in their new patch. This noise disappears after about 3 weeks.

The noise reported from patients at the end of 1996 was different in timing to those just described. Corin could not account for this noise, and we all worried that something awful might have happened in the manufacturing process that could cause premature failure of these joints. An international recall was instigated, and a thorough investigation of recalled devices was started.

Investigations showed that the probable cause of the noise was a problem with the introducer. Apparently in the interests of efficient production, a change in the order of manufacturing had occurred whereby face polishing of the cup now occurred after drilling the holes for the introducer ("animals at work"). This meant that the holes for the introducer were too close to the cup face on occasions and the impact load was transferred through the holes of the cup instead of through the face of the cup. Small burrs could be raised at the articular edge of the cup holes, and this was thought to be the reason for the noise (Figs. 1.56 and 1.57).

The few patients of mine who reported this noise in the early postoperative period all did perfectly well, and the noise typically had gone by the time of their 2–month postoperative review.

There were a number of other problems discovered in the investigation after this recall. One of these was that the components in some cases were moderately out of specification on roundness. I knew that this had occurred right from the beginning because when Harlan Amstutz started to do my resurfacing, he had all these implants measured by Harry McKellop before the implants were inserted. On a regular basis, I received phone calls from Harlan Amstutz telling me that yet again they had found some of the McMinn implants were out of round. The problem was that Harlan could never remember that there was a time difference between Los Angeles and Birmingham, and I was regularly woken up at 3 AM to be told about this out-of-round problem. I reported all these conversations to Corin, and they kept telling me that the components were fine. Thanks to Harlan's phone calls, I knew for certain that the components had been manufactured out of round long before 1996. We later had 17 new and unused McKee-Farrar and Ring metal on metal THRs measured; they were out of round also by a similar amount to that consistently reported by Harlan. There were a number

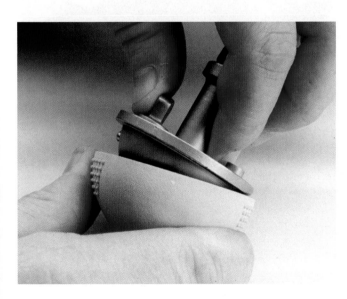

FIG. 1.56. Cup introducer being attached to acetabular component. Two locking pins hold the cup on.

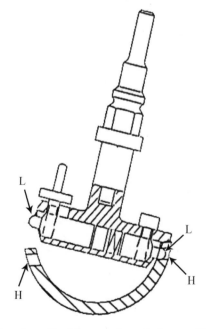

FIG. 1.57. Drawing of introducer and acetabular cup. If the holes in the cup (*H*) are too close to the cup face, then impact load will be transferred through the locking pins (*L*) to the cup hole edge, and a burr can be raised.

of other tiresome issues, but one stood out as being of potential significance. This concerned heat treatments of the metal castings; apparently there had been problems with porosity of the metal castings and a high factory scrap rate. It was described to me that a casting could look perfectly satisfactory, but when machined and polished, the articular surface would have a porosity defect and the casting would have to be scrapped. It seems that various post-casting heat treatments had been employed to attempt to get over these porosity problems. There seemed to be a certain randomness to the exact nature of the heat treatments but roughly speaking during 1994 and 1995, the implants were given single heat treatments of either hot isostatic pressing (HIP) or solution heat treatment (SHT). During 1996, the implants were given double heat treatment of both HIP and SHT. I am certain that if Peter Gibson had remained in charge, this problem would have been discussed with me given that my name was attached to the implant concerned. When I heard about this heat treatment, I looked at the literature; there were two published papers showing that heat treatment increased the wear of metal on metal bearings [11,12]. I met with Corin

and insisted that these heat treatments be stopped and that instead the implant should be manufactured like the Ring and McKee-Farrar from an as-cast structure. They refused on the grounds that they already had a number of castings in their possession that had been heat treated and they refused to scrap these castings. I pointed out that I simply could not have a device with my name attached to it where the implant had been heat treated and the available literature showed that heat treatment damaged the wear properties of the bearing. I was receiving a royalty on sales from Corin, but despite the obvious financial disadvantage, we shook hands and went our separate ways. The McMinn resurfacing double heat treated castings were used to manufacture the Cormet 2000. This was launched in 1997 and remains, I understand, double heat treated to this day.

The McMinn Hybrid Resurfacing implant continued to work very well in the early years, but time has started to show some problems (Fig. 1.58).

The mode of failure in a vast majority of the 1996 series was metallosis, osteolysis, and acetabular component loosening (Figs. 1.59 and 1.60).

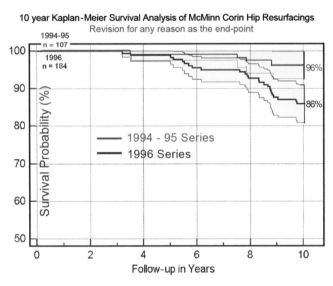

FIG. 1.58. Ten-year survival analysis showing 4% failure with single heat treated implants from 1994 and 1995 and 14% failure from double heat treated implants from 1996.

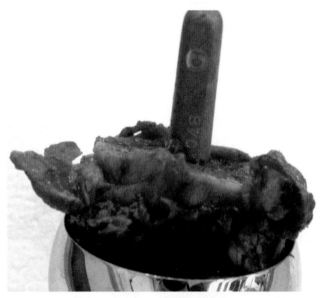

FIG. 1.59. Metallosis staining of soft tissue around femoral neck at revision of 1996 McMinn Hybrid Resurfacing. The patient had osteolysis and cup loosening.

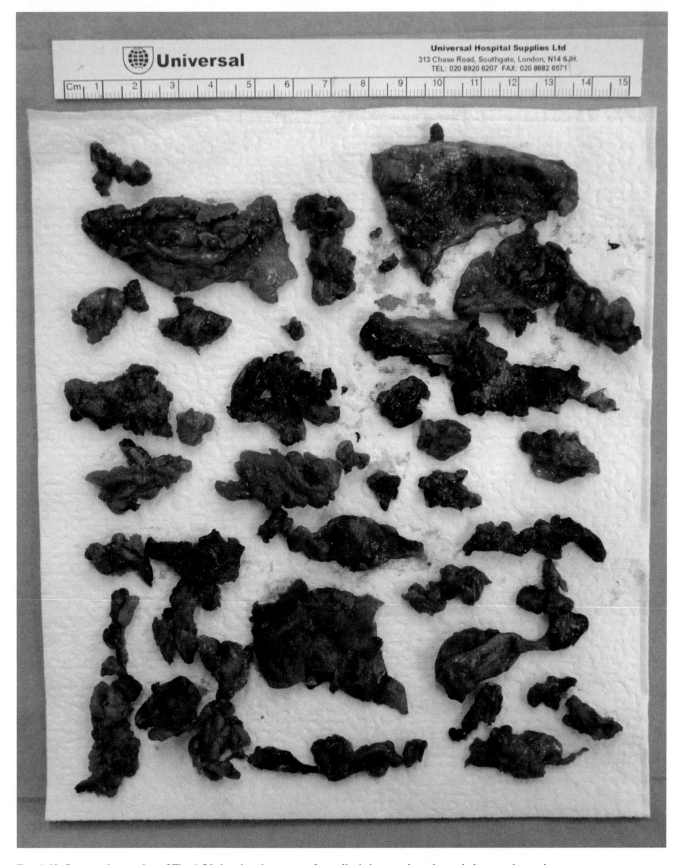

FIG. 1.60. Same patient as that of Fig. 1.56 showing the extent of metallosis in capsule and acetabular pseudomembrane.

A few patients from the 1996 series at the time of writing have still not been reviewed clinically or radiographically at 10 years even though we know that their implants are still *in situ*. At this stage, approximately 20% of the unrevised patients from the 1996 series have radiographic failure in the form of osteolysis and/or cup loosening (Fig. 1.61).

Although the divorce from Corin in 1996 was painful, I am now grateful that I did not perform more of these double heat treated implants. It should be noted on the survivorship graph of the 1996 series that failure did not become obvious until after 5.5 years. That means that if one was checking a national register or one's own results, failure of a double heat treated implant would not become obvious until after 5.5 years. On a worldwide basis, many thousands of defective implants could be inserted into patients before an obvious failure pattern was recognized. There are characteristics of the McMinn

1996 hybrid implant that could have caused earlier failure. We believe that hydroxyapatite on a substantially smooth surface is a relatively weak interface to be invaded by particulate debris like excess production of metal particles. Some of the newer implants on the market with porous coating of the acetabular component but double heat treated metal bearings may take longer before clinical failure occurs compared with my 1996 implants. However, I fear that the longevity of these implants will be at the expense of severe acetabular osteolysis.

I have heard many explanations from Corin as to why the wear of the 1996 series was so bad. They said at one stage that I had inserted the cups vertically in 1996. It would be odd for me to put in resurfacing cups satisfactorily from 1991 to 1995, then vertically during 1996, and then satisfactorily again in 1997.

The acetabular inclination angles from 1994 and 1995 to 1996 to 1997 did not change (Fig. 1.62).

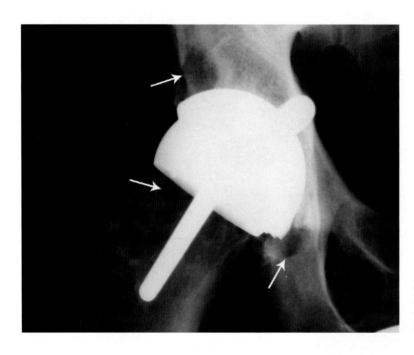

Fig. 1.61. A 35-year-old man with McMinn Hybrid Resurfacing performed in 1996. Very minor symptoms at 10-year follow-up, but radiographic osteolysis (arrows) present in pelvis and femoral neck.

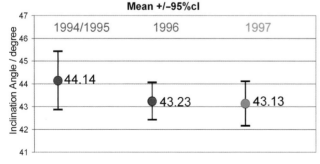

Fig. 1.62. Satisfactory cup inclination angles 1994–1995, 1996, and 1997.

In addition, a detailed wear analysis was carried out in 2002 of retrieved implants from 1996 (Fig. 1.63). Mike Tuke spent many hours carefully analyzing these implants using coordinate measuring machines (CMMs; see Chapter 3) and multiple roundness tracings. On the cups, the wear scars are colored in white, the deepest point in the wear scar is marked with a black dot, and the unworn areas are colored in black. It can be seen that in only 2 of the 9 cup explants does the wear scar extend to the cup edge (cup 2 and cup 4). However, it can be seen that the deepest point of the wear scar in all cup explants lay within the articular surface and not on the cup edge. We now know from many years of analyzing retrieved metal on metal implants that edge loading does indeed lead to marked wear of a metal on metal bearing. However, the cup wear on these edge-loaded implants is profound and localized, and the deepest point of the wear scar is right on the cup edge. The pattern of wear on these 9 cup retrievals from 1996 shows no evidence of edge loading as a cause of failure in this patient cohort.

Another reason put forward was that the introducer used in 1996 caused failure in this cohort of patients. The same introducer was used in 1994, 1995, and 1996. It is true that a small number of patients had a problem with noise in the early post-operative period as already described at the end of 1996. None of these patients however had clinical failure. In addition, if burrs at the introducer holes were the reason for failure in this cohort, one would expect wear in the region of the introducer holes. Figure 1.58 shows that only 2 of the 18 introducer holes had the wear scar encroaching onto the area of the introducer holes. Furthermore, in these two examples the wear scar only just encroaches onto the introducer holes. There is no evidence that the introducer caused failures in the 1996 cohort.

The uncomfortable fact is that the one thing that changed in 1996 was the heat treatment regimen, with the 1996 implants being double heat treated. The reader can see in the basic science chapter that pin on disk and pin on plate tests show that the wear of heat-treated cobalt chrome is higher than that of as-cast cobalt chrome. These types of tests are a test of material with the lubricant playing a small part only. If one were to judge heat treatment on the basis of these tests, then heat-treated cobalt chrome would never be used as the bearing for a metal on metal implant. There is a tendency to think of hip simulators as producing a more clinically relevant result. Perhaps surgeons equate expense of the test with clinical relevance or perhaps the apparent complexity of the machines instills

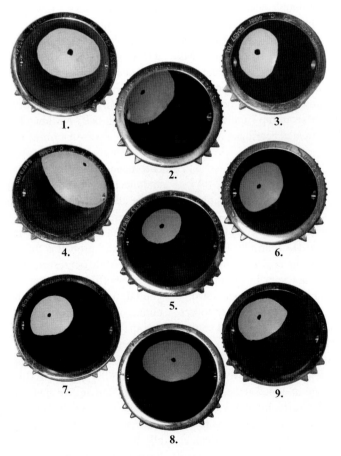

FIG. 1.63. Nine retrieved McMinn hybrid cups from revision surgery. Implants were all inserted in 1996. Wear patch is marked white, center of the wear patch is marked with a black dot, and unworn cup is black.

confidence. On hip simulators, heat-treated cobalt chrome wears no more than the as-cast material. However, one hip simulator study that purported to show no difference between as-cast and double heat treated cobalt chrome was particularly poorly controlled [13]. The mean diametral clearance of the as-cast group was 259.5 μm with the mean clearance of the double heat treated group 215 μm. The difference was highly significant (p ≤ 0.01). This lower clearance gives the heat-treated couples a fluid film advantage on a hip simulator.

It will be seen in Chapter 4 that fluid film lubrication on certain hip simulators can protect the bearing material from wear. This has important implications when testing materials with poor wear characteristics such as heat-treated cobalt chrome. It should be understood that if the bearing couple is round enough, smooth enough, and has an acceptable clearance, then it will do well on a hip simulator no matter how poor the wear properties of the material. Look at the severe clinical problems caused by the use of high wearing, low carbon containing metal on metal couples. These joints performed very well on hip simulators [14]. Read this Otto Aufranc award paper and see if you too could have been misled by this science. A simple pin on disk test would have shown the high wear of this bearing couple in a matter of days, and many patients could have been spared unnecessary early failure and revision surgery. The real-life test of double heat treated metal on metal bearings was a miserable failure, despite satisfactory simulator tests. I was unwittingly the first surgeon in the world to insert double heat treated metal on metal bearings. My patients have already paid a heavy price for this mistake, and others will continue to pay a price for many years to come. Do you seriously think that I would now accept that these awful bearings are, after all, fine on the basis of hip simulator tests, and that I would ever insert a heat-treated bearing again?

The MMT Years

My colleague Ronan Treacy, FRCS, had been using the McMinn Hybrid Resurfacing since 1994. He had constant problems with supply of enough implants from Corin. In addition, he had quality problems. He routinely tested the implants before insertion and had to reject a number of implants because the head would not spin in the cup. His confidence in the manufacturing ability of Corin was starting to ebb. During 1996, he had decided to seek another source of resurfacing implants and had made moves toward setting up an independent company. When I departed from Corin, Ronan and I joined forces in this venture. The company was called Midland Medical Technologies (MMT). Now Ronan and I had to gather a large team of able-minded people around us to develop the best hip resurfacing the world had seen hitherto. We both had total confidence in the hip resurfacing principle and, in this cause, put our families' finances and our reputations on the line.

During 1996, I had started to take an interest in how the resurfacing was manufactured. With reports of manufacturing problems, I began to realize that I could not leave things to the engineers and hope that they would fix the problems. I made trips to factories and casting houses to learn how these implants were manufactured. By 1997, therefore, I had received a good education on what to do and even more information on what not to do in relation to metal on metal bearing manufacture.

We engaged Centaur Precision in Sheffield to cast the implants, Finsbury Instruments to machine and finish the implants, Plasma Coatings to carry out HA coating of the acetabular cup, Hunts to clean and pack the finished implants, and Swann Morton to carry out sterilization.

We were very clear that we did not want to start some new experiment with the metallurgy, having developed confidence in the material used by McKee and Ring, with a successful history going back to 1960. Tim Band at Centaur was a tireless source of energy and was a key person in getting the Birmingham Hip Resurfacing developed. He took on the role of identifying the methods of casting used to make the McKee and Ring implants. We supplied him with new and used Ring and McKee implants to reverse engineer. This felt like *déjà vu* as I had gone through the same exercise with Corin in 1989. This time, however, Tim Band was in charge. He did a thorough job and produced a huge dossier of results. He was assisted by Graham Dixon, metallurgist at Centaur, and John Metcalf and Jess Crawley, materials scientists at Sheffield Hallam University.

The results of this work were clear. The historic metal on metal implants were as-cast structures.

That meant that these implants were not heat treated. All these investigators were most accommodating with their time and teaching. Ronan did not carry the same baggage as myself, but having been let down by manufacturers on my resurfacing once, I was determined to learn as much as possible from these experts. I spent hours in Sheffield learning about cobalt chrome and the effect of heat treatment on its microstructure and mechanical and wear properties.

We all believed that the implant should be as-cast like the Ring and McKee, and no postcasting heat processes would be used. This threw up some problems. How would we prevent the porosity problems that set Corin off on the wrong track with the McMinn resurfacing implant?

The Sheffield team were confident that by a combination of good design of the waxes and metal feeds, together with vacuum casting, porosity would not be a problem. Time proved that they were right.

Ronan and I were both determined to have a porous ingrowth surface on the cup. We were, however, impressed by the ability of hydroxyapatite (HA) to encourage bone to grow toward it. We had seen the large gaps left by failure of full seating of the hybrid cup fill in beautifully. However, there was accumulating evidence that HA would eventually become resorbed, and this raised concern about late cup loosening. What we really wanted was HA on a porous surface. We discussed this with the experts in HA coating and the advice was to have a coarse, porous coating. With a fine porous coating, the HA spraying can block the pores in the porous network thus removing the point of having the implant porous coated in the first place.

Also, when the pores are larger, the insides of the pores can be coated by the line-of-sight process that is involved in HA coating.

We tried various porous coatings. The BHR with sintered porous beads was investigated (Fig. 1.64). The microstructure of the cup was ruined by the sintering process, and this type of porous-coated BHR was never implanted into patients.

Interestingly, Wright have applied sintered beads to the Conserve Plus cup and DePuy have applied sintered beads to the ASR cup. We considered plasma-sprayed titanium but had two concerns. We were concerned that titanium coated onto the cobalt chrome substrate could suffer from galvanic corrosion. We were very worried about the plasma spray breaking off and entering the articulation as we had observed plasma-sprayed titanium fall off in its packaging box (Fig. 1.65). I had seen evidence of plasma-sprayed

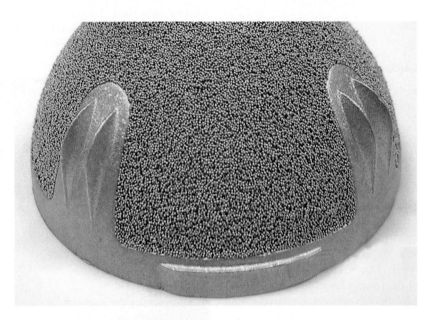

Fig. 1.64. Sintered beaded BHR cup. Because of microstructural damage of the metal, this implant was never used clinically.

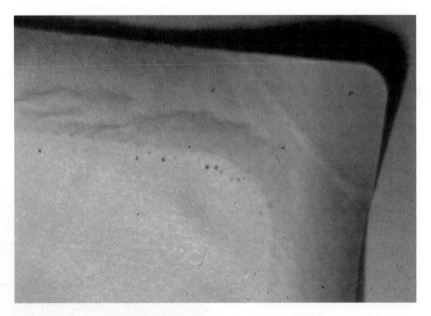

Fig. 1.65. Plasma-sprayed titanium particles in packaging box having fallen off the porous surface of an acetabular cup.

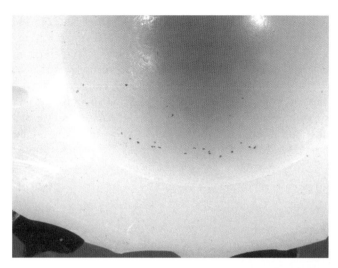

FIG. 1.66. Polyethylene liner removed at revision with embedded plasma-sprayed titanium particles. Plasma-sprayed acetabular shell was solidly fixed.

titanium coating migrate into the articulation in my revision practice (Fig. 1.66).

In view of the above, we dismissed plasma-sprayed titanium as a bad alternative for porous coating the cup. Interestingly, Corin decided to plasma spray the Cormet 2000 cup, initially with cobalt chrome and later with titanium, Biomet has plasma-sprayed titanium on the Recap resurfacing, and Zimmer has plasma sprayed titanium on the Durom cup. Elevation of blood titanium after insertion of the Durom resurfacing implant has been reported [15]. Whether this was due to galvanic corrosion on the back of the cup or particles of titanium getting into the articulation has not been clear until now (see Chapter 6). As can be seen in the retrievals section, titanium has been found ground into the articular surfaces of a retrieved Durom resurfacing. The effect of third-body titanium particles on a second-generation metal on metal bearing has been investigated in a hip simulator study. The titanium particles increased the metal on metal bearing wear by almost an order of magnitude [16].

It was decided that a cast-in porous surface would be best, and the Porocast ingrowth surface was developed (Fig. 1.67).

This was not an easy development. I landed Tim Band in trouble with the bigwigs at Centaur when I destroyed a £17,000 tank of ceramic during one of my less successful experiments. I rather liked the appearance of a tea leaf porous-coated cup, with a Harrods tea variety giving a perfect texture. Unfortunately, the tea leaves caused contamination during first dipping, destroying the tank of ceramic. Happily, success eventually followed with a much more reliable method.

Time has shown that the HA-coated Porocast BHR cup has worked very well. I have seen tremendous bone ongrowth (Fig. 1.68) and ingrowth into this cup (Fig. 1.69).

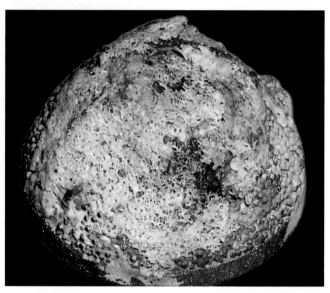

FIG. 1.68. Extensive bone on-growth. BHR cup removed at Girdle-stone excision for hematogenous infection 3 years postoperatively

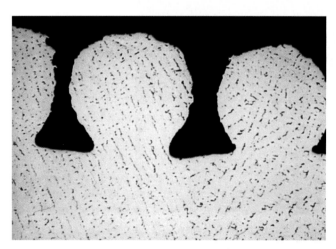

FIG. 1.67. Section through Porocast beads and cup substrate metal. Beads are integral with cup substrate metal. Carbides (dark dots) in microstructure can be seen.

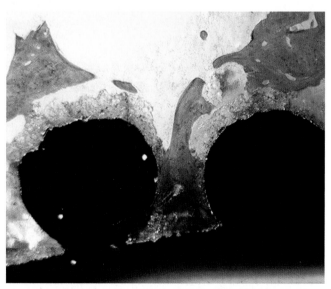

FIG. 1.69. Excellent bone ingrowth into HA on Porocast BHR surface at 6 months.

The introducer had been a problem with the McMinn Hybrid Resurfacing and a new introducer was developed with a grasping and tensioning mechanism in the introducer, locking onto cables that are prethreaded through wormholes in the cup edge (Fig. 1.70). This instrument had designed out, as far as possible, the opportunity for the introducer to damage the articulating surface of the cup.

We were not prepared to tolerate the out-of-roundness issues that kept on being brought up during the Corin years. Mike Tuke and his team at Finsbury did a great job by introducing precision manufacturing for the BHR. All the phone calls and concern about quality that existed during the Corin years disappeared at a stroke. What a joy to be able to trust your manufacturer. Clearance was another issue that had to be decided upon, and again we did not want to engage in any new experiments with patients, instead relying on the clearances used in the historic metal on metal devices (Fig. 1.71).

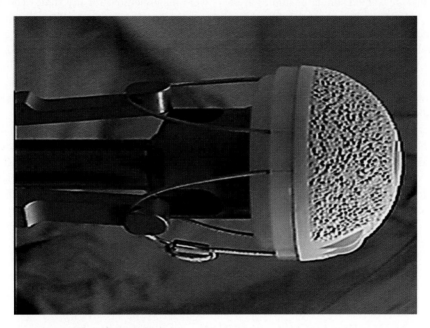

FIG. 1.70. BHR cup on introducer.

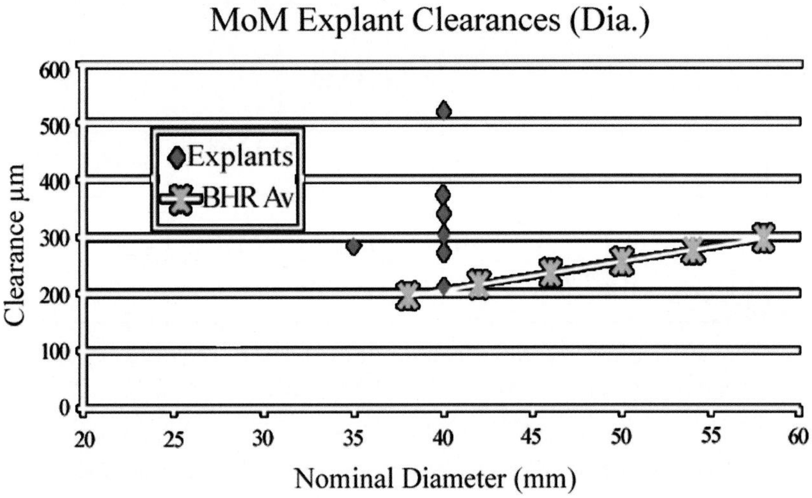

FIG. 1.71. Diametral clearances of long-term Ring and McKee-Farrar explants with measured low wear. Clearance of the BHR increases with increasing head size.

The range of clearances of the BHR was chosen from the lower end of the range of clearances from successful historic metal on metal devices.

Laboratory simulator experiments have shown that reducing the clearance reduces initial run-in wear. As already discussed, I am sceptical about laboratory simulators. Some years after the introduction of the BHR, we decided to get simulator experiments done as some of our surgeons were asking for these. A colleague and I went to see Prof. John Fisher in Leeds, and we had a tour of his laboratories. Afterwards in his office, he expressed surprise that we wanted simulator studies as the BHR device was obviously clinically successful. I explained that surgeons in some countries wanted results from these tests and hence my enquiry. He then shocked me by asking, "What do you want to show? Would you like the wear to be lower, the same or higher than other metal on metal devices? I can set the simulator to show whatever you want!" He reinforced his point by giving me a slide showing completely different wear results of the same metal on metal bearings on two different simulators. I later published this slide with his permission [17]. My colleague and I left Leeds that day rather confused about the value of hip simulators. Laboratory simulator studies will be presented later in this book for those who place reliance on these devices. My position is that if something looks good on a simulator, then it may be worthy of definitive testing in the clinical setting. I object when surgeons present suboptimal clinical results and then say; "Can't be anything to do with the bearing because the simulator results were fine!" The simulator results are a rough guide, on a good day, as to what might happen in the body. Clinical studies are reality. Conversely, if hip simulator studies produce poor results on a device that is known to work well clinically, then the hip simulator regimen needs to be examined to understand where the simulator study went wrong.

Clearance, therefore, was an issue that I considered worthy of clinical investigation. Twenty-six low-clearance BHRs were manufactured for my study. The mean diametral clearance in these implants was 98 μm, with a range 94 to 109 μm. The study was designed to remove confounding variables, and only 50-mm bearings were manufactured with this low clearance Men with unilateral hip arthritis, no other metallic devices in their bodies, and a willingness to participate in this long-term study after informed consent were regarded as suitable patients.

As will be seen in the section later in this book on metal ions, cobalt is an ion that is rapidly excreted from the body in the urine. A timed urine collection with a 24-hour measurement of cobalt excretion is labor intensive but gives an excellent measurement of daily production of metal from wear and corrosion. The graphs of Fig. 1.72 show the daily production of cobalt by the low-clearance BHRs compared with the regular-clearance BHRs.

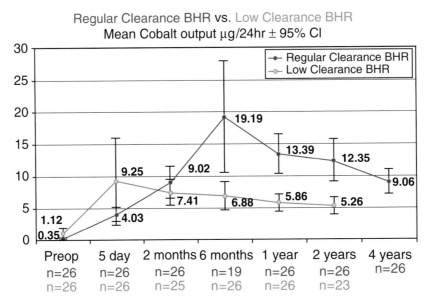

Fig. 1.72. Daily output of cobalt from regular-clearance and low-clearance BHR.

This appears to give a clear result, with the clinical study agreeing with previous hip simulator studies showing that low-clearance bearings reduce run-in wear. Interestingly, the peak production of cobalt in the regular clearance group is at 6 months with a slow decline in production to 4 years. The peak production of cobalt in the low-clearance group is at 5 days with a slower decline in production out to 2 years. It will be interesting to see when these two lines meet, if they do indeed meet, indicating an equal steady-state wear in these different clearance joints.

It might be wondered, therefore, why we have not reduced the clearance of the 50-mm-diameter bearing BHR from around 250 μm down to around 100 μm. This can easily be done from a manufacturing viewpoint. Unfortunately, there is a catch. Three patients out of the 26 low-clearance BHRs in the study have developed radiolucent lines around their cups (Fig. 1.73). This is an unusual finding for the BHR cup. An independent study of 230 BHRs with 210 complete sets of radiographs showed no radiolucent lines around the acetabular component [18]. We think that these radiolucent lines may be related to intraoperative cup deformation. A discussion of intraoperative cup deformation will be seen in later chapters; suffice it to say here that it is now known that intraoperative deformation of acetabular cups does occur. The line of deformation is from the anterior inferior iliac spine to the ischium (Fig. 1.74).

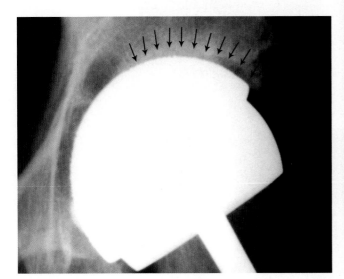

FIG. 1.73. Zone 1 and 2 radiolucent line (arrows) in low-clearance BHR cup 2 years postoperatively.

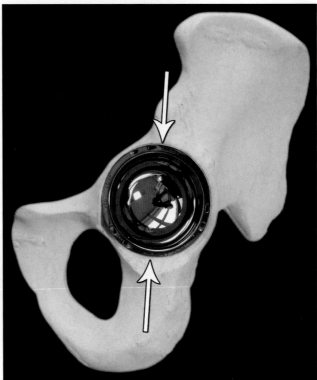

FIG. 1.74. With press-fit cementless cups, compression occurs between anterior inferior spine and ischium (arrows).

We have been able to measure intraoperative cup deformation with a special instrument and have observed cup
deformation measurements of more than 100 μm (Fig. 1.75).
Intraoperative deformation of acetabular THR cup shells has
been measured between 10 and 455 μm [19]. We speculate
that the radiolucent lines in the three patients from the low-
clearance group were due to cup deformation greater than the
clearance, thus causing gripping of the head by the deformed
cup periphery. The extent of cup deformation relates to the
quality of the patient's acetabular bone stock, the amount of
acetabular underreaming and extent of press-fit achieved, and

the deformation characteristics of the component. Only the
latter of these is under the control of the implant designers.
Excessively low clearance of a resurfacing metal on metal
device is considered dangerous. To put this in perspective, as
the BHR ball sits in the cup, the argument is about whether to
have the gap between the ball and the cup one hair's breadth or
two hairs' breadth. Two hairs' breadth gap is safer.

Thus, the ingredients for the cake were assembled, and the
first BHR was inserted in July 1997. This patient continues to
do well clinically and radiographically at the 10-year postoperative stage (Fig 1.76).

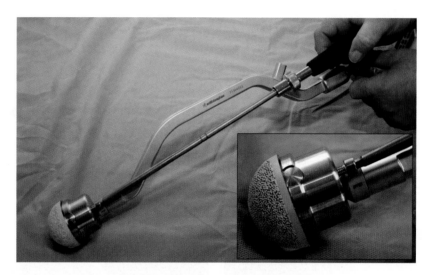

FIG. 1.75. Equipment for measurement of intraoperative cup deformation.

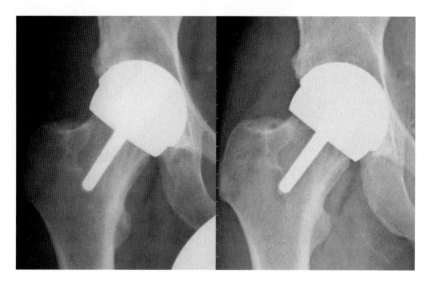

FIG. 1.76. Five-year and 10-year postoperative radiographs of first BHR patient.

Because Ronan and I were financially linked to the BHR, we were concerned that our reporting of our own results would be seen as biased. We knew very well that our results would not be biased, but it was the perception of others that mattered. We decided that an outside group should review our results; the question was who? We had an excellent research center at the Royal Orthopaedic Hospital run by Prof. Paul Pynsent, and there was an expectation that we would engage that group to carry out the independent patient follow-up. I was bothered that the Birmingham-based research group would also be seen as being our friends, and I sought another group who would definitely not be seen as our friends. For more than 100 years, the Robert Jones and Agnes Hunt Orthopaedic Hospital in Oswestry and the Royal Orthopaedic Hospital in Birmingham have competed for funding and staff and view each other as local rivals. I came to the view that the Oswestry Outcome Centre could never be regarded as our friends and that they were the perfect group to carry out an independent review of our cases. Prof. James Richardson and his group were engaged to carry out follow-up not only on Ronan's and my cases but also on the first 5000 BHRs from around the world. This decision was not popular in Birmingham and gained me some enemies, but I think in the end it was seen as an honest attempt at getting truly independent data.

More than 70,000 BHRs have been inserted in a number of countries since, with several publications showing good outcomes and investigations.

Life was never boring at MMT. Eric Isbister, Ronan Treacy, and myself carried out the BHR for 6 months before the implant was released to a wider group. We trained the company representatives properly. Every representative spent time in the operating room with Ronan and myself, and the best ones came back on multiple occasions and scrubbed in with us. We had a fantastic group of representatives who were high-quality people to start with, and the training that they received made them a valuable resource for our new surgeons performing their first few cases. When fully released, the uptake of the BHR was greater than we had ever thought likely. We had no effective competition in the early days and were able to choose the best hip surgeons across the world to take on this implant. The vast majority of these surgeons came to Birmingham for training. We discovered that the better the surgeon, the more likely they were to come for training. Really good surgeons hate failure, and any tips they can pick up to avoid problems are sought, even if it involves the inconvenience of traveling to Birmingham. We have grown to mistrust the know-all types who believe that they do not need training. Experience has shown that their results are soon found wanting, but they will always try and blame the instruments or the implant! Australia was the second biggest market outside the United Kingdom, and Harry Revelas, a BHR surgeon from South Africa, moved to Sydney to become our Australian distributor. He and his team did a wonderful job training surgeons and getting the BHR off to a successful start in Australia. We had one troublesome time when an employee had been secretly abusing company funds. We discovered very late that MMT was the owner of a luxury yacht and other items that

were a diversion from our purpose. With around 60% growth per annum, every penny the company made in the early days was ploughed back into purchase of instruments, surgeon training, and more implant stocks. With this silly diversion of funds, stocks were low and there were unhappy surgeons for several weeks until the situation was resolved. At the time of this problem, Mike Tuke temporarily assumed a management role in MMT to try and get things back on track. Finsbury and MMT had been separate companies, and I suggested to Mike that the two companies should merge. I offered a 50–50 split of shares between MMT and Finsbury, but my offer was rejected and the two companies continued to run separately. Our two nonexecutive directors, Simon Hunt and Graham Silk, spent a lot of their time guiding this happy bunch of enthusiastic amateurs in the ways of management, and now we had missed blatant misuse of funds! Simon and Graham searched out John Hatton who was appointed as the managing director of MMT. He used all his financial and people management skills to grow the company fast but at the same time taking no shortcuts that could degrade the quality of our products or services. John was a huge success, and he guided MMT into a stronger position than Ronan and I could ever have imagined. Data started to accumulate showing good results with the BHR in the hands of many surgeons. The new messages from the former malcontents at conferences were particularly amusing:

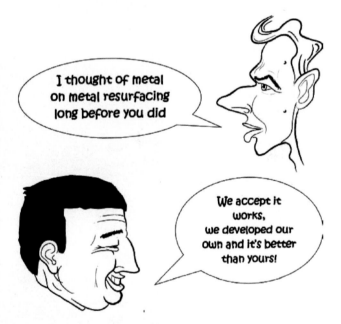

Tim Band succumbed to our offer to move from Centaur to become a director of MMT, and Brendan McGrath, Tony Alleeson, and Roger Ashton also joined as directors. We outgrew the space available at the Birmingham University Research Park and moved to new premises on the outskirts of Birmingham.

The Birmingham Mid Head Resection (BMHR) implant was developed and a radiostereometric analysis (RSA) study was started. A cemented-stem THR was developed with Richard Field, and development of a cementless THR stem with Peter Walker and Sarah Muirhead-Allwood was begun.

We started to get offers from larger companies to buy MMT. These were rejected. One major market still eluded us. We had started work to try and gain access to the United States. We hired M Squared from Washington run by Marie Marlow who were expert at building a case and putting it to the Food and Drug Administration (FDA). We discussed distribution deals with different companies in the United States, but then two offers were made to buy MMT that we could not ignore. After a lot of consideration with our agents, Kimbells[LLP], we decided to accept the offer of Smith & Nephew Ltd. The sale was completed on March 12, 2004, and announced at the San Francisco meeting of the American Academy. I gave a talk from the Smith & Nephew stand on the BHR, and the interest was so great that there was standing room only. I was asked to participate in a live Webcast to city financiers with members of the Smith & Nephew team chaired by Sir Chris O'Donnell,

chief executive officer. Ronan and I were asked to stay on for 5 years to help with the transition and also to help in gaining FDA approval. It was sad to say goodbye to Simon Hunt, Graham Silk, and John Hatton who had all done so much to ensure the success of MMT.

Smith & Nephew backed the efforts of Marie Marlow and her team with input from their regulatory affairs department. My staff at the McMinn Centre worked tirelessly to have a 100% audit of our notes and x-rays by M Squared and then make ourselves ready for a week-long audit by the FDA. The Outcome Centre in Oswestry also had the same work to prepare for audits. Smith & Nephew added 2-mm increment heads, each with two matching regular cups and each having a matching dysplasia cup. New instruments were also designed and manufactured. The BHR was now the most comprehensive resurfacing system available (Fig. 1.77).

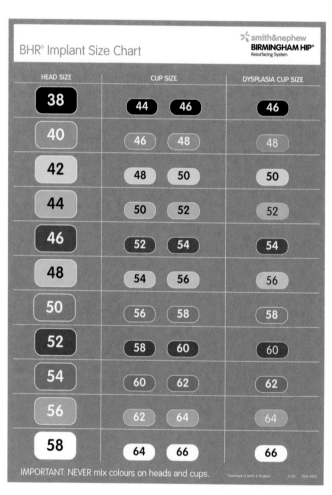

Fig. 1.77. Two-millimeter-increment Birmingham Hip Resurfacing sizing chart.

On May 9, 2006, the Birmingham Hip Resurfacing was given clearance for sale in the United States by the FDA. We all drank a toast to Marie Marlow on that day.

References

1. Swanson SAV, Freeman MAR, Heath JC. Laboratory tests on total joint replacement prostheses. J Bone Joint Surg Br 1973;55:759–773.
2. Wilson JN, Scales JT. Loosening of total hip replacements with cement fixation, clinical findings and laboratory studies. Clin Orthop 1970;72:145–160.
3. Andersson GB, Freeman MA, Swanson SA. Loosening of the cemented acetabular cup in total hip replacement. J Bone Joint Surg Br 1972;54:590–599
4. Heath JC, Freeman MA, Swanson SA. Carcinogenic properties of wear particles from prostheses made in cobalt-chromium alloy. Lancet 1971;1:564–566.
5. Mervyn Evans E, Freeman MAR, Miller AJ, Vernon-Roberts B. Metal sensitivity as a cause of bone necrosis and loosening of the prosthesis in total joint replacement. J Bone Joint Surg Br 1974;56:626–642.
6. Brown GC, Lockshin, MD, Salvati, EA, Bullough PG. Sensitivity to metal as a possible cause to sterile loosening after cobalt-chromium total hip replacement arthroplasty. J Bone Joint Surg Am 1977;59:164–168.
7. Sweetnam R. Metal sensitivity. J Bone Joint Surg Br 1974;56:601–602.
8. Charnley J. Low Friction Arthroplasty of the Hip. Berlin, Heidelberg, New York: Springer-Verlag, 1979.
9. Wagner M, Wagner H. Preliminary results of uncemented metal on metal stemmed and resurfacing hip replacement arthroplasty. Clin Orthop 1996;329S:S78–S88.
10. McMinn D, Treacy R, Lin K, Pynsent P. Metal on metal surface replacement of the hip. Clin Orthop 1996;329S:S89–S98.
11. Ahier S, Ginsburg K. Influence of carbide distribution on the wera and friction of Vitallium. Proc Inst Mech Eng 1966;181:137–139.
12. Clemow AJT, Daniell BL. The influence of microstructure on the adhesive wear resistance of Co-Cr-Mo alloy. Wear 1980;61:219–231.
13. Bowsher JG, Hussain A, Williams PA, Shelton JC. Metal-on-metal hip simulator study of increased wear particle surface area due to 'severe' patient activity. Proc Inst Mech Eng [H] 2006;220:279–287.
14. Chan FW, Bobyn JD, Medley JB, Krygier JJ, Tanzer M. The Otto Aufranc Award. Wear and lubrication of metal-on-metal hip implants. Clin Orthop Relat Res 1999;369:10–24.
15. Lavigne M, Vendittoli P-A, Roy AG. Early results of an RCT comparing conventional and resurfacing total hip arthroplasty. Presented at: International Symposium on Resurfacing of the Hip Joint, Zurich, April 2–22, 2005.
16. Lu B, Marti A, McKellop H. Wear of second generation metal on metal hip replacement. Effect of third body abrasive particles. Transactions of the Sixth World Biomaterial Congress, Kamuela, Hawaii, May 15-29, 2000, abstract 183.
17. McMinn DJW. Development of metal/metal hip resurfacing. Hip Int 2003;13:41–53.
18. Back DL, Dalziel R, Young D, Shimmin A. Early results of primary Birmingham hip resurfacings: an independent prospective study of the first 230 hips. J Bone Joint Surg Br 2005;87B:324–329.
19. Peindl RD, Squire M, Griffin WL, Mason JB, Odum S. Acetabular component deformations and press-fit loads in total hip arthroplasty. Presented at: ORS 2006, Carolinas Medical Center, Charlotte NC, OrthoCarolina, Charlotte NC, Poster 487, 2006.

2
Materials and Metallurgy

Tim J. Band

My first involvement with metal on metal bearings was in 1995. Corin Medical Ltd (Circencester, UK). asked Centaur Precision Castings Ltd (Sheffield, UK) to take over the supply of castings for the McMinn resurfacing from Trucast (Isle of Wight, UK). As the Medical Development Manager at Centaur, my engineering team and I took on that project.

Without specifications available for the device, with the exception of the material specification, ISO 5832 part 4 (formerly BS3531 and BS7252) and ASTM F75 (Tables 2.1 and 2.2), reverse engineering principles were used to identify the casting methods employed for the earlier product produced at Trucast. This included sectioning of castings to determine their grain structure and microstructure, which would allow the identification of the casting process used for the earlier product.

This forensic analysis of McMinn metal on metal hip resurfacing castings resulted in identifying that there had been a number of process methods employed in the manufacturing of these products, which had resulted in variable microstructures in the castings.

The range included the as-cast microstructure, without thermal treatment, single heat treatment of a solution heat treatment (SHT) or hot isostatic pressing (HIP), and both SHT and HIP (Fig. 2.1). The details of these treatments and their effect on the microstructure of cobalt chromium molybdenum alloy will be described later in this chapter. However, it is opportune to draw the reader's attention to the marked effect that the thermal treatment has on the microstructure, which is evidenced by the different morphology present. When these microstructural conditions had been identified, and their casting processes determined, Centaur Precision initiated the validation and approval submission documents for the McMinn metal on metal hip resurfacing castings that reproduced the structures identified in the Trucast product.

The difficulty in manufacturing the McMinn resurfacing was that the acetabular cup component had a superomedial peg that was approximately 15 mm long, 10 mm in diameter, and had splines that ran longitudinally down its length (Fig. 2.2). The convex surface of the cup also had a stippled textured surface and antirotation fins that restricted the opportunity for *gating* positions, which are an essential aspect of the investment casting process; this will also be explained later in the chapter. In order to produce as many of the surface details without the need for machining, the gating position had been located on the top of the superomedial peg as can be seen by the fan-shaped feature in the image.

This gating position created a narrow passage for the liquid metal to flow into the acetabular cup cavity and resulted in insufficient metal being available in the cup cavity after the peg metal solidified, preventing effective liquid metal *feeding* from the runner system. This resulted in microporosity, or voids, in the metal when the liquid-to-solid metal transfer occurred at the solidification temperature (Fig. 2.3).These microporosity pores, though not significantly detrimental to the mechanical properties of the casting, represented a cause of reduced manufacturing yields as negative pores can get exposed on the polished bearing surface after machining and polishing. It appears that this had been the main reason that Trucast had introduced the HIP process, which, through the application of temperature and pressure, can remove the porosity from the metal microstructure. A detailed description of the casting process and the resultant microstructures was submitted to the medical design and development team at Corin for review and subsequent approval. The dual thermal process was adopted at Centaur Precision after validation of the casting process. Mr. McMinn was not involved in any of these decisions. Centaur was a supplier to Corin, and we assumed that Corin would have made the designer aware of process changes to his implant.

It was during 1996 and early 1997 when Derek McMinn had cause to independently investigate the product produced by Corin Medical that he identified that the material of his resurfacing device had been altered without his knowledge or consent. His original request was that the material should replicate that of the successful first-generation metal on metal bearings. It was these that had provided him with the idea of reintroducing hip resurfacing with this appropriate material, which had enjoyed more than 30 years of benign clinical

TABLE 2.1. Chemical composition

Element	Compositional limits, % (*m/m*)
Chromium	26,5 to 30,0
Molybdenum	4,5 to 7,0
Nickel	1,0 max.
Iron	1,0 max.
Carbon	0,35 max.
Manganese	1,0 max.
Silicon	1,0 max.
Cobalt	Balance

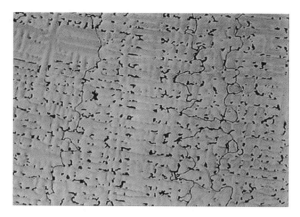

A

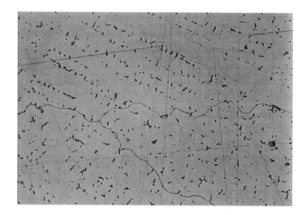

B

use. Without understanding the relevance of this change at the time, Mr. McMinn conducted a review of available literature on the subject of thermal treatments of cobalt chromium molybdenum alloy. He found that whereas these heat treatments produced an improvement in mechanical properties such as fatigue strength, and rendered the material easier to machine, a big downside was that they led to a reduction in its wear properties. Of course, it was the wear properties of the alloy that had been the attraction of this material. For a variety of reasons, the McMinn resurfacing hip prosthesis was withdrawn from use, and the fate of these prostheses is described elsewhere in this book.

If one considered introducing another metal on metal bearing at this time, you could have been excused for thinking that the limitation of the specification, with regard to material, was one of bulk chemical composition only, as there were a number of material wear test reports from reputable test houses suggesting that most variations and combinations of CoCrMo alloy would provide comparable durability. It was even suggested that the carbon content of the alloy, that is to say, high-carbon (C>0.2%) or low-carbon (C<0.07%) alloys,

TABLE 2.2. Chemical composition

Element	Composition, % (Mass/Mass)	
	min	max
Chromium	27.00	30.00
Molybdenum	5.00	7.00
Nickel	…	0.50
Iron	…	0.75
Carbon	…	0.35
Silicon	…	1.00
Manganese	…	1.00
Tungsten	…	0.20
Phosphorous	…	0.020
Sulfur	…	0.010
Nitrogen	…	0.25
Aluminum	…	0.10
Titanium	…	0.10
Boron	…	0.010
Cobalt[A]	balance	balance

[A] Approximately equal to the difference of 100% and the sum percentage of the other specified elements. The percentage of the cobalt difference is not required to be reported.

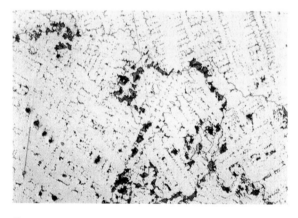

C

FIG. 2.1. (A) As-cast. (B) Single solution heat treatment (SHT). (C) Hot isostatic pressing (HIP).

behaved with the same performance in hip simulators [1]. This helped to support the introduction of future bearings, as CoCrMo alloy is more easily machined if the carbon content is low or if the carbon is not allowed to precipitate in a coarse form during casting solidification.

When the design of the Birmingham Hip Resurfacing (BHR) device commenced, it included the formalizing of a

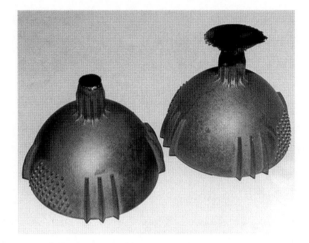

FIG. 2.2. McMinn resurfacing acetabular cup casting.

detailed specification that included material, microstructural, and geometric characterization of both the femoral head and acetabular cup components. On this occasion, when Midland Medical Technologies (MMT) provided specimens of the first-generation metal on metal devices that had worked well for many decades, they insisted upon a detailed forensic analysis.

The forensic study of these first-generation metal on metal bearings, the Ring and McKee-Farrar devices (Fig. 2.4), included bulk chemical analysis, surface examination and characterization to determine the surface topography and the wear mechanism of the material, inspection and measurement of profiles to determine the sphericity, clearance (difference between the head and cup size), wear of the articulating surfaces, and sectioning of the articulating surfaces to examine and determine the metallurgical structure of the components.

It was important to consider, while conducting the forensic analysis, that the first-generation metal on metal devices had been produced as two-piece components that were welded together to allow the head to be a hollow component, reducing the component weight and eliminating the difficulties in

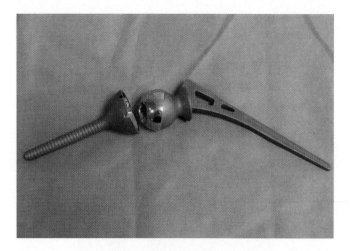

A

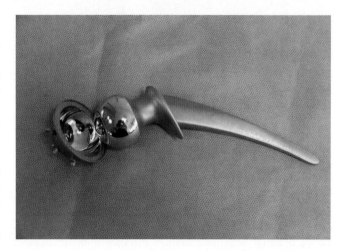

B

FIG. 2.4. (A) Ring metal on metal hip prosthesis. (B) McKeeFarrar metal on metal hip prosthesis.

producing large thick sections during the casting process. The weld line that joined the head cap to the stem was a narrow band close to the equator of the femoral bearing and away from the intended articulation area (Fig. 2.5). The original welding would have used a filler wire produced from cobalt chrome alloy, whereas contemporary welding of two-piece femoral devices uses electron beam welding (EBW), which melts and fuses positive ribs produced on the host component to avoid *sinking* of the casting profile during welding.

The forensic analysis of these devices took place between Centaur Precision and the Materials Research Institute (MRI) at the Sheffield Hallam University, where there was a combined resource of experts in the fields of engineering of orthopedic devices, investment casting, and metallurgy. Particularly helpful in this exercise were Graham Dixon, chief metallurgist at Centaur, and John Metcalf and Dr. Jess Cawley, who were scientists at MRI. Bulk chemical analysis identified the material as cobalt chromium molybdenum alloy, where the

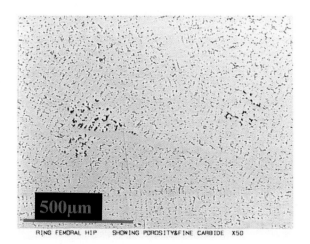

RING FEMORAL HIP   SHOWING POROSITY&FINE CARBIDE X50

FIG 2.3. Micrograph showing microporosity in the microstructure.

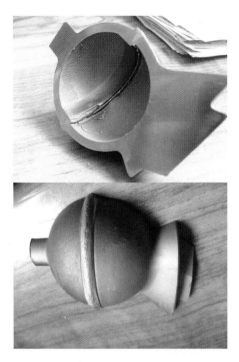

Fig. 2.5. Cross section of a two-piece assembly of the hollow femoral device in an electron beam welded condition.

chromium content was ~28% to 30%, molybdenum content was ~5% to 7%, carbon was 0.20% to 0.35% by weight, and the balance was cobalt. Other elements in smaller amounts were identified as nickel, silicon, manganese, nitrogen, and iron with other trace elements such as aluminum, titanium, sulfur, and phosphorus. The microstructural characteristics of the material, identified through metallography, revealed a biphasic structure (Fig. 2.6). This was where the matrix of the material, rich in cobalt with chromium and molybdenum, supported a second metallurgical phase carbide that was rich in chromium, molybdenum, and carbon.

The carbide phase had a coarse block morphology and was similar to Chinese script in its shape (Fig. 2.7). This was due to the fact that the carbide particulate is the last liquid to solidify

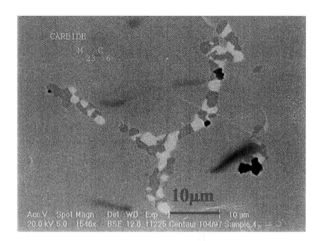

Fig. 2.7. Micrograph showing as-cast, block carbide in the interdendritic pattern.

in the casting process as it is the lowest melting point solute in the interdendrite spaces. The solidification process of this alloy system will be described in more detail later in this chapter.

Surface characterization using low-power optical microscopy identified surfaces that were predominately measured as a negative skew, where there were more scratches than asperities on the surface, in an area that had experienced wear. The scratches on the worn areas of approximately 2 to 3 μm in width were indications of an abrasive wear process as the scratches were seen to be in the intercarbide spacings of the matrix material. These were most probably due to fractured carbide particles acting as third-body wear components as the wear process evolved (Fig. 2.8). There was evidence that the carbide component resisted abrasive wear, in that it can be seen on micrographs that scratches terminate when they meet a carbide in the matrix (Fig. 2.9).

At the same time, in areas where no wear had been experienced, such as the inferior medial zone of the femoral head, the surfaces were found to be in their original manufactured condition of more than 30 years earlier and were found to have a positive skew, with more asperities than scratches on the surface. This phenomenon is described as *relief polishing* in manufacturing terms and is the term used to describe a softer matrix material being worn at a faster rate than is a

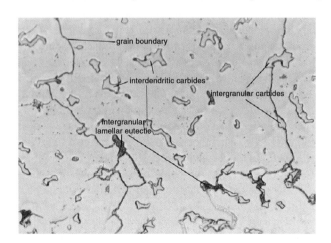

Fig. 2.6. As-cast microstructure showing biphasic structure of carbide and matrix.

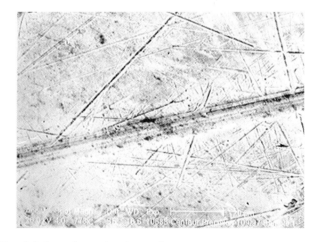

Fig. 2.8. Scratches on bearing surface.

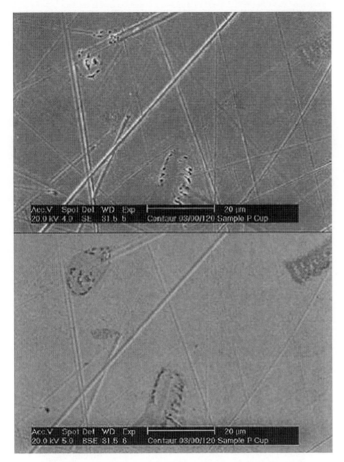

FIG. 2.9. Termination of scratches at carbide junctions.

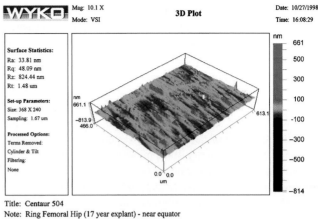

Title: Centaur 504
Note: Ring Femoral Hip (17 year explant) - near equator

FIG. 2.10. Noncontact profilometry of the as-cast surface showing asperities coincidental with the carbide of 100 nm.

harder second metallurgical phase that stands proud of the matrix surface due to its resistance to wear. This is similar to the hard rings and knots found in hardwoods when polishing takes place resulting in high points on the polished surface.

To conduct further analysis of the surfaces, an analytical technique called noncontact surface profilometry was used to measure the surface contours at a nanometric level and to provide a representation of the surface in three-dimensional images (Fig. 2.10).

These measurements confirmed that the unworn, as manufactured, surfaces had peaks of up to 100 nm (0.1 μm, or 0.0001 mm) that were coincidental with the carbide distribution seen in the optical micrographs. On the worn surfaces, the scratches were easily identified. It could be seen that the scratch edges had small ridges indicating that the material had undergone plastic deformation rather than having had a strip of material removed, which occurs in the machining process. The CoCrMo alloy system had already been described as having a *self-polishing* capability, which was further confirmed when evidence of multiple scratch paths crossing each other showed a softening of the ridges at the edge of the earliest scratch on the micrograph by the passage of a later scratch. This can also be seen on Figs. 2.8 and 2.9.

More extensive metallurgical examination took place by examining the bearing surfaces using scanning electron microscopy (SEM). Many weeks, days, and hours were spent at MRI in Sheffield examining these precious retrieved specimens that held the key to the durable bearing solution. When examining the material using secondary electron imaging, there is an opportunity to see surface discontinuities and some topographical features. However, this technique does not measure height, depth, or give any indication of whether or not one is looking at a positive or negative feature on the surface. It was always important to consider this in context with the earlier examination to avoid confusion or misinterpretation. By looking at the same field of view but using backscatter electron imaging (BSE), it was possible to see the contrast in atomic mass of the elements in the microstructure and therefore determine the presence, morphology, and distribution of the metallurgical phases in the microstructure. Through elemental mapping, it was determined that the carbide phase in this biphasic material was rich in chromium, molybdenum, and carbon and that the matrix was predominately cobalt, chromium, and molybdenum, the latter two elements being in lower concentrations than in the carbide phase. The contrast in atomic mass between the chromium-rich and the molybdenum-rich carbide phase can be seen in Fig. 2.11, which was

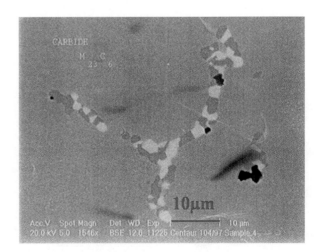

FIG. 2.11. Micrograph showing as-cast, block carbide with molybdenum-rich (light phase) and chromium-rich (dark phase) areas in the carbide.

previously used to show the Chinese script form of the carbide, where the molybdenum is lighter in contrast, because of its heavier atomic mass, when compared with chromium or the surrounding matrix. The carbide phase within the matrix was determined, by phase proportion analysis to occupy between 4% and 5% of the field of view and was of a large block morphology. The size of the carbides were observed to be 2 to 3 μm wide and 10 to 30 μm long, following the pattern of the dendritic structure of the matrix. It was comforting to see the consistency and similarity of the microstructures of these first-generation metal on metal bearings as this was leading toward the development of a sensible material specification.

Further detailed metallurgical analysis of the bearing material was carried out by sectioning the material and preparing specimens for microstructural examination. Care was taken when examining the femoral devices to ensure that observations were made on representative sections of the two-piece assembly previously described. It was by using transmission electron microscopy (TEM) that the real structure of the material could be determined, which was extremely important in determining how these components had been manufactured more than 30 years earlier. The bright-field images recorded during TEM examination revealed that the matrix was a face-centered-cubic, austenitic structure and that the carbide was an $M_{23}C_6$ type carbide, where M represents the metal elements of Cr and Mo, and C represents carbon (Fig. 2.12).

The atoms of chromium, cobalt, and molybdenum are of a similar size, with goldschmidt atomic radii of ~130 to 140 angstroms (Å), and at temperatures below ~1230°C form a solid-state solution where they arrange themselves in an organized face-centered-cubic structure, or lattice, but with random element positioning within the structure (Fig. 2.13). The carbon atom is approximately half the size of these other atoms and is described as an interstitial atom that occupies discontinuities, vacancies, or faults in the lattice. This was

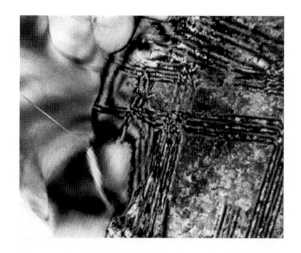

A

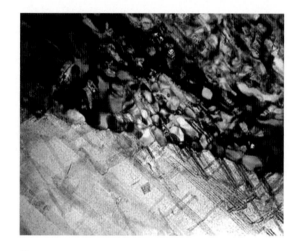

B

FIG. 2.12. (A) Bright-field TEM image of the matrix in as-cast CoCr. (B) Bright-field TEM image of the carbide phase in as-cast CoCr.

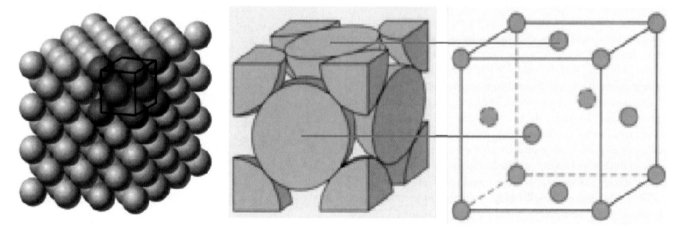

FIG. 2.13. Atoms in a face-centered-cubic (FCC) lattice structure.

further confirmed when the electron diffraction patterns and kikuchi lines, recorded during electron backscatter detection (EBSD), where electrons are passed through a thin film of the material, were solved through identifying the planes and orientations of the atoms in the structure (Fig. 2.14).

Although CoCr is predominately a face-centered-cubic, austenitic alloy system, it has been hypothesized that during work-hardening (which can occur during final stages of the machining and finishing processes as well as during articulation) of the bearing surface, a metallurgical phase change occurs where the face-centered-cubic structure is modified into a hexagonal close-packed (HCP) structure. Because of the extremely narrow affected zone, it is necessary to use TEM to determine this change. Although this transformation in cobalt alloys is not well understood and cannot be precisely

controlled, it remains a variable contributor to the wear process of CoCr bearing materials.

It was quite remarkable how similar the metallurgical characteristics of these first-generation metal on metal bearings were. The forensic analysis had identified that the devices had been produced in high-carbon cobalt chromium alloy and from the investment casting process. The casting process of the high-carbon-containing alloy had allowed sufficient time for the precipitation of the large block carbides, which suggested that no *forced cooling* of the casting took place after the metal pouring process. A forced cooling process is a post-cast technique often employed to develop a finer grain structure in casting alloys, for improved mechanical and fatigue strength, and shortens the solidification range (time to cross between liquidus and solidus temperature and phases), which reduces the time for carbides to precipitate. The evidence of low wear, of the order $2\,\mu m$ of linear wear per year *in vivo*, lower wear on the cup than on the head, and a comparable microstructure on both articulating surfaces suggested that the femoral head device had been marginally subservient to the acetabular cup device. This is most likely due to the nature of a polar bearing contact, with the contact surface area of the head articulating on a larger equivalent contact surface area of the cup, demonstrating that the parity in microstructure had not been a subservient variable in the articulating pair.

Having identified these material, microstructural, and geometric characteristics from the retrievals, it was possible to develop a specification for the controlling features of the BHR device. The formalizing of a specification at this stage would ensure that product conformance and repeatability would be ensured through the application of quality accredited manufacturing and inspection processes, which had not been in place when the original metal on metal bearings were produced. It had been, in part, due to the variability in the manufacturing processes employed more than 30 years before these devices were examined that a number of early failures had been experienced. The product dimensional and geometric variability had resulted in suboptimal bearing conditions, developing high frictional torques, loosening, and wear. The development of a specification based on the forensic analysis, determining the critical factors leading to the good long-term clinical results of the first-generation bearings, was intuitively the right approach as there would be no "new" variables in the design that could not be linked to a prior accepted experience in clinical use. Any variation to these characteristics would have to be considered untried and untested, and therefore their introduction would have to be considered a risk factor to the longevity and benign clinical acceptance of the bearing.

The characteristics of the forensic studies of the successful first-generation metal on metal bearings were that they were produced from high-carbon-containing cobalt chromium molybdenum alloy and were produced in the as-cast microstructural condition. Both bearing components of the articulation were found to be produced in the same metallurgical condition with a cobalt, chromium, molybdenum matrix

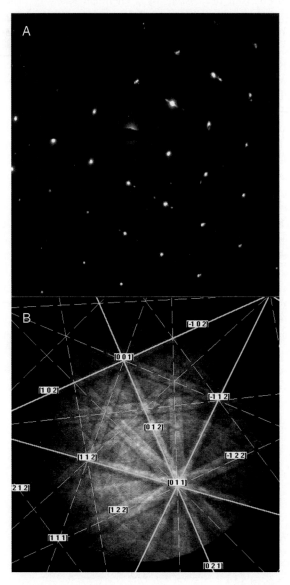

FIG. 2.14. (A) Electron diffraction pattern of face-centered-cubic CoCr and (B) solved kikuchi lines to diffraction pattern of carbide.

supporting interdendritic block carbides of $M_{23}C_6$. The atoms are both ionically and covalently bonded in the carbide precipitate phase.

Casting Method

The first-generation metal on metal bearing components, such as the Ring, McKee-Farrar, Huggler, and Muller devices, were produced from the investment casting process. The investment casting process is one of the oldest metal-forming processes in history with origins dating back more than 4000 years. For those readers with further interest, I recommend a concise text by Beeley and Smart, entitled *Investment Casting* (ISBN 0 901716 66 9). The term *investment casting* is derived from the characteristic use of mobile ceramic slurries, or *investments*, to form molds with extremely smooth surfaces. Another description of the process is *the lost wax process*, where the facsimile, or copy, of the final design is produced from a wax pattern that is sacrificed later in the process after it has been used to produce a cavity inside the ceramic mold.

A major advantage of the casting process is that detailed features can be produced, which reduces significant machining time and costs of the final device. The process begins by producing a facsimile of the final component in wax. This wax pattern can be produced by machining a cavity into a wax pattern tool, or die, which allows molten wax to be injected into the cavity to form the pattern shape (Fig. 2.15).

Investment casting engineers have to consider the complexity of the shapes, and details to be cast in, to design the wax pattern tool to allow the wax pattern to be produced and removed from the tool cavity without distortion of the form. Detailed surfaces, passages, and or channels in the casting can be produced using either soluble wax cores or ceramic cores, but the

relative simplicity of the detail on the first-generation metal on metal bearings did not require any complex tooling or core design to be used. If ceramic or soluble cores are used, then they are produced as prefabricated objects with a core print having similar constraints as a casting gate. The core print is used to locate the core inside the wax pattern tool so that when the wax is injected into the tool cavity, the wax surrounds the core except for the print, which is located outside the tool cavity, and the core becomes a secure feature inside the wax pattern. In the case of soluble wax cores, these are dissolved out of the wax pattern. The resultant recessed feature, or cavity, is invested in the standard shelling process, whereas in the case of a ceramic core, the core print/wax pattern junction is sealed prior to investment. Then, after dewaxing, the ceramic core is located in the ceramic shell awaiting the pouring of molten metal around the core feature. This ceramic material is later removed from the casting by a chemical leaching process, leaving the casting with detailed features that otherwise would not be producible or would be very costly to machine. Ceramic cores are used to produce the introducer threaded holes on the BHR acetabular cup. The core print locations can be seen in the wax pattern tool shown in Fig. 2.15, and the core prints can be seen on the wax pattern shown in Fig. 2.16.

The investment casting engineer must also determine how the metal will flow from the runner system to the wax pattern and has to design a feeder connection between the two, which is known as a *gate* (Fig. 2.16). The gate has to allow sufficient metal to flow into the pattern cavity from the runner before it freezes, during solidification of the metal during casting, to reduce the formation of microporosity.

The gate position also affects the grain structure of the casting during solidification, because normally under ambient cooling conditions, the last section to solidify is the hottest position in the system. If this is the gate area, then where it contacts the casting, the grain size will be large, which represents a weaker structure than a fine or equiaxed grain structure. It is therefore important to ensure that the gate position is not at, or in close proximity to, an area of significant high stress in the design, where the highest

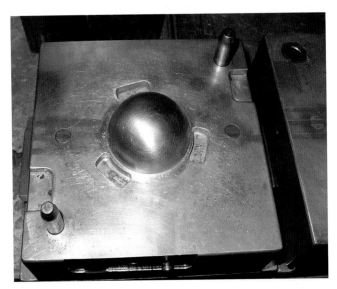

Fig. 2.15. View inside a wax pattern tool cavity of an acetabular cup with three ceramic core print locations.

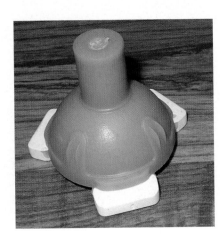

Fig. 2.16. A wax pattern of an acetabular cup showing the gate on the convex surface and three ceramic core prints.

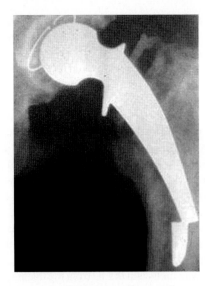

FIG. 2.17. As-cast femoral hip stem showing fracture at the distal third.

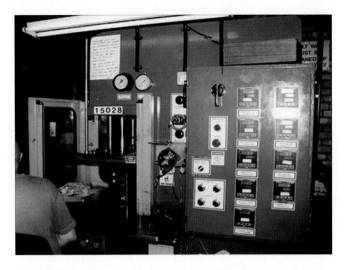

FIG. 2.18. Wax injection machine, or press, injecting wax into a wax pattern tool.

fatigue strength in the casting would be required. An example of such a position would be the lower third of a narrow cast femoral stemmed prosthesis, which over time has proved to be the inherent weak point of a femoral stem under the tortional loading at the hip joint. An example of a femoral stem device that failed in its lower distal third because of low fatigue strength properties in the as-cast condition is shown in Fig. 2.17.

As well as identifying the optimal structural position, the engineer must also consider how easily the gate can be removed after casting and how easily the casting profile can be restored. Having identified the gating position on the component design, the engineer can design the wax pattern tool. This tool will contain the cavity of the wax pattern shape and its gate or gate pad if the overall shape is too complex for a simple tool split. The tool has to allow the injection of liquid wax into the cavity and then allow the wax pattern to be removed. The cavity is split, usually along a line of symmetry of the pattern, and this split is replicated in the wax pattern tool. In the case of the Ring prosthesis, the femoral component tool cavity was produced by having half of the medial lateral profile of the stem in each half of the tool. This included approximately half of the femoral head and the fenestrations, or holes, in the proximal stem, which were also produced in each half of the tool. The recess in the femoral head was produced by a sliding metal core, which produced a 2- to 3-mm wall thickness in the femoral head. The two halves of the wax pattern tool were held close together by placing tapered dowels in the corner of the tool to ensure accurate alignment of both cavities in both halves of the tool. Any malpositioning of the tool cavities results in a mismatch between the two halves of the pattern, and there may also be evidence of a die line on the split line position on the pattern. The liquid wax, at temperatures ~60°C to 70°C, is injected into the wax pattern tool through a small-diameter hole in the side of the tool (Fig. 2.18) and is usually routed through a sprue to the wax pattern gate.

This allows the wax sprue to be removed without significant damage to the wax pattern. As the lost wax, investment casting process is capable of faithfully producing the features on the wax pattern, a thorough inspection and repair of the wax patterns takes place prior to further processing.

Before I explain the next stage of the investment casting process, it is necessary to be aware that the wax pattern is approximately 2% larger than the required final metal casting as there are a number of expansions and contractions that take place throughout this process. The first contraction experienced is when the liquid wax is injected into the tool cavity and the warm wax contacts the cooler metal tool. This contraction is of the order 0.5% but is dependent upon the actual process parameters at the foundry and upon the specific geometry and section thickness of the component. Clearly, a thinner section thickness will solidify faster than will a thicker section and therefore maintain its injected size. Also, complex geometries will restrict certain contractions due to solid metal tooling inserts, such as the fenestrations on the Ring prosthesis.

After the inspection of the wax patterns, they are assembled onto a wax runner system by welding them to the runner by melting the gate using hot pallet knives or gas flames. The wax runner is a wax tree where the branches are connected to a funnel that eventually forms a pour cup to allow liquid metal to enter the ceramic mold (shell) cavity. It is imperative that the junction between the gate and the runner is sealed to prevent the penetration of liquid ceramic into the wax assembly, which occurs at a later stage in the process. The wax patterns are arranged on an appropriately designed runner system to ensure that they are close enough to allow an economic mold size, but separated sufficiently to ensure that they do not insulate each other during cooling after metal casting to affect the required microstructure. In the inside of the wax pour cup, there is a nut that has been secured in place by producing, or injecting, the wax runner system around the nut, in much the same way as the wax pattern is produced. Once the wax assembly is complete, the mold can be transferred to the shelling, or investment, area.

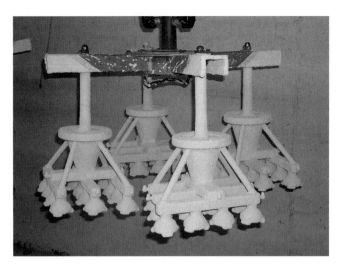

FIG. 2.19. Wax assemblies supported by a robotic arm for shelling.

A metal pole is screwed into the nut in the wax pour cup, which allows the mold to be manipulated by an operator. Historically, the shelling process was a manual operation. More recently, robotic systems have been introduced that provide more consistency and greater mold size and economies of scale to be enjoyed (Fig. 2.19). Ceramic shell molds are made up of three components: the binder, the filler, and the stucco materials. The binders are usually made with silica, a ceramic material, and are either water or alcohol based. Filler and stucco materials are used in a wide range of combinations including silica sand, alumino-silicates, alumina and zirconium silicates. The process of shelling, or investing, the wax assembly involves immersing the mold into liquid ceramic and then applying a coat of solid ceramic, or stucco, onto the liquid layer.

Each coating is allowed to dry before applying the subsequent coat, and the process continues until the shell coating is approximately 4- to 5-mm thick all over the wax mold. The first coat is critical for achieving fine detail on a casting surface and can influence the resultant grain structure of the casting if any grain nucleation additions are made to the coating. It has been demonstrated that additions of cobalt aluminate in the

first coat, or face coat, can initiate grain growth when the CoCr alloy meets the shell surface, resulting in a finer grain size and structure than would otherwise result. This can be useful if high fatigue strength properties are required on the final casting. The subsequent coats, which can be 10 or more further coats, have coarser textures and are used to develop a harder, stronger shell. The time between shell coatings is dependent upon the specific parameters specified by the foundry producing the components. A typical drying time for each coat is of the order 4 hours with a total shelling time of 2 to 3 days. When the final seal coat is applied, there is no stucco applied to the surface, which allows the final coat to be of a smooth texture sealing the ceramic particulates on the surface.

The shells, still containing wax assemblies, are moved to the dewaxing process where, inside an autoclave, they are subjected to steam temperatures of 150°C to 180°C. At this temperature, the wax melts and drains from the opening of the pour cup leaving an empty shell with residual wax on the shell surface. Vents are designed on the runner system to allow wax to escape from the patterns and runner system to reduce the risk of cracking the shell due to the differential in thermal expansion between the wax and the shell materials. After dewaxing, the shells are flash-fired in a gas-fired oven to burn the residual wax, leaving the shell clean and empty (Fig. 2.20). Careful selection of waxes with low ash contents are used to reduce the risk of residual impurities remaining in the shell. A thorough inspection of the shell takes place to identify any cracks and vents that require repairing, using a refractory cement to seal the shell prior to the casting process. It is important to ensure that there are no impurities inside the shell cavity prior to casting as these may become inclusions in the metal once the casting process commences. In contemporary practice, a refractory filter is fitted to the mold mouth to allow a filtering of inclusions that may be carried over in the molten metal. This process was unlikely to have occurred during the manufacturing of the first-generation metal on metal bearings.

The inspected shell is placed into a gas-fired preheat furnace where it is soaked at a temperature of ~1050° C for an hour or more (Figs. 2.21 and 2.22).

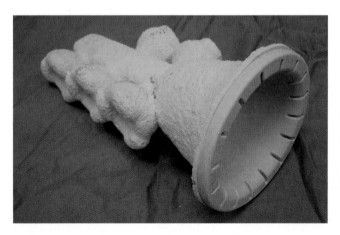

FIG. 2.20. Ceramic shell after dewaxing and flash-firing.

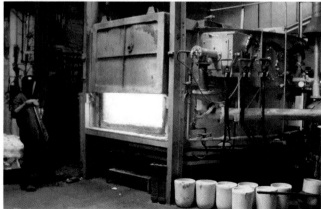

FIG. 2.21. Preheat furnace.

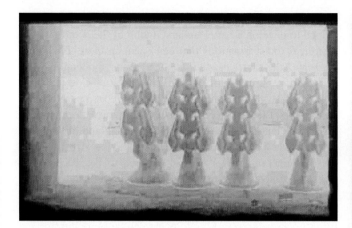

FIG. 2.22. Molds at temperature (~1000°C) in preheat furnace.

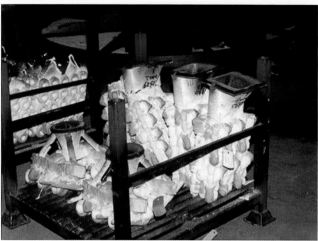

FIG. 2.24. Molds on foundry cooling rack after casting.

The temperature of the preheat process is generally above 1000°C where the ceramic material is sintered and undergoes a phase change from its green state and is rendered inert to the molten metal that will be poured into the shell. While the shell is being preheated, a billet of CoCr alloy, cut to the required weight, is being melted in an induction furnace in a preformed refractory crucible. As the CoCr alloy contains highly reactive elements such as titanium, it is important to protect the metal from oxygen in the atmosphere by melting under an inert gas atmosphere or in a vacuum chamber. Once the alloy reaches the foundry-specified temperature, usually above 1550°C, which is measured in real-time using a thermocouple, the shell is taken from the preheat furnace and placed upside down, so that the pour cup is like a funnel, in the casting furnace. In the case of a vacuum furnace, the mold is placed in a mold chamber, which can be evacuated prior to entering the casting chamber, and in the case of an inert gas cover rollover process, the mold is placed above the molten metal. When the shell is adequately protected, in either process, the metal is transferred to the shell by pouring the liquid metal (see Fig. 2.23). This process takes a few seconds, and the shell, full of metal, can be removed from

the casting stage and placed on a foundry rack and allowed to cool (Fig. 2.24).

It is during this cooling process that the microstructure of the casting will form. As the metal is at a much higher temperature than is the shell (1550°C compared with 1000°C), cooling starts at the surface of the shell-metal interface.

Nucleation of grains starts by the precipitation of dendrite arms that grow, like Christmas trees, into the liquid metal (Fig. 2.25).

The solidification process starts at the liquidus temperature (~1395°C for CoCr alloy) and finishes when the solidus temperature (~1230°C for CoCr alloy) is reached. The liquidus and solidus temperatures vary with subtle differences in chemical composition of the alloy and are often only applicable in what is called *equilibrium* conditions where environmental cooling influences are reduced. The dendrite structures are predominately rich in the higher melting point elements and can be seen as *coring* in the as-cast microstructure. As

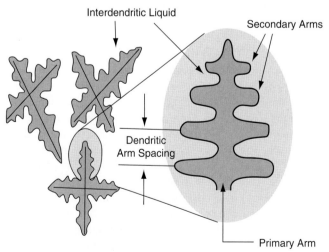

FIG. 2.25. Dendritic pattern formed during the solidification from liquid metal.

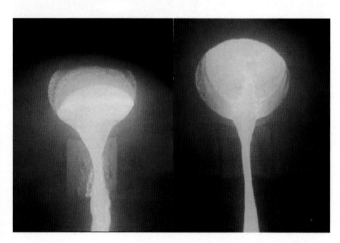

FIG. 2.23. (A, B) Molten metal pouring from the crucible (~1560°C).

the total system continues to cool and the dendrite arms continue to grow, the solid phase dominates the volume in the mold cavity, and the residual liquid between the dendrite structures is rich in the lower melting point elements. When these residuals solidify, they form predominately as the interdendritic carbide phase, rich in chromium, molybdenum, and carbon, and form in the Chinese script morphology previously described. Upon complete solidification, the metal component has contracted from the shell cavity size to a size approximately 2% smaller than the starting wax pattern.

The shell material cracks during the final cooling process and is removed using a short vibratory process followed by blasting the casting surface using stainless steel shot where the surface texture permits. Once the connecting gate between the casting and the runner can be clearly seen, the individual castings can be removed using rotating cutting wheels or gas cutting techniques. In all cases, great care is taken to avoid damaging the castings as repair by welding is usually not permitted in the case of medical devices. Once separated from the runner, each casting can have its gate reduced in size, or formed to the casting profile. Traceability of each casting to its respective manufacturing history is maintained, and vibro-etching can be used to permanently identify the castings.

The metal castings can be inspected to specified criteria and can include visual, gauging, fluorescent penetrant (crack detection), and radiographic inspection methods. Rejected castings and residual runner system alloy pieces are reverted into new billets for future casting production. Metallurgical examination can also be carried out by macro grain etching the casting surface to reveal the grain structure or sectioning and etching to reveal grain boundaries and metallurgical phases in the microstructure.

Thermal Treatments of Cast Alloys

As described earlier in this chapter, the McMinn metal on metal resurfacing hip raw-material castings had been produced in the as-cast (not heat treated) microstructural condition and/or subjected to variable thermal treatments, including SHT, HIP, and both SHT and HIP conditions (Fig. 2.1). The reason for employing these treatments was to reduce and/or remove microporosity from the microstructure when HIP is employed and to homogenize the microstructure to reduce residual casting stresses when SHT is employed. Annealing the material at temperatures below the eutectic temperature of the alloy prevents the carbides from melting and produces an equalization of the dendritic segregation, without the loss of tensile properties. This process is normally carried out at temperatures around 1170°C. HIP was introduced in the 1980s as a method of improving the fatigue strength properties of alloys used to produce components for the aerospace industry where complex shapes and light weights were commonplace, putting high demands on the alloys employed. Cobalt-containing alloys have been extensively used in the aerospace industry

since the 1930s by the Austenal Company (Warsaw, IN). This helped to develop a better understanding of the complex metallurgical transformations that can occur in these alloys and facilitated their later usage in medical grade applications.

The typical process for thermally heat treating CoCr castings is to preheat a gas-fired furnace to the required temperature and then to load the castings in an appropriate formation on racking, dependent upon the size of each casting and the number to be processed together. For medical device–size castings, it is not uncommon for several hundred to be processed at the same time. These can of course be different devices but produced from the same alloy type. The furnace types vary between suppliers of the process. An image of a contemporary furnace can be seen in Fig. 2.26. As can be seen, the furnace volume is approximately 1.5 m × 2 m × 1.5 m.

As the thermal processes are time, temperature, and furnace position dependent, all of which have their own process tolerances, the variation in the resultant microstructures can be extensive.

The typical parameters used for the HIP process of cast CoCrMo alloy are 1200°C for 4 hours in an inert atmosphere followed by a gas fan quench at a relatively slow cooling rate. This thermal treatment is carried out at a high pressure of 103 MPa, which is sufficient to squeeze the micropores out of the microstructure provided that they are not connected to the casting surface. The reason for this relatively slow cooling process is to avoid significant damage to the refractory lining due to the expansion and contraction of the refractory bricks in the furnace walls, floors, and ceilings. The resultant effect on the microstructure is that at this time and temperature, there is sufficient time for the metallurgical phases in the microstructure (carbide precipitates and matrix) to reach a temperature close enough to the solidus temperature (~1230°C)—which is the temperature at which the solid metal starts to melt and become a liquid phase—to start a diffusion process and movement of

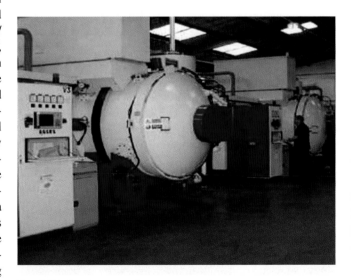

Fig. 2.26. Contemporary heat treatment furnace.

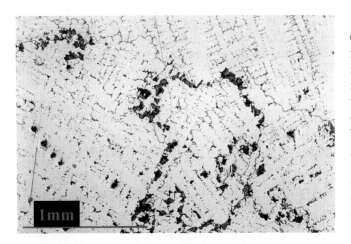

FIG. 2.27. Microstructure of hot isostatic pressed CoCr showing lamellar carbide at grain boundaries.

atoms within the microstructure. At this process temperature, there is a diffusion of the chromium, molybdenum, and carbon atoms from the carbide precipitate into the surrounding face-centered-cubic lattice of the matrix, in the case of Cr and Mo, and into the interstitial spaces in the lattice, in the case of C. As the alloy cools from the process temperature, there is an opportunity for reprecipitation of the carbides. However, they form predominately at the grain boundaries and are not re-formed as the original as-cast morphology. The marked effect that this has on the carbides is that they are reduced in overall size from the "blocky" Chinese script form to smaller, fine, agglomerate carbides that have a lower mechanical stability in the supporting matrix, whereas the matrix itself has larger intercarbide areas, the effect of which will be discussed later. There is also evidence of the formation of lamellar carbides, which are lineated in pattern and found at the grain boundaries (Fig. 2.27).

In this microstructural condition, the mechanical properties of the alloy are generally below those required by ISO 5832 part 4 (Table 2.3), and subsequent treatments, such as SHT, are employed, where a faster quenching rate can be achieved to restore the required mechanical properties. After the reduction in carbide, grain size can increase due to the reduction in grain boundary pinning, which is enjoyed by the presence of grain boundary carbides. This also increases the ductility of the material. The subsequent heat treatments that follow HIP do not further influence the microporosity but can significantly alter the already modified carbides.

TABLE 2.3. Mechanical properties

Tensile strength	Proof stress of nonproportional elongation	Percentage elongation after fracture[1]
R_m min. MPa	$R_{p0,2}$ min. MPa	A min.
665	450	8

[1] Gauge length = 5,65 $\sqrt{S_o}$ or 50 mm, where S_o is the original cross-sectional area, in square millimetres.

The typical parameters used for the SHT process of cast CoCrMo alloy are 1200°C for 4 hours in an inert atmosphere followed by a rapid gas fan quench to 800°C in less than 8 minutes (50°C per minute). Unlike the HIP process, there is no requirement for a significant pressure in the chamber other than to maintain an inert gas atmosphere to prevent oxidation of the castings due to the reaction with oxygen at temperature. This is achieved by heating in a vacuum chamber. The inert gases used are typically argon or nitrogen and partial pressures of 2.7 to 5.3 mbar. As the temperature is similar to that employed in the HIP process, the effect on the carbides is to continue their diffusion into the matrix. With the rapid gas fan quench cooling, their reprecipitation is restricted, resulting in much of the carbide remaining in the matrix solution. When a CoCr alloy casting has been heat treated and its carbide morphology altered, further subsequent heat treatments diffuse the remaining carbides at a more significant rate. This results in a dramatic reduction in the phase proportion (volume fraction) of the carbide phase in the matrix. The measurement of the amount of carbide present in a microstructure is carried out by identifying a field of interest and capturing it on a micrograph at an appropriate magnification. Using imaging analysis techniques (e.g., Image Pro Plus), it is possible to identify the carbide phase by its contrast against the matrix on optical or SEM images (Figs. 2.28 and 2.29).

These identified contrast areas are then calculated as a percentage against the total *field of view* area.

The significant effect on the carbide morphology after a single thermal treatment of 1200°C for 4 hours can be seen in Fig. 2.30, where the phase proportion has been halved. It can be seen at this higher magnification that the diffusion of chromium and molybdenum from the carbide results in the stable block morphology being transformed into a fine, dispersed morphology, which is less mechanically stable and exposes more area of the matrix.

The reducing amount of carbide phase observed after a single thermal heat treatment over time is expressed as the Larson-Miller parameter (Fig. 2.31). As can be seen, the higher the temperature and the longer the time at which the casting is exposed to the temperature, the more significant the reduction in carbide phase becomes.

Therefore, if a CoCr casting is exposed to multiple thermal heat treatments at the solutionizing temperatures, the resultant microstructures will have small, fine, dispersed carbides with a low carbide phase proportion and more surface area of the matrix exposed as seen in Fig. 2.30. The significance of these modifications is that the finer dispersed carbides are less mechanically stable within the supporting matrix, because they are smaller and more easily extracted during articulation against another surface, and that the larger areas of matrix exposed are at a higher risk of adhesive wear against the counterface of the bearing. I have previously mentioned a number of studies that show the significance of the carbide phase and its resistance to wear [2–7]. However, it is interesting to consider that a number of other studies have

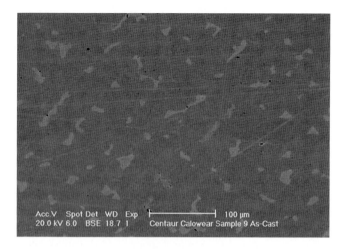

A

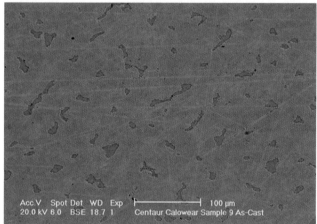

B

 5%

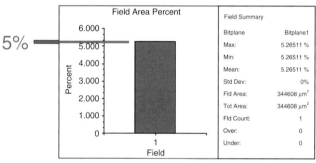

C

FIG. 2.28. Image analysis used to quantify the carbide phase in the field of view in an as-cast microstructure.

failed to identify the relationship between the reduction in carbides in the microstructure and the wear rate of the bearings. This is most probably because, during hip simulator studies, the articulating surfaces are protected by the generation of a fluid film as the components are both optimally positioned in relation to one another and that they are in continuous motion promoting the entrainment of fluid. When CoCr materials

are tested for their wear resistance using pin on plate or pin on disk methods, there is a statistically significant difference identified in the wear properties with the as-cast, block carbide having the lowest wear. The subject of wear testing and results are described later in this book.

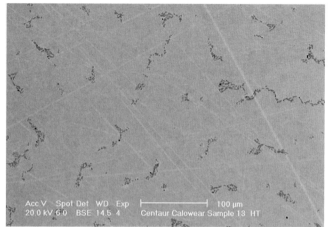

A

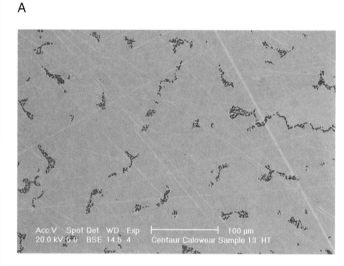

B

2.4%

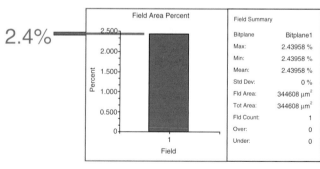

C

FIG. 2.29. Image analysis used to quantify the carbide phase in the field of view in a heat-treated microstructure. After a single heat treatment, the phase proportion is reduced by 50%.

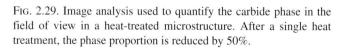

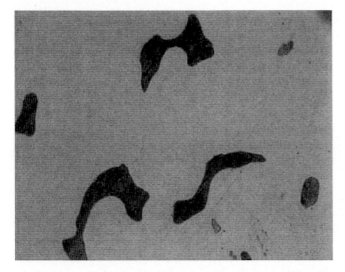

A

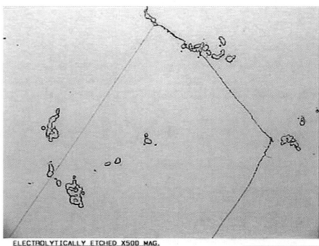

ELECTROLYTICALLY ETCHED X500 MAG.

FIG. 2.32. CoCr cast alloy after HIP and SHT.

Other examples of contemporary metal on metal bearings are shown in Figs. 2.32 and 2.33 where essentially a material containing high carbon >0.2%) with the same bulk chemistry has been subjected to post-cast thermal treatments and the carbide structure has been disintegrated.

As well as the previously described thermal treatments, other processes such as sintering, by which beads are attached to the convex surface of an acetabular cup device, are employed in the production of some orthopedic devices. This high-temperature process also modifies the microstructure through a diffusion process of the carbides. Another point worthy of mention is that these thermal treatments were not used in the first-generation metal on metal bearings, and therefore there is no long-term clinical experience to complement their use.

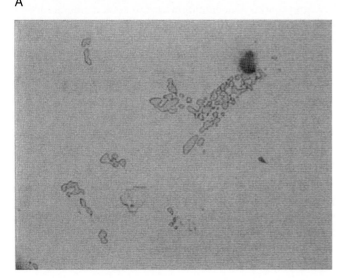

B

FIG. 2.30. (A) High magnification of carbide phase in the as-cast block and (B) fine dispersed, particulate, morphology after a single thermal treatment at 1170°C for 4 hours.

The reduction in carbide size and the exposure of matrix surfaces subject these structures to a significant risk of adhesive wear when matrix contact occurs in the bearing between the articulating surfaces. The distraction of the smaller carbides from the supporting matrix occurs more easily when compared with the as-cast microstructure.

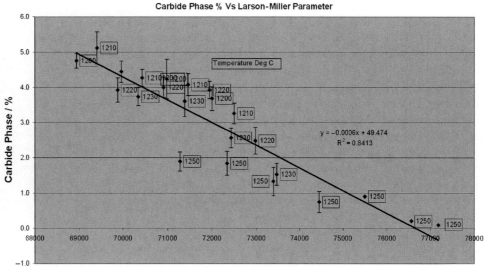

FIG. 2.31. Carbide phase % versus Larson-Miller paramter.

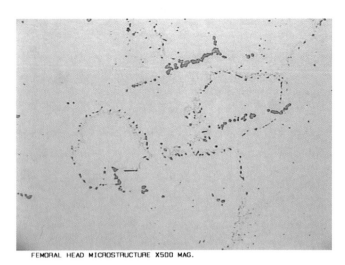

FEMORAL HEAD MICROSTRUCTURE X500 MAG.

Fɪɢ. 2.33. CoCr cast alloy after sintering, HIP and SHT.

The Development of the Birmingham Hip Resurfacing Device

When I first met Derek McMinn in 1995, I was the proud owner of a full head of hair. After my involvement in the transfer of the McMinn metal on metal resurfacing from Trucast to Centaur, which has been described earlier, I was involved in the development of the Birmingham Hip Resurfacing (BHR) device. My initial task was to characterize the metallurgical features of the first-generation metal on metal devices and to establish a bearing material specification based on these characteristics, which led to the long-term clinical success of the CoCr metal on metal bearings. This, as previously described, was to specify the BHR in CoCrMo alloy to ISO 5832 part 4 chemistry in the high carbon grade and in the as-cast microstructural condition. The objective was to employ state-of-the-art foundry practices and to replicate the coarse block carbide morphology in the as-cast condition. Without the benefit of employing the HIP process to reduce any casting voids, or microporosity, the gating design of both the femoral and acetabular components required efficient feeding capabilities.

I was also tasked with the development of an integrally cast surface texture on the convex surface of the acetabular cup to negate the need for any thermal processes to attach a porous surface, which would significantly modify the as-cast microstructure. Derek McMinn was dogmatic and adamant about this due to his previous unsatisfactory experience with the McMinn resurfacing device. It was this part of the project that made the highest demands and brings back the most memories of late nights, pondering, and hard work. The development of this surface included many late-night meetings with Derek, where I listened to numerous descriptions of what the "ideal" surface texture would look like. I also need to add the fact that none of them was capable of being produced through

the conventional wax pattern tooling methods, which was due to the fact that the surface texture was to be produced as an undercut feature to produce a mechanical interlock for the resultant bone on-growth. Derek made many "visits" to the foundry in Sheffield. Initially, his aim was to learn everything about cobalt chrome and the casting process. He then started to get his hands dirty by joining workers on the factory floor in every stage of the casting process. We had never before seen a surgeon with this level of interest. None of us had the heart to tell him that everything he touched had to be scrapped as he was "untrained"! It must also be stated that cobalt chrome alloy has not proven itself to be an effective osseo-integrating material, unlike titanium alloys.

Mr. McMinn's preference was to have a beaded surface texture with a defined bead spacing to permit adequately sized pedestals of bone to grow between and underneath the equator of the beads under the positive influence of hydroxyapatite. Our intention was to stick a suitable material to the outside of the blank wax pattern surface, which could then be invested in the shelling process. I wanted to see if wax beads could be produced in 1-mm-diameter spheres by dripping molten wax into cold water, but this idea was met with great despair at the foundry. I was later informed, by reputable and reliable sources at Centaur, that there was no such medium available that would allow such a surface to be produced.

My meetings with Mr. McMinn identified a number of other bead-shaped mediums such as icing sugar decorative beads and even poppy seeds! These were trialed by sticking them to wax patterns with large flat surfaces or other shapes (Fig. 2.34), but their shortcomings were soon identified if they were either soluble, in the case of sugar-based materials, or absorbent and explosive, in the case of poppy seeds, when they were immersed in the investment slurries or fired off in the flash-fire furnaces.

The resultant cast surfaces were far from optimal. Other suggestions included intricate structures produced by sprinkling

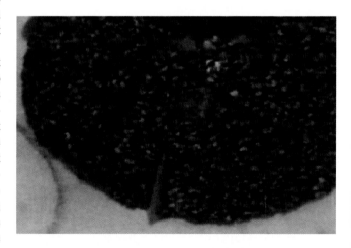

Fɪɢ. 2.34. Wax pattern covered in poppy seeds.

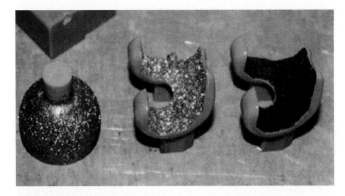

FIG. 2.35. Wax pattern covered in decorative glitter.

decorative glitter particles or even tea leaves onto the surfaces of waxes to test the resultant cast surfaces (Figs. 2.35 and 2.36).

This iterative process of "design, try, and test" became a regular activity, and it is worthy of note that I was delighted to receive the support of Dave Skupien, Bob Bruce, and the late John Harris, who were part of the Centaur management, in the pursuit of a final objective. One particular incident that left me with a real problem was when Derek convinced me that we were on the edge of identifying the final surface texture, which involved the use of tea leaves from Harrods tea, blend 20. How on earth would I be able to get hold of Harrods tea leaves in South Yorkshire? Anyway, we continued to produce a number of wax patterns covered in Harrods tea leaves, and I persuaded colleagues in the operations department at Centaur to process these components only to find that the isoferulic acid in the tea leaves reacted with the ceramic slurry resulting in the contamination, discoloration, and wastage of an expensive slurry. Imagine, a casting engineer not knowing that! The resultant surface texture was actually not too bad, however. We had even considered building a metal *master* that could be used to produce a rubber mold to place inside the wax pattern tool, injected with wax, and then peeled off the surface, but this was beyond our development timescale.

It was by pure coincidence that I was visiting another business contact at the Casting Technologies Institute (CTI) in Sheffield, where they operate a polystyrene pattern casting process, that I stumbled upon large volumes of polystyrene beads of roughly 1 mm in diameter. These beads, it turned out, were the pre-expanded beads used to produce the polystyrene patterns in the CTI casting process. I couldn't wait to return to my own process with a container full of these beads and "test" how they might perform under the Centaur casting process. Finally, we had a breakthrough in our development program, and these beads produced a surface texture exactly as Mr. McMinn had originally requested (Fig. 2.37).

There was of course a whole series of other process issues to overcome, but we had finally identified a suitable material for what was to become trademarked as Porocast.

To complement the polystyrene beaded surface, it was necessary to develop a bonding technique and a leachable face coat to invest this undercut surface (Fig. 2.38).

The bonding technique is not discussed here, and my only reference is to the adoption of a primary investment coating that has a capability of being leached by an alkali solution, a number of which are available to investment casting foundries with a design need. As the standard method of shell removal, blasting, is a line-of-sight process, it is not capable of removing the face coat from under the beaded texture, and so an effective chemical process is required to remove the residual shell. Just

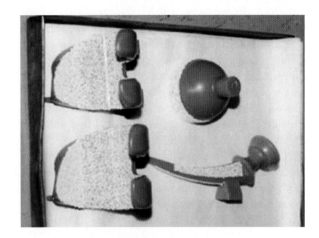

A

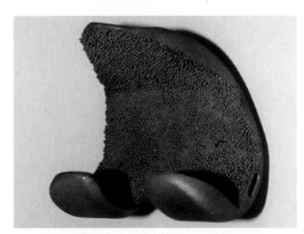

B

FIG. 2.37. (A) Wax patterns covered in polystyrene beads; (B) the resultant cast surface.

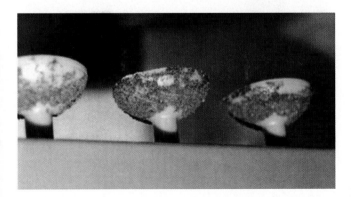

FIG. 2.36. Wax pattern covered in tea leaves on a wax runner.

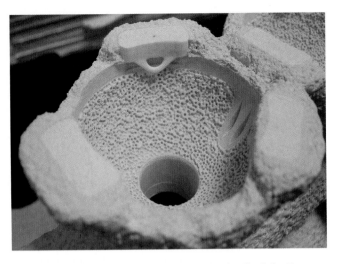

FIG. 2.38. A section of a shell showing the detail of the Porocast structure.

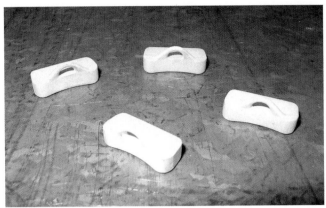

FIG. 2.40. Ceramic core used to produce the cast in introducer threaded wormholes.

as the leachable face coat processes are widely available to the casting community, so are the chemical leaching processes.

The third development activity for the BHR acetabular component casting was to produce the tunnels, or wormholes, which allow the threading of the introducer wires into the thin wall section of the casting on the face of the cup. The use of ceramic cores to produce detailed features in a CoCr casting was not new to Centaur as previous developments had included producing a ceramic core with a detailed M8 thread that reduced significant time, difficulty, and cost in the finish machining of a femoral knee device (Fig. 2.39).

This allowed for the attachment of augmentation blocks on the inner surface of the knee component. As that particular ceramic core was performing well, it appeared logical to use that ceramic material type to produce a ceramic core capable of producing the 1.75-mm-diameter holes in the BHR cup for

threading the introducer wires through. The critical aspect of the ceramic core for this feature was that the threaded hole needed to match the radius of the cup peripheral face, dictated by the radius and the wall thickness, match the curvature of the cup, dictated by the external and internal radii, and for one ceramic core to complement each size of cup. Another small challenge! A small team of engineers from Centaur, Finsbury (Leatherhead, UK), and Certech (Kettering, UK) (ceramic core suppliers) worked on the final design, which ended up looking like a small stirrup (Fig. 2.40). The resultant ceramic core allowed an optimal position for the wormhole, or tunnel, so that the cavity was central to the casting section in all planes.

The development of the femoral head casting was rather less challenging than that of the acetabular cup as its external surface was to be extensively machined, which means that a gating design could take advantage of that activity. The gate therefore was positioned centrally on the zenith of the head sphere and was large enough in diameter to effectively feed the casting without microporosity. An inner core was produced

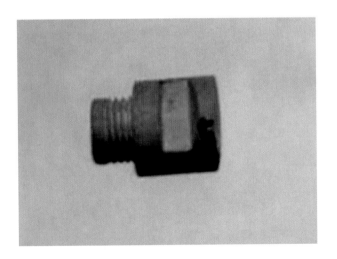

A

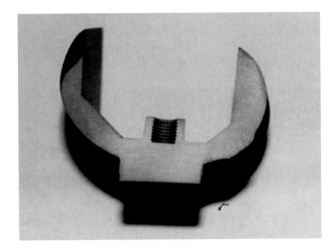

B

FIG. 2.39. (A) Ceramic core used to produce an M8 thread in a femoral knee; (B) cross section of the resultant cast form.

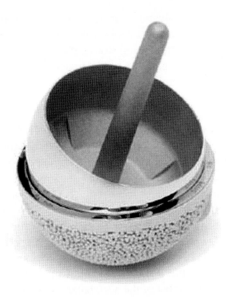

Fig. 2.41. The internal detail of the femoral head casting produced on the casting without machining.

in the wax pattern tool to create the internal profile, stem, and cement pockets (Fig. 2.41).

Once the casting process was determined, which included the design of the wax pattern and gating, the wax assembly, shelling technique, casting technique, finishing methods, and inspection methods, the casting validation process took place. Initially, we employed bizarre logistical processes that included the transportation of wax assemblies across South Yorkshire for the shell investment to take place at a development site, while Centaur was developing an in-house leachable face coat. More hair loss! The final casting process was effectively validated and locked down to ensure continued compliance with the product specification, and all characteristics of the castings met with Mr. McMinn's expectations. We had produced a casting system that replicated the excellent material properties of the first-generation metal on metal bearings with an integrally cast in-growth structure and an efficient introducer system that allowed a thin wall casting section cup to be gripped without encroaching on the important articulation surface of the bearing (Figs. 2.42 and 2.43).

Summary

In the preceding sections, I have covered the forensic analysis of successful long-term retrieved metal on metal implants, detailed descriptions of a number of manufacturing and technical processes, the development of the BHR device, and microstructural changes in CoCr alloy due to thermal processes and its subsequent effect on wear. I will summarize this chapter in the following section bringing the salient points together from each of the topics covered to establish their combined significance.

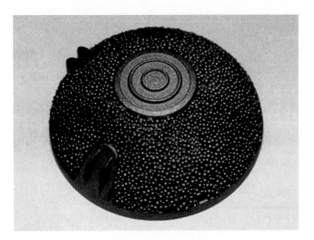

A

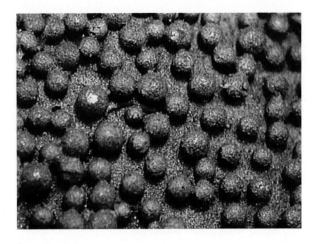

B

Fig. 2.42. (A) BHR cup with Porocast surface; (B) high magnification of beaded surface.

The critical factors that had provided such an excellent performance in the first-generation metal on metal bearings were that the CoCr microstructure was produced in its highest wear-resistant condition, with large block carbides protecting the metal surfaces from adhesive wear (Figure 2.30A), both articulating surfaces were similar, reducing the risk of having a subservient component and articulating pair, and the manufactured geometry resulted in sphericities and clearances that would allow at least partial fluid film to occur during articulation of the bearing. As the fatigue strength failures of long-stemmed devices did not occur until later in the implants (fatigue is a cyclic effect on a structure that involves elastic or plastic bending or movement over time and under load), the use of as-cast microstructural condition was fortuitous for the bearing properties of the material and allowed the experience of CoCr as a metal on metal bearing to continue.

The McMinn metal on metal resurfacing device was produced and implanted between 1994 and 1996, and part of its material, microstructural evolution has already been described in detail. The significance of this device is that the product

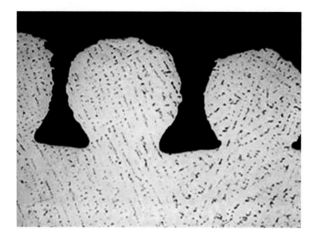

A

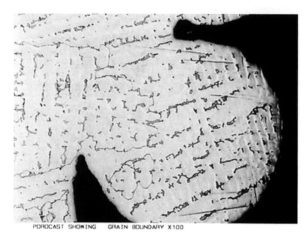

B

FIG. 2.43. (A) Cross section through Porocast beads; (B) high magnification of cross section through a single bead.

produced in 1996 had a microstructure that was based on high fatigue strength, high manufacturing yield (no scrap due to casting microporosity), and easiest machining condition (Fig. 2.32 as an example) and has behaved differently than those devices produced and implanted in 1994 and 1995. The microstructure generally had small dispersed carbides and large areas of matrix exposed between the carbides, however due to the variability in thermal treatments, evidence on some retrievals from this group show a higher diffusion of carbide. Of course, there are a number of causes of implant failure, septic or aseptic, which result in the need for revision, and when investigating a revision it is important to determine what role the implant materials and or design have played in the cause. The details of the implant cohorts, including revision rates and causes of revision, are described by other authors in this book.

The microstructures of the retrieved devices from the McMinn cohorts implanted in 1994–1996 were examined to determine if there was any relationship between the material of the device and the cause of revision (i.e., metal-losis-induced osteolysis). Because the product implanted was taken from implant stocks (including finished goods, work-in-progress and casting stock), it appears that products implanted in 1996 included products that were produced in 1995, or earlier, leading to combinations of microstructures articulating against each other and artificially increasing the cohort size for 1996, therefore understating the revision rate. It was interesting to see in those devices revised for metal-losis-induced osteolysis that there was a direct relationship between the microstructure of the device and the linear wear rate measured, where low-carbide-containing devices had higher wear when both bearing surfaces were in parity. It can also be seen that the higher-carbide-containing microstructure protects the device from the counterface, which becomes subservient, whether it is a femoral head or an acetabular cup component. This is in contrast with the previously reported observation that the linear wear rate of the femoral component is higher than that of the acetabular component when the microstructures are in parity (e.g., first-generation metal on metal bearings and BHR). Of course, if the femoral device is protected by being produced in a higher-carbide-containing microstructure, the total wear of the bearing will be lower than when both surfaces are low carbide as it is the linear wear of the head that is most easily identified due to the localized position of the smaller wear patch and ease of measurement of a convex object.

The lower-carbide-containing alloy (carbon <0.07%) microstructures have a greater risk of experiencing adhesive wear on asperities in the matrix on both bearing surfaces, which occurs at a nanometric level, than do the higher-carbide-containing bearings where the large block carbides, because of their higher hardness, reduce the occurrence of adhesive wear. It is the biphasic nature of the hard carbides in the softer matrix that provides the CoCr alloy with its excellent wear properties. I remember attending an excellent seminar on "Tribology in Practice" at the National Physical Laboratory in the United Kingdom, where it was described by Neale and Gee that "for loaded metal-on-metal contacts some lubrication is essential to avoid seizure and wear. The optimum structure is then one in which there are small dispersed hard areas in the surface to carry the load, supported in a strong but softer matrix, which wears to form recesses around the hard areas, and in which lubricant can be retained. In the case of piston rings and cylinder liners which are made from cast iron, this is achieved by adding phosphorus, vanadium to chromium to create localized hard areas of phosphate or metal carbides." It occurred to me that it was serendipity that the as-cast CoCr microstructures produced for the first-generation metal on metal bearings had an inherent protection to adhesive wear, due to these large block carbides, and had allowed these bearings to perform. Low-carbide-containing bearing surfaces, where high material loss had been experienced, evidenced adhesive wear when their articulating surfaces were scratch-free and did not have particulate available (i.e., carbide particulate) for abrasive third-body wear scratches to form.

Although there are other design factors that can contribute to the failure of a metal on metal bearing device, the material condition is of fundamental importance to the longevity of these devices, which are intended to be *in situ* for many decades, and there are already reports, both written and anecdotal, suggesting that the use of mixed microstructures or low-carbide-containing bearings are leading to early failure of these devices [8–14]. The use of low-carbon alloys, which do not have sufficient carbon to produce carbides and where there is no inherent protection against adhesive wear, are no longer used for metal on metal bearings, however high-carbon-containing alloys that have been thermally treated, reducing the carbide content and behaving like low-carbon alloys, continue to be used. The problem with the risk of high wear in the bearing material due to microstructural differences in the *in vivo* situation (i.e., in the patient and outside the laboratory) is that it does not manifest itself until the midterm time period. Any bearing material wear risks must be considered as latent risks and should be a consideration when choosing a bearing material for use in orthopedics.

References

1. Medley J et al. Engineering issues and wear performance of metal on metal hip implants. 1997.
2. Ahier S, Ginsburg K. Influence of carbide distribution on the wear and friction of Vitallium. Proc Inst Mech Eng 1966;181:137–139.
3. Clemow AJT, Daniell BL. The influence of microstructure on the adhesive wear resistance of a Co-Cr-Mo alloy. Wear 1980;61:219–231.
4. Wang KK, Wang A, Gustavson LJ. Metal on metal wear testing of chrome cobalt alloys. In: Digesi JA, Kennedy RL, Pillar R, eds. Cobalt-Based Alloys for Bio-Medical Applications. ASTM STP 1365: Wear Characterization. West Conshohocken, PA: ASTM, 1999:135–144.
5. Que L. Effect of heat treatments on the microstructure, hardness and wear resistance of the as-cast and forged Cobalt-chromium implant alloys. Presented at the Symposium on Cobalt-Based Alloys for Bio-Medical Applications, November 3–4, 1998, Norfolk, Virginia, USA.
6. Varano R, Bobyn JD, Medley JB, Yue S. Does alloy heat treatment influence metal-on-metal wear? Poster no. 1399 presented at the 49th Annual Meeting of the Orthopaedic Research Society, New Orleans, Louisiana, USA; 2003.
7. Cawley J, Metcalf JEP, Jones AH, Band TJ, Skupien DS. A tribological study of cobalt chromium alloys used in metal-on-metal resurfacing hip arthroplasty. Wear 2003;255:999–1006.
8. McMinn D et al. Hip resurfacing—how metal on metal articulations have come full circle, IMechE June 2002.
9. MacDonald et al. Metal on metal versus metal on polyethylene liners in total hip arthroplasty: clinical and metal ion results of a prospective randomized clinical trial. AOA 2002;601:27–34.
10. Pfister et al. Metal ion levels from low and high carbon metal-on-metal bearings. Presented at the 7th Swiss Orthopaedic Congress, Laussane, Switzerland, 19–22 June 2002.
11. McMinn D, et al. Development of metal/metal hip resurfacing. Hip Int 2003;13;41–53.
12. Park Y-S et al. Early ostolysis following second-generation metal-on-metal hip replacement. J Bone Joint Surg Am 2005; 87:1515–1521.
13. Kovac S et al. Survivorship and retrieval analysis of sikomet metal-on-metal total hip replacements at a mean of seven years. J Bone Joint Surg Am 2006;88:1173–1182.
14. Nolan JF et al. Metal on metal hip replacement. Presented at the British Hip Society Meeting, Leeds, March 2007.

3
Machining Processes

Roger W.F. Ashton

Machining and Finishing

Manufacturers of the first-generation metal on metal bearings had little guidance as to the limits, clearances, and geometric tolerances that would be required for best performance of the bearing system. Neither did they have the benefit of the development of cutting tool materials for this metallurgical system. They did, however, have access to the required metal forming and machining processes even if these did not have the benefit of modern computer controls or analysis techniques.

Suitably accurate methods for the production of optical devices have existed for a number of centuries, and even though these methods were laborious (hence these days not very cost effective), they were easily capable of producing parts that would meet the current specifications. What would not have been available would have been the methods to reliably control the processes. This is evident in the variability seen in some early devices, where the metrology required in the production environment has clearly developed at a slower rate than the processes themselves. However, it was the geometry of these devices, which enjoyed a benign long-term clinical record, that was later used to define the design specification and hence the manufacturing controls.

Effect of Metallurgical Condition on Machining

The metallurgical condition of the as-cast raw material largely dictates the sequence of machining operations. The carbide distribution is uniform throughout the material, but the grain size and distribution of casting inclusions varies toward the outer surface of the casting. Although their presence has been shown to not adversely affect the function of the bearing, it is preferred that casting inclusions, which predominate in the upper 0.5 mm of the raw casting, are removed. This is a bulk material removal operation where the part is generally turned.

The material, being in the as-cast condition, can be prone to occasional subsurface microporosity. This is in the form of microscopic tensile cracks that are caused by the volume change occurring during cooling. If the cast component is subject to high cyclic tensile loads, these may become growth points for fatigue cracks. It was an attempt to minimize this phenomenon in conventional femoral stems, which are subject to cyclic bending loads, that led metallurgists and engineers to apply hot isostatic pressing techniques to most cast devices. This reduced the microporosity and improved their structural strength and machinability. However, as the Birmingham Hip Resurfacing (BHR) device is a bearing element rather than a structural member, the untreated metallurgy is selected for its wear properties.

The volume changes that occur in the casting process, during solidification, also result in a level of residual stress in the material. This has little effect on the mechanical properties of the bearing elements but must be considered during the machining processes. Removal of material during machining will result in some relaxation and dimensional changes at the moment of machining. Hence all bulk material removal operations must be complete before the superfinishing of bearing surfaces, otherwise the bearing geometry will be compromised leading to high bearing wear, especially during the run-in period.

This is graphically demonstrated when preparing samples for wear evaluation, where some machining may be required on the finished component prior to testing. This can cause distortions through stress relaxation as well as clamping that can greatly affect the wear performance.

During the high deformation rates of machining and in particular turning, the alloy exhibits a degree of work hardening. This effect is likely to be present but less marked during the superfinishing operations. It may also occur in service. It has been suggested that this has an effect on the wear mechanisms, particularly abrasive wear, and is due to a local phase transformation. This is difficult to verify as the affected layer is very thin and hence examination of the transformation is only possible through x-ray diffraction (by TEM).

Available Standards and Measuring Methods

ISO 7206-2 makes an attempt to specify parameters such as surface roughness average, sphericity, and radial clearance for metallic, ceramic, femoral, and acetabular components. Its scope assumes that the acetabular component is "plastic" or that the femoral component contacts the biological acetabulum. As a result, the values and tolerances stated for the bearing are massively large and hence not at all relevant. The standard also attempts to state a measurement method for these values. As the actual values used during manufacture of the bearing couple are very much smaller than those stated in the standard (between 10% and 20%), the methods outlined are also of little relevance. This has resulted in the development of an inspection protocol specific to the BHR using measuring equipment capable of a much improved resolution and more relevant specification.

In broad terms, the key parameters for the control of machining of the bearing couple are clearly size (this controls the clearance of the bearing), roundness or sphericity (which influences the contact conditions in the bearing), and surface finish (which influences the initial lubrication conditions).

For the person who is not involved in the manufacturing processes, it is hard to appreciate the tolerances and control limits specified. ISO 7206-2 intimates that form on a femoral head should be controlled to 10 μm. The actual value used on the BHR is 2 μm, and to ensure compliance during manufacture, maximum control limits of 1 μm may be used. A view of the relative size of a micrometer can be seen in Fig. 3.1. In macroscopic terms, if one wanted to control the earth to this level of roundness, then all high ground more than 250 m above sea level would have to be leveled. To achieve the same finish, then, most irregularities greater than 2.5 m would have to be removed. Sadly, the earth is actually 40 km out-of-round.

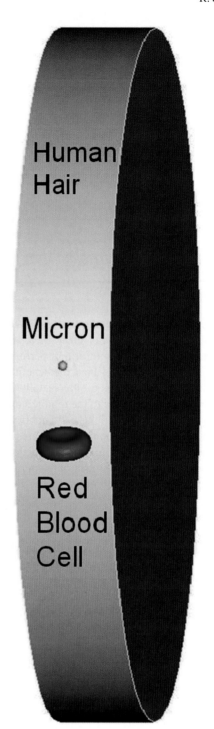

FIG. 3.1.

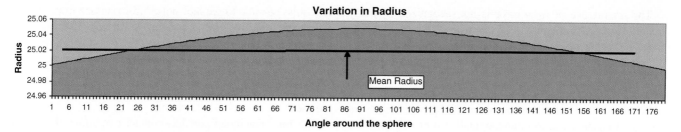

Fig. 3.2.

In reality, radius, form, and finish interact. For a bearing, they are increasingly detailed ways of looking at the same thing. A radius measurement of a sphere is a single value giving a "best-fit" size over many contact points on the entire available surface. If the sphere is actually the shape of an egg, then a simple radius measurement assumes it is a billiard ball of mean size. (Some manufacturers consider eggs and billiard balls to be very similar.) Figure 3.2 shows variation in radius around the sphere being expressed as a single "best-fit" value. These measurements require a resolution of the order 3 μm (3/1000 mm), hence coordinate measuring machines (CMM) are used.

To better control conditions in the bearing, then form needs to be considered. A roundness or sphericity value is obtained by gathering a large number of measured points from the surface of the bearing, best fitting a circle or sphere through them, then expressing the maximum deviation of the actual measured points around the perfect best-fit circle or sphere (RONT) (Fig. 3.3). If this form value is correctly specified and small enough, it prevents eggs being mistaken for billiard balls. In effect, roundness is used to ensure that the curvature of the contact point and hence the effective diameter is controlled. Figure 3.4 shows this variation in radius around the sphere being expressed linearly as form error. These measurements are of a resolution of the order 0.1 μm (1/10,000 mm), hence roundness machines are used.

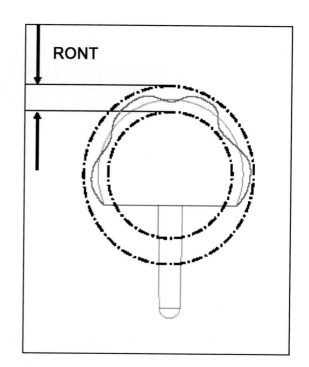

Fig. 3.3.

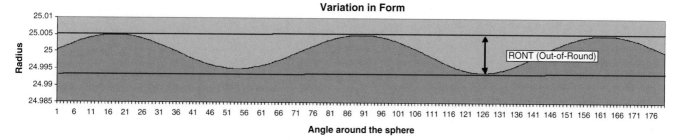

Fig. 3.4.

The importance of form error is not recognized by many manufacturers. Its effects can be surprising. One such device, from a manufacturer who based their bearing performance claims largely on their "low" clearance, exhibited sufficient form error for the effective clearance to vary by 230 μm depending on the point of bearing contact *in vivo*.

Whereas form measurements control shape variations of medium frequency and medium amplitude, surface finish is the expression of the high frequency and small amplitude variation.

It is quite possible to see the "noise" from surface finish on the form measurements. The engineering world tends to express the finish as a roughness average (Ra) (Fig. 3.5), filtering out the lower-frequency effects of form and diameter. These measurements are of a resolution of the order 5 nm (5/1,000,000 mm), hence surface contact profilometers or optical interferometers are used.

The final machined part has contact conditions that are a composite of all these measured features (Fig. 3.6).

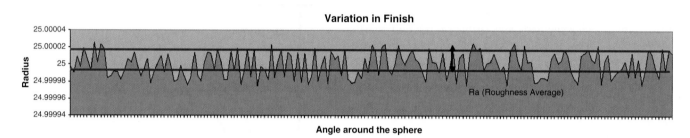

Fig. 3.5.

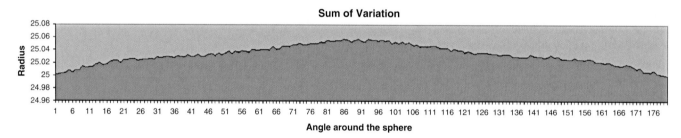

Fig. 3.6.

Although it is possible to find specialist equipment capable of simultaneously measuring this full range, it is invariably hugely expensive, so the task has historically been devolved to specific machines:

Diameters: Coordinate measuring machines and hand-held equipment (Fig. 3.7)
Form: Roundness machines (Fig. 3.8)
Finish: Surface contacting profilometers and optical interferometers (Fig. 3.9)

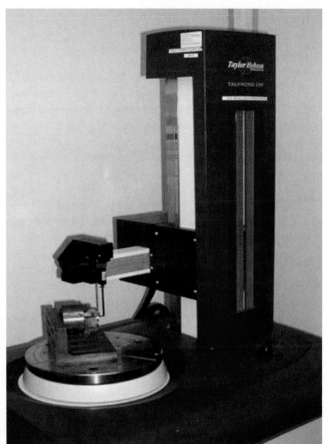

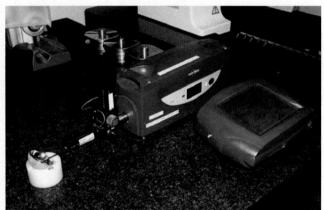

Fig. 3.8.

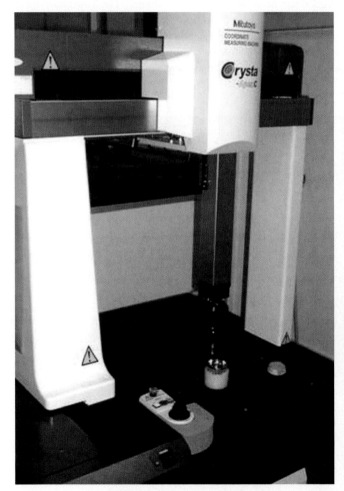

Fig. 3.7.

Fig. 3.9.

Machining Operations

Turning

Turning is the process used to produce cylindrical components in a lathe. It can be controlled manually or by using computer-controlled (CNC) machines. When turning, an axisymmetric piece of raw material is rotated and a cutting tool is traversed along two axes of motion to produce precise diameters and depths and forms. Turning can be either on the outside of the cylinder or on the inside (also known as boring) to produce tubular components to various geometries.

The machining properties of the alloy in the as-cast condition limit the effectiveness of intermittent cuts and light finishing cuts. This encourages the machinist to attempt to achieve finished size in larger steps than he would otherwise be inclined to do. As the tool wear rate is considerable, achieving close dimensional accuracy as well as good surface finish by turning is very difficult. As a result, turning is used to provide the machined feed-stock for subsequent operations

more capable of producing the required surface finishes and geometric accuracies. Notwithstanding this, excessive variations and lack of control at this stage can introduce some undesirable effects on the finished product. Excessive removal rates or badly selected tool geometries can encourage tensile failures in the material especially at the grain boundaries as seen in Fig. 3.10.

The resurfacing componentry presents additional complications. Parts of the cross section of the head are quite small relative to the material to be removed and the cutting forces required. The result is that there is slight deformation of the component under cutting loads. Typically, after turning, the head could be 20 µm out-of-round relative to a 2-µm finished specification. This excessive form variation has to be corrected by a subsequent honing and polishing operations, described under the heading of "Superfinishing." The cup component presents additional distortion challenges. The section at the periphery is slender and hence prone to distortion on fixturing in the turning machines. In addition, the internal form modifies through stress relaxation as the casting runners are removed.

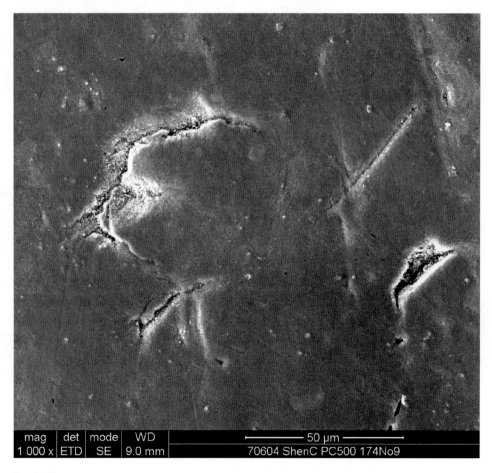

Fig. 3.10.

Superfinishing

There are many variants of superfinishing operations—and the definition is by no means standard. For the purposes of this discussion, all are assumed to be cutting by abrasion.

Lapping is a machining operation, in which two surfaces are rubbed together with an abrasive between them, by hand movement or by way of a machine. This process has been developed for use in many applications such as in the optics and bearing industries. In its simplest form, lapping typically involves rubbing a hard work-piece material, such as a glass lens, against a former, such as iron or glass itself (also known as the "lap"), with an abrasive, such as aluminum oxide, emery, silicon carbide, diamond, and so forth, in between them. This produces microscopic conchoidal fractures (like knapped flint) as the abrasive rolls about between the two surfaces and removes material from both. Figure 3.11 shows silicon carbide powder of the kind used in both honing wheels and as loose abrasive.

The other form of lapping involves a softer material for the lap, which is "charged" with the abrasive. The lap is then used to cut a harder material—the work-piece. The abrasive embeds within the softer material, which holds it and permits it to score across and cut the harder material. Taken to the finer limit, this will produce a polished surface such as a polishing cloth on a femoral head, or polishing pitch upon glass. These processes are analogous to the abrasive wear mechanisms occurring *in vivo*.

Taking the principle of embedded abrasives in another direction, a grinding wheel consists of fine abrasive particles (usually aluminum oxide or silicon carbide) captured in softer supporting matrix. This wheel as it wears provides a constantly renewing source of abrasive cutting edges. Grinding is normally considered a high-speed process involving the generation of localized heating and sparks. The process of honing is a hybrid of grinding and lapping, whereby the hone, as well as providing supported abrasive particles, also releases abrasive particles into the interface. It is generally considered to be a lower-speed process having little potential effect on the surface properties of the material.

These abrasive processes are more generally applied to the machining of flat and cylindrical surfaces. It is possible, with the application of appropriate tool geometries and motions, to apply them to the machining of spherical surfaces, both convex and concave.

Spherical Honing

In contrast with most short-stroke cylindrical and flat honing operations, rotating abrasive cup-wheels are used. The work-piece, in this case a femoral head, is rotated about its stem axis (Fig. 3.12). The abrasive wheel, rotating in the opposite direction to the work-piece, is presented at an appropriate angle defined by the normal to the chord between pole and end surface of the head.

The bore diameter of the cup-wheel is defined by the length of the chord. As the wheel wears, it is advanced in a direction toward the center of the sphere. Thus, the wheel can be considered to be self-dressing, in that wear should have no impact on the geometric configuration. It can be seen that the cutting area of the cup-wheel remains in full ring contact with the work-piece. This produces a "cross-hatch" effect of fine machining lines.

The theory of this process is elegant, and provided that the manufacturing limits in terms of roundness are wide enough, then the process performs as described. The geometric specification of the BHR has roundness limits of less than $2\,\mu m$. At this level, the process has had to be refined considerably in order to achieve process stability.

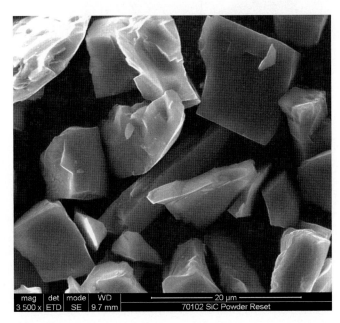

Fig. 3.11.

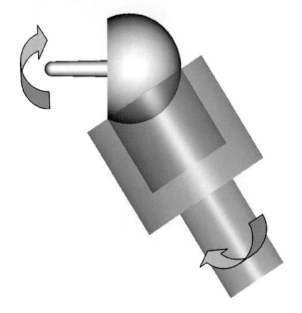

Fig. 3.12.

Development of the BHR Sphere Honing Process

The effect of the roundness limit on the manufacturing processes of the BHR was probably not realized when the processes were first established. It is always the goal of the manufacturing engineer to establish repeatability of process. Their desire is that when the process is started today, they will expect the same result as the day before and the day after. Statistically, and with measurable dimensions, this may be expressed as the process potential—how much of a statistical variation one can expect on a particular measurable value relative to the tolerances on that value. This approach only considers a dimensional output. Just as importantly, the engineer requires that the "recipe" to achieve that dimensional stability should remain exactly the same. This stable recipe may include machining speeds and feeds, cutting tool and abrasive specifications, raw material condition, and so on. Without this approach, the manufacturing process becomes a craft. The process to more fully understand the honing operation, and hence stabilize it, has been evolving over a number of years.

Exploring Geometric Effects of Sphere Honing

Theoretically, the sphere honing process should produce a perfect sphere. Perfection requires no errors in alignment, perfect raw material, no distortion of tools or work-pieces during operation—and hence no cutting forces. This results in no parts being produced.

The polar or R,θ plot represents a cross-sectional scan of the manufactured sphere in a plane through the stem axis (Fig. 3.13).

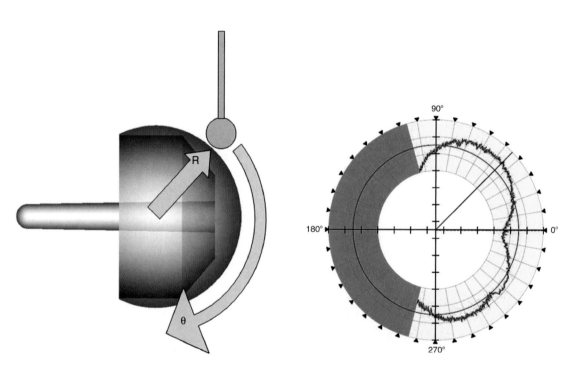

Fig. 3.13.

The plot shows deviations relative to a perfect circle that are calculated by a least squares fit through all the data points in the graph. The deviations can then be scaled in the R direction to aid visualization of error from the true circle. This representation can be used not only to explore the parameters controlling the manufactured shape but also to examine the performance effects of varying geometries and allow assessment of linear wear levels both in test specimens and explanted parts.

The "apple" shape shown is characteristic of the cross-hatch honing technique on an external sphere. What is important is the amount of deviation from the perfect circle, and this can be influenced by a number of factors.

Parameters affecting manufactured shape have been studied in more detail in a three-dimensional simulation of the metal removal process. For example, when distortion is introduced to the honing wheel in response to the cutting pressures, the degree of out-of-roundness found in the simulation work-piece is found to be similar and proportional to the wheel distortion introduced. (This is represented in Fig. 3.14 by the scaled length of the porcupine vectors shown.) The rigidity of the work-piece relative to the applied pressure on the honing wheel will lead to a varying degree of nonuniform elastic deformation of the work-piece. This complements the wheel distortion. As both wheel distortion and work-piece distortion are a function of applied honing load, it is clear that machining rate and wheel cutting efficiency can affect the final geometry of the finished part. Most other geometric misalignments tend only to affect final work-piece size, although in practice, more consistent form results are obtained by carefully controlling the manner in which the wheel first comes into contact with the work-piece at the start of the machining operation.

It is possible to improve honing wheel rigidity by various means including increasing the outside diameter of the wheel. This, however, has a number of contrary effects. First, the cutting area of the wheel is increased, affecting the wheel breakdown rate and hence the rate at which new abrasive is exposed. This leads to wheel "blocking," where used abrasive and debris block the pores in the wheel preventing any new edges being exposed. Second, when the wheel is used in a self-dressing mode (i.e., is allowed to adopt the shape of the last work-piece; Fig. 3.15), then some shape aberrations occur on the pole of the part. This can be controlled through wheel redressing.

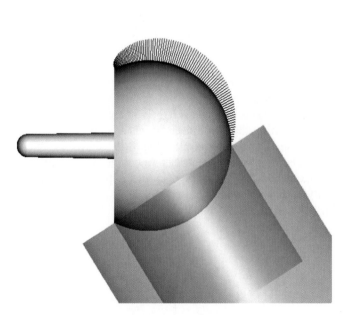

FIG. 3.14.

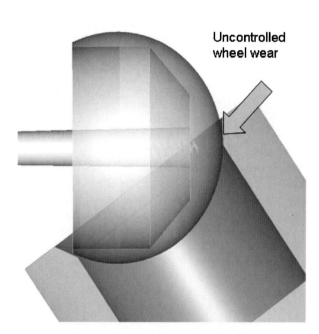

FIG. 3.15.

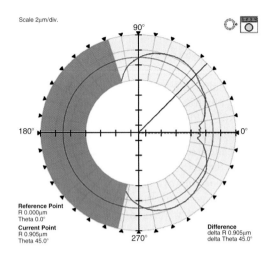

Fig. 3.16.

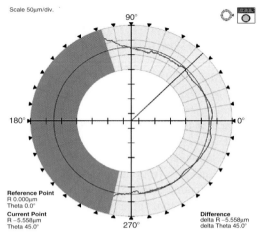

Fig. 3.18.

In Fig. 3.16, the wheel shape and approach angle have not been controlled. This gives rise to varying effects in the pole area, some of which can affect wear behavior.

Lack of attention to detail on this aspect of process set-up can lead to interesting results, many of which have been observed in components produced by other manufacturers of metal on metal parts (Fig. 3.17). These devices still have the appropriate visual appearance despite their curious geometry.

The characteristic apple shape of cross-hatch honing at least reassures us that work-piece and wheel are in alignment. In cases where poorly maintained honing machines are used, the two working axes may not intersect. It is possible to observe the effects of honing on only one side of the wheel. In Fig. 3.18, the apple shape gives way to a shape with two intersecting radii without a common center. It is possible to introduce some flexibility in either the work-piece or wheel mountings thus allowing the two working axes to self-align. This can have some unfortunate effects as the resonant frequency of the system can be altered to such an extent that "chatter" may occur (uncontrolled vibration of the system leading to poor surface finish and dubious results).

Flexibility in the system that allows the working axes to coincide explains why it is possible to achieve very good results by hand honing of spheres. By this method, the honing wheel is held on a powered device such as a drill. The wheel is brought into contact with the counterrotating work-piece and pressure is applied. Angular alignment errors that give rise to pole aberrations are reduced by manual oscillation of the wheel so that the pole is constantly covered and uncovered by the wheel.

This process can give fine results in skilled hands but has the obvious drawbacks of cost, repeatability, and dependence on craft skills.

The concentration has been so far on the polar roundness values and shape in the plane through the stem axis. Roundness in the equatorial plane is largely influenced by the bearings supporting the work-piece or wheel spindles and their interaction. The equatorial plot (Fig. 3.19) shows the effect of spindle run-out or eccentricity where the spindle speed is approximately four times the work-piece speed. This type of analysis can sometimes be used to analyze spindle and bearing behavior in the machine tool.

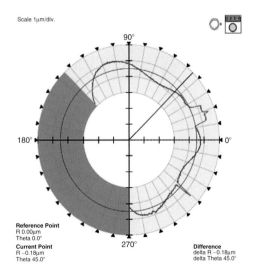

Fig. 3.17.

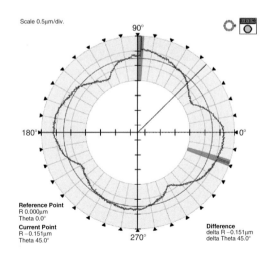

Fig. 3.19.

The surface finish that can be produced with spherical honing depends primarily on the work-piece material and the fineness of the abrasive in the wheel used—although various other machining parameters also come into play to a lesser extent. Some manufacturers make attempts to produce the finished product surface finish during this operation, which is possible provided absolute cleanliness is maintained and their surface appearance standards allow occasional sweeping machining marks caused by stray abrasive or other particulates.

In general, the manufacturer will repeat this honing operation with increasingly fine grades of abrasive wheel in order to achieve the appropriate balance of material removal, geometric form, and surface finish. The finest grades of these wheels contain abrasive particles with average grit sizes of the order 5 µm, but as the grading process for superfine abrasive is difficult, there tends to be a large distribution about the average (up to 20 µm at times). This indicates why final finishing with this type of process can be difficult; the abrasive particle used is 100 times larger than the maximum final surface roughness average (0.050 Ra). Unless it is carefully captured in its support matrix, this will result in very visible scratches as it breaks free and becomes entrained between wheel and work-piece.

If the visible scratches are sufficiently spaced, then they have little effect on the roughness average. It is therefore quite possible to satisfy the ISO standard value of 0.05 Ra with this process. However, as tribologists strive for fluid film perfection through decreased roughness average, and as most surgeons would find the appearance of such parts to be unacceptable, further finishing techniques need to be employed.

Final Finishing

It is a principle of large metal on metal bearings that they optimally operate in a "mixed" lubrication regime. Their mode of operation hovers between asperity contact and motion on a fluid film. It is not possible for such a bearing system to remain in fluid film mode at all times, and a full fluid film occurs only at the extremes of speed, viscosity, and lack of load. Largely, wear by whatever mechanism only occurs when the surfaces contact. If one then compares the relative magnitude of wear in use (2 µm during run-in) with the depth of the surface finish represented by the Ra (10 nm say), then the layer where the manufacturer did their finishing work will have departed after about 1 month in operation. This leaves the native material to self-polish without the aid of expensive abrasives and special manufacturing techniques.

A feature of this cobalt chrome system is that even after sustaining quite severe damage, or if "poor" surface finishes are presented to each other, the surface finish can recover with use through a burnishing process of contact with itself. Hence the role of the manufacturer is largely to optimize the start-up conditions of the bearing; that is, to minimize the production of wear debris during that period before the bearing adopts its activity specific steady-state shape and surface finish.

To this end, it is necessary to target a surface finish and texture that will most quickly be transformed to the run-in condition while producing the least-wear products. It stands to reason, therefore, that the manufacturer should target a roughness average of approximately 15 nM or better.

At great magnification, the topography of the run-in surface in this material is generally characterized by a predominance of plateaus interspersed by V-shaped valleys (Fig. 3.20). This type of topography is denoted by its negative "skew" value (Rsk).

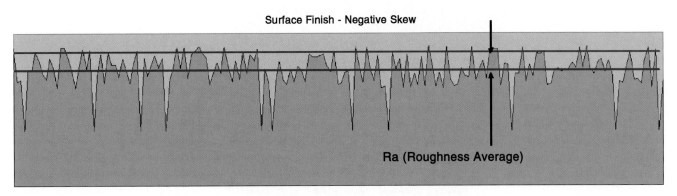

FIG. 3.20.

By this notation, wide valleys, interspersed by occasional high peaks, would have a positive skew value (Fig. 3.21). Where valleys and peaks are in equal number and magnitude, the skew is zero. To best approximate the average run-in part, the skew value should be just below zero. The polishing process employed dictates both the Ra and Rsk values.

As previously described, the morphology of the as-cast cobalt chrome alloy is characterized by a uniform matrix containing approximately 5% or more (by area) of chromium-rich blocky carbides. These carbides are harder and somewhat resistant to wear compared with the surrounding matrix. Where the polishing processes are not controlled, the less wear-resistant matrix can be removed from around the carbide, leaving the carbide elevated. In extreme cases, the carbide can dislodge and be "plucked" from the surface, leaving a small hole, sometimes visible to the naked eye, measuring approximately 30 μm across. High-speed polishing processes such as buff-polishing can be more prone to this phenomenon.

Rigidly supported diamond impregnated cloths, running at lower speeds, are less prone to this, and they also tend toward a negative skew finish—although the perceived lustre of this type of finishing is slightly lower.

All polishing processes remove material; in the case of localized buff-polishing, up to 1 μm in 5 seconds. It is therefore critical to control the duration and uniformity of application otherwise the geometric form will be compromised. As high lustre is perceived as high precision, there is a temptation to overpolish components to the detriment of their function. This can be seen on various manufacturers' components in the form of extreme "relief polishing" (a raised stipple effect seen under magnification), plucked carbides, and high out-of-roundness values. (Figure 3.22 shows a relief-polished surface as measured by optical interferometry. The height scale is greatly exaggerated for visualization purposes.)

Surface Finish - Positive Skew

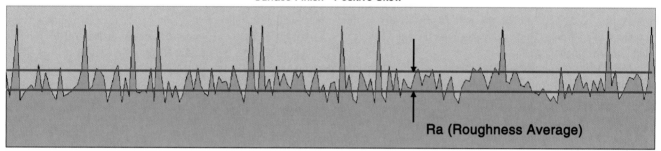

Ra (Roughness Average)

Fig. 3.21.

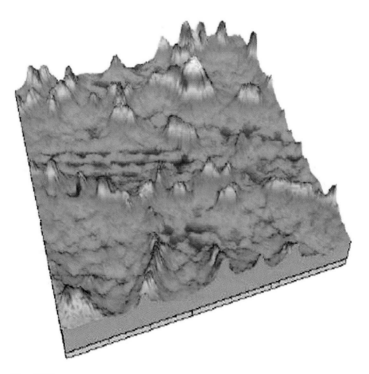

Fig. 3.22.

Conclusion

In Chapter 1, Derek McMinn has already alluded to the constraints that the BHR device placed upon its manufacturing processes. The geometric specification is demanding while the cobalt alloy system, selected for its wear properties, is necessarily in the worst possible condition to facilitate metal removal. It would be expedient to make modifications to the manufacturing processes to reduce some of these difficulties. The addition of heat treatments would improve metal cutting properties and reduce the effort required to produce the surface finish, and relaxation of the geometric specification to "normal" levels would reduce machining times and levels of inspection. Intimate knowledge of the process characteristics and their impact on the device performance is central to future improvements in the bearing technology. It is fortunate that this resurfacing system has always been processed in an environment where the manufacturing, design, and testing are closely interlinked so that the manufacturing elements that contribute to the device's excellent clinical history are never overlooked.

4
Hip Joint Tribology

Amir Kamali

According to the ASM International handbook, *tribology* is defined as the science and technology of interacting surfaces in relative motion and all practices related thereto. It includes the study of wear, friction, and lubrication.

Wear and Wear Mechanisms

Wear is defined as the progressive removal of material from contacting surfaces in relative motion. The wear mechanisms in metal-on-metal bearings are as follows:

Adhesive wear occurs by the transfer of material from one surface to another when two surfaces articulate against each other under load. The transferred material could break off and act as third-body particles resulting in abrasive wear.

Abrasive wear occurs when material is removed from a surface by hard asperities on the counterface and hard particles (third body) trapped between the two contact surfaces.

Corrosive wear occurs by the combination of mechanical wear and chemical reaction. Corrosion is the mechanism by which metal ions are released, and as this process is less understood than the other wear mechanisms, more details have been provided in Chapter 5.

It should be pointed out that in metal on metal bearings, all the above-mentioned wear mechanisms could occur simultaneously but at different rates.

Friction and Lubrication

Friction describes the force that opposes motion between articulating surfaces. Lubrication between the bearing surfaces of hip implants and its effect on friction generated during articulation is commonly illustrated by a Stribeck diagram, as shown in Fig. 4.1.

The Stribeck curve is traditionally depicted in three phases. When the thickness of the fluid film is less than or equal to

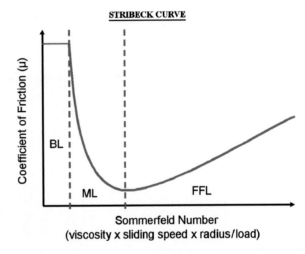

FIG. 4.1. Stribeck curve showing lubrication regimes and their effect on friction.

the average surface roughness of the articulating surfaces, boundary lubrication (BL) is achieved. In this phase, the asperities of the articulating surfaces are in contact at all times. As the thickness of the fluid film increases, the articulating surfaces become separated from each other. There is a transition stage called mixed lubrication (ML), where there is a combination of fluid film and boundary lubrication. As it can be observed in Fig. 4.1, the coefficient of friction continues decreasing until full fluid film lubrication (FFL) is generated, where the articulating surfaces are separated by the lubricant.

Tribology Testing Using Hip Simulators

Tribological testing has been carried out for decades in order to predict the longevity of different designs of hip prostheses. Hip wear simulators have been used extensively by researchers to determine the wear of implants under conditions that are considered to be relatively close to the normal walking cycle. However, *in vitro* hip simulator studies have consistently reported wear rates that are lower than those reported in *in vivo* studies.

Because of the uninterrupted and identical motions per cycle in hip simulators, the joints will be operating in exaggerated lubrication conditions most of the time, which would protect the bearing surfaces. However, *in vivo*, the extensive range of motion (including stop-start motion), high force, and microseparation between the articulating surfaces would break down the fluid film lubrication in metal on metal bearings resulting in the implant operating in less favorable lubrication regimes and consequently generating higher wear than in *in vitro* samples.

Despite the differences between the *in vitro* wear simulator testing conditions and *in vivo* conditions of the metal on metal implants, the morphologic analysis of the components after wear simulation has shown comparable wear morphology/mechanisms to the clinically retrieved metal on metal hip implants, as shown in Fig. 4.2.

There are a number of different hip simulators available in the market, as shown in Fig. 4.3.

One of the most popular hip simulators that is currently used to predict the long-term performance of hip implants is the MTS machine (orbital type or biaxial rocking motion). In this hip joint simulator, the femoral head is mounted at an angle of 23 degrees to the horizontal, resulting in ±23 degrees of flexion/extension and ±23 degrees of abduction/adduction of the implant. The average sliding distance in an orbital-type hip simulator under the above-mentioned conditions has been reported by Wang et al. [1] to be $1.045D$, where D is the diameter of the femoral head. Hence, the sliding distance for a 50-mm femoral head per cycle translates to 52.3 mm. As the tests are normally carried out at 1 Hz, the sliding speed per cycles is going to be 52.3 mm/s. However, the average sliding distance in a natural hip joint on average is $0.67D$, which for a 50-mm femoral head, the average sliding distance per cycle and sliding speed translates to approximately 33.5 mm

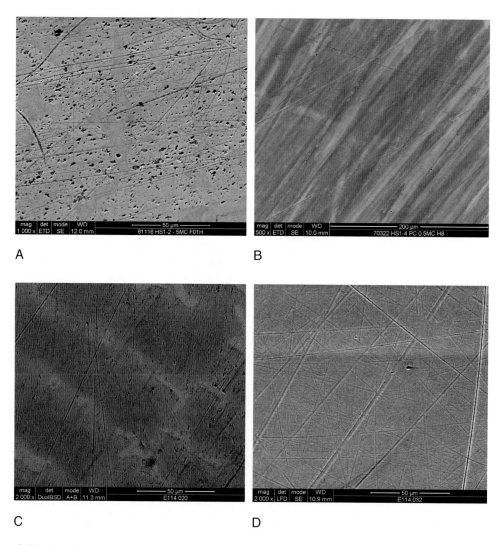

A   B

C   D

FIG. 4.2. Wear morphology/mechanisms of hip simulator tested and retrieved implants. (A) Hip simulator, corrosion wear. (B) Hip simulator, abrasive wear. (C) Retrieved implant, corrosion wear. (D) Retrieved implant, abrasive wear.

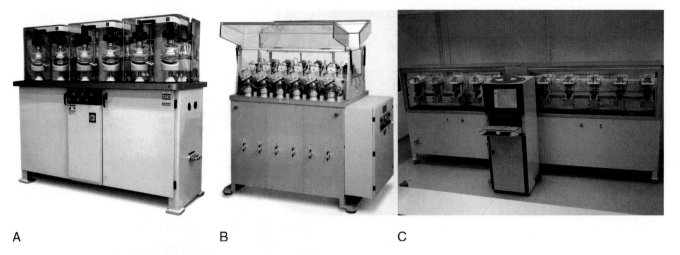

FIG. 4.3. A selection of the hip simulators available on the market: (A) MTS, (B) AMTI, (C) SimSol.

and 33.5 mm/s, respectively. Hence, the orbital-type hip simulator would produce a 56% increase in the sliding distance per cycle in comparison with that generated by the natural hip joint. The significant increase in sliding distance and sliding speed would improve the lubrication and consequently reduce the contact between the articulating surfaces.

A number of researchers have reported no significant difference between the wear generated by various CoCr alloy microstructures in hip joint simulator studies. However, as mentioned previously, the excessive fluid film lubrication generated between the articulating surfaces of metal on metal bearings in hip simulators would reduce the effect of material microstructure on wear of the implants, as the contact between the components is artificially minimized. The effect of material microstructure on wear is clear when the lubricant in the test is not separating the two articulating surfaces. This can be achieved by using pin-on-plate or pin-on-disk machines. These machines are used for material screening purposes, and it has been shown in a number of studies that as-cast high-carbon CoCr alloy microstructure is superior in terms of wear resistance to other CoCr alloy microstructures. In one of the more recent pin-on-disc studies, Kinbrum et al. [2] demonstrated that the microstructure and in particular the carbide volume fraction present in the material is critical to the tribological performance of metal on metal devices. The authors had a series of as-cast (high carbide), single heat treated (medium carbide), and double heat treated (low carbide) CoCr alloy pins and disks. The single and double heat treatments had been carried out in order to reduce the carbide volume fraction in the material. The results are presented in Fig. 4.4.

It can clearly be observed in Fig. 4.4 that the as-cast material has greater wear resistance when compared with single and double heat treated materials.

It should be pointed out that it is not advisable to compare wear results generated at different laboratories and/or hip simulators as factors such as the kinetics, kinematics, synchronization

between the load and motion, the fluid test medium and its degradation with time may differ greatly from one center to another, all of which would affect the wear results. Also, measurement techniques (i.e., gravimetric or volumetric wear measurements) are other factors that may influence the wear results.

It is also important to mention that one of the most significant factors affecting the wear of implants *in vitro* is the correct test setup and component alignment. In a series of hip simulator studies by Dowson et al. [3] and Isaac et al. [4], the researchers showed that low-clearance (83–129 μm) components generate significantly lower wear than do the high-clearance (254–307 μm) components. A series of pictures of the hip simulator stations has been published, showing that within the first 150,000 cycles of the test, the lubricant (newborn calf serum) for the high-clearance joints had gone black due to the high wear of the components. It was also reported that there were no significant changes in the color of the serum used in the stations with low-clearance joints.

Similar hip simulator studies have been carried out at Smith & Nephew's Implant Development Centre (IDC) on 50-mm

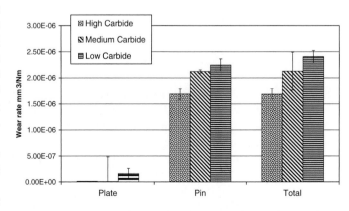

FIG. 4.4. Comparison of the CoCr alloy wear with varying carbide volume fraction.

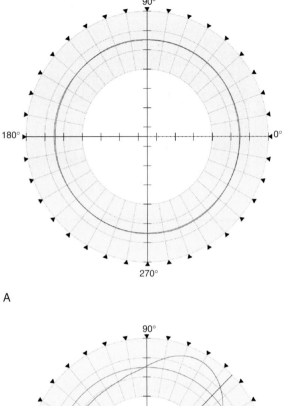

A

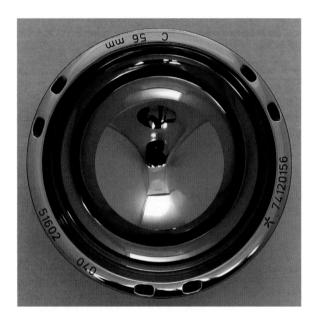

A

et al. [3], the authors stated that "the acetabular components were modified to remove fixation surfaces that would have hindered component location and measurements." Although this practice may have made it easier for the researchers to mount the components in their hip simulators, unfortunately, as any modification to the fixation surfaces, it would have also deformed the cups during the removal of the fixation surfaces. Also, this process could release the residual stresses within the material, which in turn would deform the cups even further. From a manufacturing point of view, this type of material removal should never be carried out without consideration of the final bearing geometry. In order to demonstrate this phe-

B

Fig. 4.5. Equatorial roundness measurements shown (A) before and (B) after the removal of fixation surfaces.

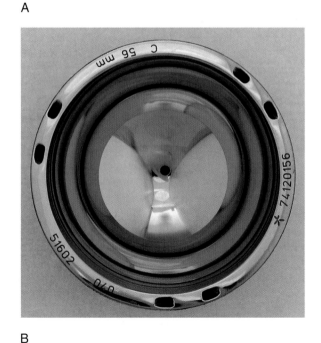

B

Fig 4.6. Photographs of a cup (A) before and (B) after the removal of its fixation surfaces.

Birmingham Hip Resurfacing (BHR) devices with approximately 250-μm clearances without observing any significant discoloration of the fluid lubricant. It should be pointed out that irrespective of the clearance, minor discoloration will occur in lubricant during the early stages of wear tests due to the generation of more wear debris (running-in phase) compared with the latter stages of the test (steady-state phase) and also due to the degradation of the fluid lubricant (newborn calf serum).

Further studies were carried out by the IDC to find out how the researchers managed to get such profound metal staining from the BHR. In close examination of the study by Dowson

nomenon, the IDC repeated this type of maneuver and then carried out a similar hip simulator study. In this study, five 50-mm BHR devices with 240- to 250-μm clearances were tested. The fixation surfaces of three cups were removed, and the other two cups were tested without the removal of their fixation surfaces. A series of roundness measurements was carried out before and after the removal of the fixation surfaces of the cups to determine the amount of cup deformation (Fig. 4.5).

It is clear from the above measurements that the cups are significantly deformed (compressed by approximately 180 μm from their original shapes) due to the fixation removal process. This amount of artificial deformation would have a detrimen-

tal effect on the implant wear. Although cup deformation can clearly be observed using a roundness machine, it is extremely difficult to detect this with the naked eye, as shown in Fig. 4.6.

After the removal of the fixation surfaces, the implants were tested in a ProSim multi-axis hip wear simulator. The simulator was stopped every 10,000 cycles and photographs taken of each station. This procedure was repeated, and pictures of the stations were taken until 150,000 cycles, as shown in Fig. 4.7. The lubricant was then changed at 150,000 cycles, and the test was continued until 300,000 cycles. The machine was stopped every 50,000 cycles for photographs to be taken of each station, as shown in Fig. 4.8.

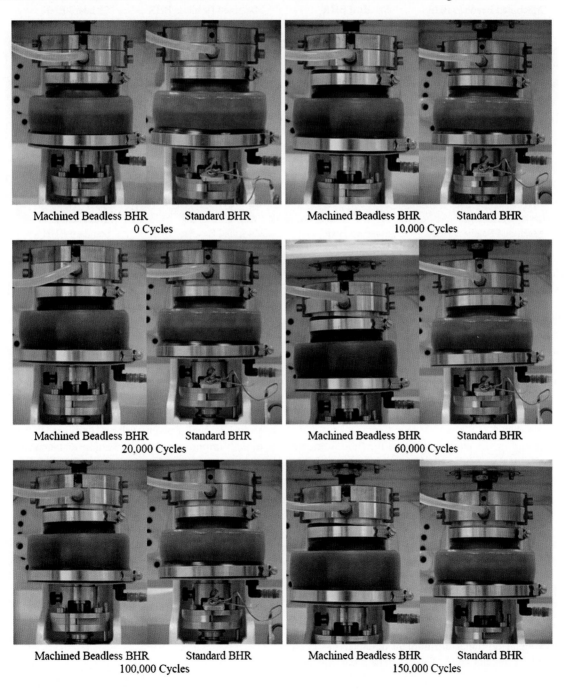

Fig. 4.7. Photographs of representative stations up to 150,000 cycles of wear testing before serum change (left, BHR cup with removed fixation surfaces; right, standard BHR cup).

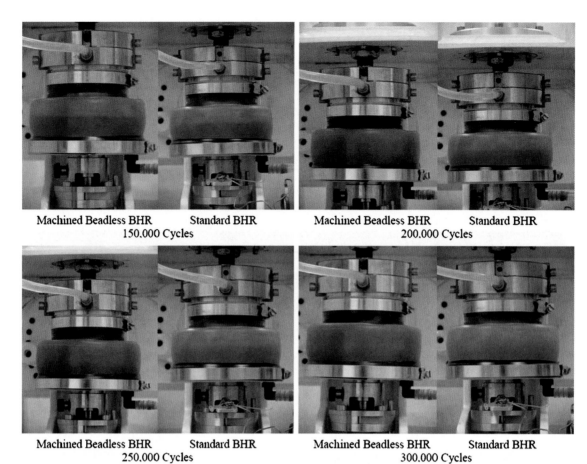

FIG. 4.8. Photographs of representative stations up to 300,000 cycles of wear testing before serum change (left, BHR cup with removed fixation surfaces; right, standard BHR cup).

The color of the serum in the stations with the BHR that had the fixation surfaces removed from the backs of the cups showed similar discolorations to the ones published by Dowson et al. [3] and Isaac et al. [4]. This study has clearly demonstrated the importance of test setup in hip simulator studies and its effect on implant wear. It should be pointed out that test protocols should always consider the final representative features of a product.

It is clear from Fig. 4.8 photographs that the fluid lubricant in the station with the standard BHR device has not visibly changed color during the second 150,000 cycles of the test. However, the station with the BHR with removed fixation surfaces continues to show darkening of the fluid lubricant.

The Effect of Diameter on the Tribology of a Metal on Metal Implant

The effect of metal on metal hip implant diameter has been examined, and the results are as follows. The wear equation states that:

$$V = K \times L \times x,\qquad(4.1)$$

where V is the volume of wear (mm³), K is the wear factor (mm³/N·m), L is load (N), and x is the sliding distance (m) covered during the test. Thus wear increases as any of these parameters increases and vice versa. K, the wear factor, is related to the probability of producing a wear particle, so under different conditions of surface cleanliness or the chemical nature of the surfaces, K will vary and so will the wear rate. However, for a given load and a given surface condition, the wear volume is directly proportional to the sliding distance, which in turn is directly proportional to the radius of the joint. Thus greater wear volumes arise from larger heads. Hence, a large head (e.g., 50 mm diameter) would wear more than a small head (e.g., 38 mm diameter) provided that K and L did not vary.

However, if we use larger head diameters in the presence of a lubricant, then there is an increased chance of fluid-film lubrication and thus a reduced probability of producing a wear particle (as K reduces) because the surfaces do not make contact except occasionally. Thus from a fluid-film lubrication point of view, the smaller head represents the worst-case scenario in terms of wear as K would be largest for the smaller head.

The equation governing the film thickness is as follows:

$$\frac{h_{\min}}{R_X} = 2.798 \left[\frac{\eta u}{E' R_X}\right]^{0.65} \left[\frac{L}{E' R_x^2}\right]^{-0.21}\qquad(4.2)$$

E' and R_x are defined as below:

$$R_x = \frac{R_1 R_2}{R_1 - R_2}. \qquad (4.3)$$

In equation (4.3), R_1 and R_2 is the radius of the cup and the head respectively.

$$\frac{1}{E'} = \frac{1}{2} \left[\frac{1 - \sigma_1^2}{E_1} + \frac{1 - \sigma_2^2}{E_2} \right] \qquad (4.4)$$

In equation (4.4), E_1 and E_2 are the Young's modulus of the cup and the head, respectively, and σ_1 and σ_2 are the Poisson's ratio of the cup and the head, respectively.

It is generally considered that fluid film lubrication occurs when the fluid-film thickness is three times larger than the combined surface roughness of the articulating surfaces. Theoretical calculations using equation (4.5) are used to determine the lubrication regimes generated between the bearing surfaces:

$$\lambda \left(Lambda\ Value \right) = \frac{h_{min}}{Surface\ roughness\ of\ the\ articulating\ surfaces} \qquad (4.5)$$

$1 > \lambda$	Boundary lubrication
$1 < \lambda < 3$	Mixed lubrication
$3 < \lambda$	Fluid film lubrication

However, it is not as simple as this. Surfaces that have the same surface roughness can have peaks and valleys that are very differently distributed. Surfaces with a positive skewness in the distribution of surface asperities are less easy to lubricate with fluid film lubrication as the peaks of the surface roughness can penetrate the fluid film more readily. Surfaces with a negative skewness have more valleys than peaks and are easier to lubricate with fluid film mechanisms. This is explained in more detail in the "Superfinishing" section in Chapter 3.

Another important factor in producing fluid-film lubrication is the clearance between the ball and socket of the resurfacing device. The effects of this can be seen in equation (4.3) where R_x is dependent on the radial clearance, $R_1 - R_2$. If $R_1 - R_2$ is very small, then the fluid film thickness becomes greater and K should reduce. However if the clearance ($R_1 - R_2$) becomes too small, then the risk of the two surfaces "clamping" through cup deformation increases.

Theoretical Calculations

In order to assess what might be happening in the different sizes and clearance of components, calculations have been performed on a range of products.

38-mm-Diameter BHR Head

If we calculate the film thickness using a typical synovial fluid viscosity of 0.01 Pa¢s, an entraining velocity of 0.02 m/s, $E¢ = 2.3 \times 10^{11}$, and relative radius of curvatures based on

implanted clearances of 130 µm and 260 µm, then the range of film thicknesses is from 0.085 µm to 0.05 µm giving λ values of between 2.4 and 1.4 (for a combined surface roughness of 0.035 µm).

Thus, the theoretical predictions are that for a 38-mm femoral head with the smallest specified diametral clearance, the joint will be close to fluid film lubrication ($\lambda = 2.4$ rather than 3 for full fluid film), but at the higher clearance, more asperity contact would be expected as the λ value is calculated at only 1.4.

50-mm-Diameter BHR Head

Again the viscosity was chosen as 0.01 Pa¢s $E¢ = 2.3 \times 10^{11}$, the entraining velocity in this case is 0.026 m/s, and hence for an implanted clearance of 190 µm, the film thickness is 0.115 µm and for an implanted clearance of 320 µm the film thickness is 0.077 µm. Hence the λ values again vary from 3.3 to 2.2 indicating that the joints operate about the fluid level, but with some asperity contact depending on the clearance.

Small-diameter heads (in this case 38 mm) do not produce a sufficiently thick film of lubricant to separate the surfaces. Thus this would be the worst-case scenario for reducing K in the wear equation. However, as we know that some asperities penetrate fluid film and cause metal on metal wear, then for smaller heads, the sliding distance (x) is the shortest, consequently the wear volume will also be small. Thus the small head is the best-case situation for metal on metal direct wear. In the large-diameter heads (in this case 50 mm), the opposite of this would be true. The film thicknesses would be greater, thus reducing K, as x would be greater.

On balance, it would be expected that the wear rates would be similar at all diametral sizes because of these two competing factors (K and x).

Experimental Work

Hip simulator studies have been carried out at Durham University investigating the effects of head sizes on the wear of the implants. BHR 38-mm and 50-mm devices were tested in the Durham hip function wear simulator I for 5 million cycles each. These studies showed no statistically significant differences between the wear rates generated by the 38- and 50-mm BHR devices (1.32 and 1.08 mm³/million cycles, respectively). Bowsher et al. [5] have also demonstrated in a hip simulator study that running-in wear did not correlate with joint diameter.

The experimental results are in agreement with the theoretical calculations. When a larger-diameter (50 mm) joint has been used, the surface will have traveled faster than that of a smaller-diameter (38 mm) joint causing a thicker fluid film to develop. Fluid film lubrication will prevent asperities touching and therefore little wear will be accumulated.

With the smaller-diameter joint (38 mm), a thinner fluid film will be generated, as the surface will move more slowly, however there will be less wear due to the shorter sliding distance of the smaller-diameter head. The above theoretical calculations and the experimental studies have shown that the effect of head sizes in wear of implants is insignificant.

The Effect of Clearance on the Tribology of a Metal on Metal Implant

In vitro friction and hip simulator studies continue to be conducted to determine the optimum clearance for a given bearing diameter. There has been a consistent trend in these studies showing that low clearance in a bearing improves the lubrication between the articulating surfaces and consequently reduces the friction and wear generated between the bearings. However, if we consider friction hip simulator studies, most of them have employed bovine serum (BS) or bovine serum with added carboxy methyl cellulose (CMC) as the lubricant, as this combination is believed to simulate the viscosity of synovial fluid. In real life, as soon as the joint is implanted, the joint is actually bathed in blood and not even synovial fluid. Blood contains macromolecules and cells that measure 5 to 20 μm or more. The effect of these on friction is not fully understood.

Also, none of the previous friction studies have taken cup deformation, which occurs during cup implantation and may also occur during physiologic loading *in vivo*, into consideration. It should be pointed out that intraoperative measurements of the BHR devices have shown up to more than 100 μm of cup deflection immediately after implantation. Cementless cup designs in metal on metal hip resurfacing devices generally depend on a good primary press-fit fixation, which stabilizes the components in the early postoperative period. This allows bony ingrowth or ongrowth to occur, which in turn provides durable long-term fixation. However, press-fitting the cup into the acetabulum generates nonuniform compressive stresses on the cup and consequently causes nonuniform cup deformation. That in turn may result in equatorial contact, high frictional torque, and femoral head seizure. Increased bearing friction in the early weeks and months after implantation can lead to micromotion and has the potential to prevent effective bony ingrowth from occurring. Therefore, friction in the early postoperative period can be critical to the long-term success of joint fixation.

Concerns were raised by McMinn et al. [6] in a clinicoradiologic study of metal on metal bearings with closely controlled 100-μm clearance. A progressive radiolucent line indicated by the arrows in Fig. 4.9 around the acetabular component, seen in some of these cases at follow-up, raises the possibility that increased friction is affecting component fixation. It should

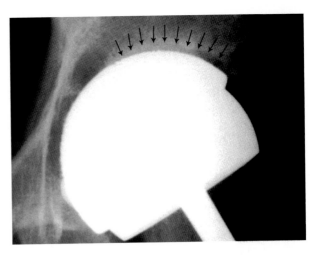

FIG 4.9. A 2-year postoperative radiograph of a patient with a low-clearance BHR, showing a progressive radiolucent line around zones 1 and 2 of the acetabular component (arrows), suggesting increased friction and micromotion resulting in poor fixation.

be pointed out that this phenomenon has not been observed in devices with regular (higher) clearances.

In order to identify the optimum clearance for a given bearing diameter and to understand the above-mentioned phenomenon, a series of friction simulator tests under physiologically relevant conditions was carried out by the author.

Initially, six BHR devices with various diametral clearances (80 to 306 μm) were tested in a hip friction simulator to determine the friction between the bearing surfaces. The components were tested in whole and clotted blood (viscosity 0.0083 and 0.0108 Pa·s, respectively), which are the primary lubricants during the early postoperative period and also in BS + CMC and BS + CMC + hyaluronic acid (HA) with viscosity of 0.01 Pa.s. The results are presented in Fig. 4.10.

When serum-based lubricants are used, it can be observed that as the clearance increases, the friction between the articulating surfaces also increases. A slight increase in friction was noted when HA was added to the serum, as shown in Fig. 4.10, which may have been generated due to the shearing of the HA molecules. Statistical analysis showed that this difference was not significant (p > 0.05).

However, when physiologically relevant lubricants such as whole and clotted blood are used, the friction between the bearings with low clearances (80 and 135 μm) is significantly increased (p < 0.05) in comparison with those generated in serum-based lubricants. It can also be observed that as the clearance is increased, the friction is reduced, following the opposite trend to that of the serum-based lubricants.

The components were then deflected by 25 to 35 μm using a two-points pinching action and tested in clotted blood, which is the primary lubricant during the early postoperative period. The results for this test are presented in Fig. 4.11.

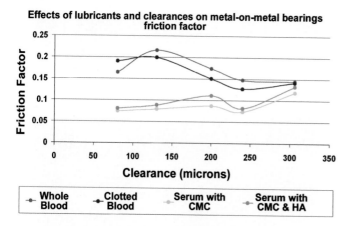

FIG. 4.10. Effect of clearance and lubricant on friction factor.

The results presented in Fig. 4.11 show that for the reduced-clearance components, friction was significantly increased ($p < 0.05$) when the cups were deflected by only 30 μm. However, for the components with higher clearances, the friction did not change before and after deflection. It is postulated that the larger clearances can accommodate the amount of distortion introduced to the cups in this study.

It has been reported that reduced clearance results in reduced friction. However, factors such as cellular and macromolecular shear and cup deflection that can affect friction in these bearings *in vivo* have not been specifically investigated *in vitro* before. Progressive radiolucent lines that appeared in a few patients with low-clearance bearings alerted us to the need to study this issue of increased friction in these bearings.

The results of this study suggest that reduced clearance bearings have the potential to generate high friction especially in the early weeks after implantation when cup deflection has occurred due to press-fitting of the cup into the acetabulum and the presence of whole and clotted blood as lubricant. Friction factors in higher clearance bearings

are much reduced in comparison. The increase in friction results in increased frictional torque at the implant-bone interface, which could in turn cause cup loosening and increased wear.

The Effect of Cup Orientation on the Tribology of a Metal on Metal Implant

There is increasing evidence from retrieval studies that cup positioning, particularly inclination angle, has a significant impact on the wear of metal on metal bearings [7,8]. The effect is identified by *edge wear* on the peripheral edge of the cup component. Also, correct orientation of the implant is essential for maximizing its range of motion as well as preventing impingement and dislocation [9,10].

A hip simulator study was carried out by the IDC to compare the effect of cup orientation on the wear performance of BHR devices.

The wear test was performed in a 10 station ProSim hip joint simulator. A series of 50 mm BHR devices was tested in this study. The bearings were divided into three groups (n = 3/group) with various cup orientations and one control sample. Thereby, the distance between the wear patch of the bearings and the superior edge of the cup was different for each group. This would then allow investigation of changes to the contact and lubrication between the articulating surfaces and consequently wear of the implants. All the implants were mounted in an anatomical position. The cup orientations are as follows (Fig. 4.12):

Group A: The edge of the wear patch at maximum flexion is 19 degrees away from the edge of the cup (n = 3).
Group B: The edge of the wear patch at maximum flexion is 8 degrees away from the edge of the cup (n = 3).
Group C: The edge of the wear patch at maximum flexion is 5 degrees away from the edge of the cup (n = 3).

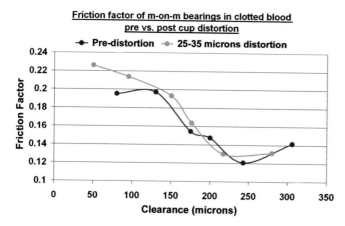

FIG. 4.11. Effect of cup deflection on friction in clotted blood.

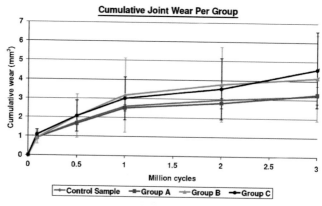

FIG. 4.12. Average cumulative wear volume loss of BHR bearings with varying cup orientations and slow walking speeds.

Control sample: The edge of the wear patch at maximum flexion is 38 degrees away from the edge of the cup (n = 1).

The lubricant in this study was newborn calf serum with 0.2% sodium azide concentration, which was diluted with de-ionized water to achieve average protein concentration of 20 g/L. The flexion/extension and internal/external rotation of the implants were +30 degrees/−15 degrees and ±10 degrees, respectively. Paul-type stance phase loading with a maximum load of 3000 N and a standard International Standards Organization (ISO) swing phase load of 300 N were applied to the implants. The frequency was 1 Hz.

The average cumulative wear volumes for the three BHR groups at various orientations plus a control sample are presented in Fig. 4.12.

As it can be observed, the devices showed the typical characteristics of wear for metal on metal joints, with a high wear rate during the initial running in period (0 to 1 Mc) followed by a lower steady-state wear rate between 1 and 3 Mc.

At 2 million cycles, one implant in group C (implant no. 9) exhibited extremely high wear. This was caused by neck (head holder) impingement, resulting in head articulation against the edge of the cup. It is interesting to note that edge articulation caused a 60-fold increase in wear generated between 2 and 3 Mc (8.74 mm³) in comparison with that generated between 1 and 2 Mc (0.15 mm³) for implant no. 9, as shown in Fig. 4.13. The wear result of implant no. 9 was excluded from this study after 2 million cycles of testing.

The joints showed no significant difference between the groups during their running-in period, nor was there any significant difference during the steady-state period of the test between the groups (p > 0.05). Hence, when articulation occurred within the bearing surfaces of the implants, no significant differences in wear rates were observed between the groups implanted at various alignments.

The surface measurements in this study showed an increase in average surface roughness of the heads and cups combined

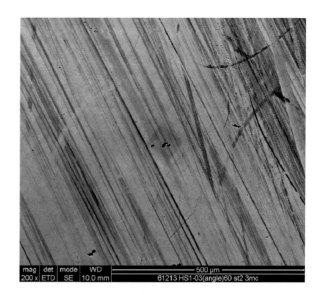

FIG 4.14. SEM image of typical abrasive wear characteristics on the articulating surfaces.

with the significant reduction in the average skewness of the test samples, clearly indicating the diminishing of peaks and increasing valleys on the surface of both cups and heads during the initial 90,000 cycles of the test (approximately 1 month *in vivo*). This is due to the abrasive wear mechanism that occurs between the articulating surfaces, as shown in Fig. 4.14.

In conclusion, no significant differences were observed between the wear rates of the groups when articulation occurred within the bearing surfaces of the implants. However, a significant increase in wear rate was measured in one of the joints when articulation occurred on the edge of the cup. These findings suggest that the wear rate will not be affected by cup orientation as long as the articulation occurs within the bearing surfaces of the implant. However, edge loading/articulation will increase the wear of the implant significantly, which in turn may result in osteolysis and/or aseptic loosening of metal-on-metal bearings.

Summary

Tribological testing using hip wear and friction simulators continues to be carried out in order to investigate the performance and to predict the longevity of different designs of hip prosthesis. Despite their limitations, these machines are efficient tools for basic research and are essential in improving our understanding of the wear, friction, and lubrication generated by the metal on metal bearings. However, it should be pointed out that, in order to generate meaningful data, it is crucial that the test setup in hip simulator studies is correct and that the final representative features of the products have been considered in the test protocol.

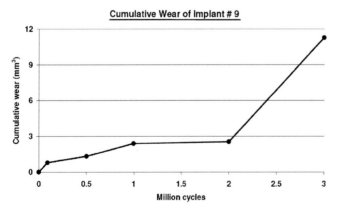

FIG 4.13. Cumulative wear volume loss of implant no. 9 in group C.

Acknowledgments. The author would like to thank Dr. A. Hussain and Mr. J.T. Daniel for their assistance with the experimental studies.

References

1. Wang A., Sun D.C., Yau S.S, Edwards B., Sokol M., Essner A., Polineni V.K., Stark C., Dumbleton J.H. (1999). Orientation softening in the deformation and wear of ultra-high molecular weight polyethylene. Wear 203–204, 230–241.
2. Kinbrum A., Unsworth T., Kamali A. The wear of high carbon metal-on-metal bearings after different heat treatments. 54th Annual Meeting of the Orthopaedic Research Society. Transactions Vol. 33, San Francisco, CA, 2008.
3. Dowson D., Hardaker C., Flett M., Isaac G. (2004). A hip joint simulator study of the performance of metal-on-metal joints, Part II: Design. J Arthroplasty 19(Suppl. 3), 124–130.
4. Isaac G., Hardaker C., Hadley M., Dowson D., Williams S., Fisher J. Effect of clearance on wear and metal ion levels in large diameter metal-on-metal bearings in a hip joint simulator. 53rd Annual Meeting of the Orthopaedic Research Society. Transactions Vol.32, San Diego, CA, 2007.
5. Bowsher J.G., Hussain A., Nevelos J.E., Shelton J.C. The importance of head diameter on minimising metal on metal hip wear. 50th Annual Meeting of the Orthopaedic Research Society. Transactions Vol. 29, San Francisco, CA, 2004.
6. McMinn D. and Daniel J. (2006). History and modern concepts in surface replacement. Proc IMechE Part H: J. Eng Med. Special Issue Paper, 220, 239–251.
7. Brodner W., Gruble A., Jankovsky R., Meisinger V., Lehr S., Gottsauner- Wolf F. (2004). Cup inclination and serum concentration of cobalt and chromium after metal-on-metal total hip arthroplasty. J Arthroplasty 19, 66–70.
8. Campbell P., DeHann R., DeSmet K. (2006). Implant retrieval analysis of hybrid metal-on-metal surface arthroplasty. 52nd Annual Meeting of the Orthopaedic Research Society. Transactions Vol. 31, Chicago, IL, 2006.
9. D'Lima D.D., Urquhart A.G., Buehler K.O., Walker R.H., Colwell C.W., Jr. (2000). The effect of the orientation of the acetabular and femoral components on the range of motion of the hip at different head-neck ratios. J Bone Joint Surg Am. 82 (3), 315–321.
10. Kummer F.J., Shah S., Lyer S., DiCesare P.E. (1999). The effect of acetabular cup orientations on limiting hip orientation. J Arthroplasty 14, 509–513.

5

Corrosion and Its Contribution to Metal Release

Joseph Daniel and Amir Kamali

Generation of wear particles and metal ions are the main concerns associated with metal on metal bearings. The following section provides the reader with an understanding of how wear debris and the wear process contribute to generation of metal ions.

The conversion of metal into soluble metal ions always occurs through a process of oxidative degradation. When a metal is placed in a wet, aerated environment, it will oxidize unless it is a noble metal such as gold. It may corrode by dissolving into the environment releasing metal ions, which can be represented by a simple empiric equation:

$$M \rightarrow M^{n+} + ne^-,$$

where n is the valency of the metal.

Alternatively, it may *passivate* by forming a protective metallic-oxide (MO) film on the surface of the metal preventing further corrosion. These *passive* films are typically a few nanometers thick (a few atomic layers):

$$M + H_2O \rightarrow MO + 2H^+ + 2e\cdot$$

Both corrosion and passivation reactions are described as *anodic* reactions. They produce free electrons that must be consumed in *cathodic* (reduction) reactions in an adjacent portion of the metal involving the reduction of water and reduction of oxygen. The rate of electron production (anodic processes) must be equal to their rate of consumption (cathodic). The internal environment in the body including the pH, the abundance of free chlorides, peroxides, and proteins in the tissues, and the dissolved oxygen favor oxidation (corrosion). With reference to the CoCr alloy surfaces and particulate debris in the body, chromium leads to the formation of a protective Cr-rich passive oxide around a metallic implant, which ensures a low general corrosion rate. The function of molybdenum is to promote resistance to localized corrosion.

Localized Corrosion

In a metal cavity or pit, oxygen is quickly used up, so the cavity acts as an anode and the external surface as a cathode (Fig. 5.1). Metal dissolves in the pit forming metal ions. Chloride ions are drawn in for charge balance. Hydrolysis leads to acidification and formation of concentrated acidic metal chloride solution, which tends to favor further dissolution and prevents repassivation. Different types of localized corrosion are of clinical relevance.

Inside the cavity, if metal ions are produced at a rate faster than they can escape, the aggressive environment is maintained and corrosion continues resulting in *pit growth*. If ions escape at a rate faster than they are produced, the solution dilutes until repassivation is possible resulting in *pit death*.

Crevice corrosion works through a similar mechanism. A tight crevice makes escape of ions difficult and an aggressive solution develops easily in a small volume.

Two dissimilar metals in direct contact with each other and bathed in an electrolyte solution allow the flow of electrons from the more reactive (base) metal to the more noble metal, resulting in a corrosive attack on the base metal (anode) through a process called *galvanic corrosion*. This phenomenon can occur in situations such as a stainless steel stem being used with either a titanium alloy femoral head or a cobalt alloy head.

Mechanically Enhanced Corrosion

Fretting corrosion (e.g., modular junctions, cement-stem interface) is also called mechanically enhanced crevice corrosion. The enclosed space maintains an aggressive environment, and the micromotion breaks down any attempted passivation resulting in bursts of dissolution. Given the fact that patients are walking around, most apparent crevice corrosion will really have some mechanical enhancement.

Tribocorrosion is the most relevant mechanism working in a metal on metal bearing situation. Macroscopic movement between articulating surfaces breaks down the passive film in places through wear, resulting in a burst of dissolution. Constant movement of fluid prevents the build-up of a chemically aggressive environment and allows repassivation. Continuing bearing movement breaks down the passive film again, and the cycle continues repeatedly making dissolution and release

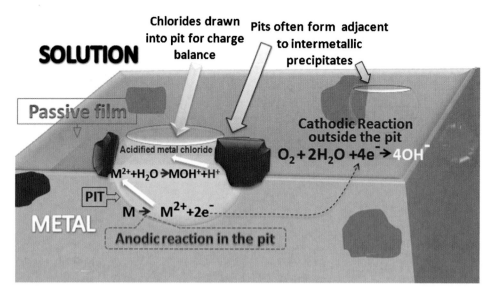

FIG. 5.1. Pitting corrosion.

of metal ions a function of both the corrosion resistance as well as the wear resistance of the material.

Finally, wear particles released at the time of wear can also corrode. However, wear particles also produce passive films and therefore undergo a very slow rate of dissolution, although by virtue of their large surface area, collective dissolution from the particles may be high. It is also known that particles are phagocytosed by macrophages and other leukocytes and that the intracellular environment can further promote corrosion. The interaction between cells and these particles continues to be a subject of investigation.

Role of Metallurgy in Corrosion

Any change in the homogeneity of the protective elements (Cr, Mo) can in principle lead to change in corrosion susceptibility. Chromium and molybdenum are preferentially drawn into the carbide residues from the surrounding matrix during the solidification process of their manufacture as seen earlier (Chapter 2) leading to a relative depletion of these elements in the zone immediately surrounding the residues. This can affect passive corrosion susceptibility. However, these carbide residues protect against wear and therefore potentially reduce the overall tribocorrosion effect.

Clinical Relevance of Corrosion

Several studies have shown the presence of corrosion products such as chromium-rich precipitates in modular junction tapers, synovial fluid, capsular tissue, and in disseminated sites [1]. Furthermore, demonstration of elevated metal ion levels in the blood and urine of patients with artificial hips in the early weeks and months and their persistence in later years suggests that this electrochemical degradation is an ongoing process. These metal ions are effectively cleared by the renal excretory system, and a dynamic balance is reached with time between metal released from the device and that excreted in urine, allowing a steady state of blood levels to be maintained in the long-term, as will be seen in Chapter 13. In particular, cobalt has been found to have a short half-life of around 24 hours. Daily output of cobalt in urine thus provides a good noninvasive measure of the combined *in vivo* processes of bearing wear and corrosion, and is useful as an excellent surrogate measure of overall bearing performance *in vivo*.

References

1. Jacobs JJ, Gilbert JL, Urban RM. Corrosion of metal orthopaedic implants [review]. J Bone Joint Surg Am 1998;80:268–282.

6
Retrieval Analysis

Tim J. Band, Roger W.F. Ashton, and Amir Kamali

Retrievals

Although the evolution, design, and development of the Birmingham Hip Resurfacing (BHR) have been described in detail in Chapters 1 and 2, it is important to comment on the performance of the device after implantation. The clinical success and results of the BHR are also described in detail in this book and reflect the mid-term to long-term survival rate of the prosthesis. At the time of writing, the BHR device has an Orthopaedic Data Evaluation Panel (ODEP) rating of 7A indicating that there is a minimum of 7-year follow-up data, which satisfies the highest requirements for follow-up, including Kaplan-Meier survival. ODEP provides an independent assessment of clinical outcomes data on the compliance of devices with National Institute of Clinical Excellence (NICE) benchmarks for the effectiveness of primary total hip prostheses, which includes hip resurfacing.

Of course, those devices that are implanted and continue to provide an excellent outcome for the patient cannot be accessed for examination, and they continue to increase the time *in vivo* for effective clinical follow-up. When the unfortunate event of revision surgery occurs, for whatever reason, it provides an opportunity for the devices to be examined to determine how they have been performing, which can often assist in identifying possible causes of the revision. The examination of retrieved devices includes visual inspection, measurement of size and profiles, and a review of the x-rays of the devices *in situ* to determine if the implant position was a contributor to any alteration to the design performance of the bearing. The BHR device enjoys a high survival rate, which means that the number of revised prostheses that become available for examination is small. Manufacturers of the BHR have always made efforts to ensure that BHR devices that have been revised are examined. Just in the way that the first-generation devices were examined forensically, examination of the BHR explants provides valuable information about the performance of the bearing.

Before we describe what has been observed during the examination of the BHR and other explants, it is necessary to comment that at the time of writing, the predominant cause of revision surgery for the BHR device is for femoral neck fracture, which represents more than half of all the revisions. The mode of failure for femoral neck fracture is multifactorial including varus positioned femoral devices, notched lateral neck cortex, poor bone quality, and/or a combination of these. As described by Kishida et al. [1], in their Dual Energy X-Ray Absoriometry (DEXA) bone scan test study, there is a significant increase in bone mineral density in the femoral neck from around 6 months after the primary operation, which appears to offer increased protection from femoral neck fracture. When explants are examined from this early implanted period, there is very little information that can be ascertained as the articulation has generally had limited activity while the patient is convalescing after surgery. Of more interest for bearing performance monitoring are the explants available from longer periods of *in vivo* experience as these provide an indication of how the bearing works under physiologic conditions.

The difficulty of determining the activity that has been experienced by the bearing lies in estimating the number of cycles that may have occurred over time. For many years, prior to the introduction of metal on metal hip resurfacing, the estimate of the number of cycles that a hip articulates each year was based on work by Dowson et al. [2] who estimated the hip to articulate approximately 1 million cycles per year. This allowed the total wear measured on an explant bearing to be divided by the number of years implanted to express the total wear as an annual wear rate (i.e.. micrometers or millimeters per year). It is speculated that the patient group used for this early study were hosts of traditional total hip prostheses and of a lower activity level than the younger, more active patients who are candidates for metal on metal hip resurfacing devices at time of writing. More recent studies by Schmalzried et al. [3] and Daniel et al. [4] have higher numbers of articulations per year, which are closer to 2 million or 2.5 million cycles per year.

The examination of BHR explants has confirmed that the general appearance of the bearing, which has a high lustre polished surface finish, after its *in vivo* experience is not dulled, which is as observed on the first-generation metal on metal devices over a longer period of time. With the exception of scratches as a result of removing the devices, the bearings have no visible evidence of abrasive wear. When higher-magnification inspection is carried out, it has been observed that the bearing surfaces have scratches between 2 and 3 μm wide in the intercarbide spacings of the matrix material, again resembling the evidence observed on the first-generation metal on metal devices. These confirmed the wear process as one of an abrasive mechanism as previously discussed.

The measurement of BHR explants when plotted as time *in vivo* (time between primary surgery and revision) and the linear wear rate in micrometers (total measured wear divided by number of years *in vivo*) shows that there is small spread in the results, probably due to variable activity in patients, and so forth, with a line of best fit showing annual wear rates of 2 to 3 μm per year (Fig. 6.1). This linear wear rate is comparable with those measured on the first-generation metal on metal devices examined, even though they had enjoyed a significantly longer period *in vivo*, which reduces the effect of any "run-in" wear over time. Another observation of these wear measurements is that there are a number of devices with higher wear rates than those of the general population, which, upon more detailed analysis, have evidence of atypical wear patterns (e.g., the devices plotted at 8.1 million and 11.7 million cycles in Fig. 6.1). These devices with atypical wear patterns and an explanation for their higher wear rates were not excluded from the data set that has been used to calculate the average linear wear rate and line of best fit for the BHR. The atypical wear patterns include evidence that the femoral head device had articulated at, or on, the edge of the acetabular cup component due to an incorrect positioning of the two articulating surfaces in relation to one another. The malpositioned component was observed to be the acetabular cup and involved both the inclination and version angles of the device after implantation. This results in increased wear of the bearing and is described in more detail later in this section. Evidenced by the examination of these BHR explants, the bearing is performing in good parity with, and better than, the first-generation metal on metal bearings, which had enjoyed a

benign long-term experience, upon which the BHR specification was developed. The only instances when wear has been identified at higher levels than this is when there have been confounding factors, such as implant position, which have led to an atypical wear process.

Having discussed the analysis of the BHR retrievals, it is important to introduce other factors that can lead to high wear in a metal on metal bearing produced in CoCr alloy. The McMinn metal on metal hip resurfacing devices that were revised for metallosis-induced osteolysis, produced in 1996, have already been discussed, and it was observed in those cases that a reduction in the carbide phase, due to thermal processing, had adversely affected the wear performance. It was also observed on the device pair with the lowest carbide phase that the wear process appeared to be of an adhesive mechanism, which was evidenced by it having the highest wear and wear patches without evidence of abrasive wear scratches. The burden of increased wear debris from these devices as a consequence of higher wear reacted with periprosthetic tissue resulting in metallosis and osteolysis. In contrast with some laboratory studies, the examination of metal on metal bearings that have been obtained through revision surgery, and therefore experienced physiologic forces and motions, the microstructure, and specifically carbide phase proportion, have been contributors to high wear. The following sections in this chapter will discuss other design features and implant orientation and their contribution to reduced bearing performance using case studies as illustrations.

To complement the physical examination of explanted devices, it is useful to have access to other details about the device. This is of particular importance if one is to determine if the device has contributed to the cause of revision. Full information describing the *in vivo* conditions is not often available, so the process is usually one of forensics. In cases where the failure is, for example, early neck fracture, then wear values are so small that they can be difficult to resolve from the original manufactured shape. However, other observations can be made including the verification of microstructure, changes to the surface texture, and so forth,

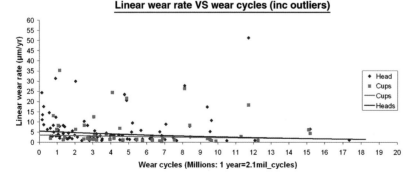

FIG. 6.1. Linear wear rate of BHR versus number of cycles using an estimate of 2.1 million cycles per year *in vivo*

which are of broader scientific interest in the context of the explant population as a whole but sometimes cannot provide the conclusion for a specific revision case.

Methodology

Indication of Wear Levels

As the original mass of the implanted device is not available, wear assessments can only be made by scanning the bearing profile and comparing this to the original manufactured shape. The method is that described for the assessment of geometric form during the manufacturing process, using roundness machines, profilometers, and, when wear is large enough, three-dimensional coordinate measuring machines.

For a good assessment, it is essential that an unworn portion of the bearing surface can be identified. This is usually possible, but in some cases when wear is generalized over the entire surface, wear measurement may be inconclusive. With these cases, and with the benefit of experience in this field, it is possible make a judgment as to the position and direction of largest wear and hence gain an indication of device positioning.

Microscopy

Determination of contact area: Through stereomicroscopy, it is usually possible to determine the areas on the bearing surface that have been in contact. Outside this area, the original polished texture is sometimes visible. On the boundaries, some deposits may be seen, and then in the contact areas, the texture can give an indication of the dominant wear mechanism. Once the contact area has been determined, further localized scanning electron microscopy (SEM) can be used to confirm the wear mechanism or to identify the composition of any foreign material in the bearing.

Microstructure: As the worn bearing surfaces are usually still in a highly polished condition, it may be possible to view the microstructure without sectioning and repolishing. However, staining or etching is required in order to make an assessment of phase proportion.

Device Positioning

Where x-rays are available, it is possible to make an approximate radiographic assessment of device position and hence determine whether this has contributed to the wear on the device. For the acetabular side, this provides information on approximate inclination and version angles. (Note that retroversion and anteversion cannot truly be distinguished by this method.) The values ascertained are *radiographic* and must not be confused with *anatomic* or *operative* definitions.

To illustrate the application of the above methods, the following is a series of case studies from this explant population focusing on the engineering bearing performance.

Case 1: Corin McMinn Device Implanted 1996; Explanted at 5 Years 1 Month

On visual inspection, the femoral head component still had tissue on its inner surface with evidence of metallosis (dark staining) (Figs. 6.2 and 6.3). Fine scratches were observed generally over the bearing surface particularly on the "wear" zones. The stem was removed to permit examination using the scanning electron microscope.

Further optical and SEM examinations revealed a monophasic structure on the head (Fig. 6.4), and the cup microstructure consisted of particulate agglomerated carbides plus lamellae carbides at the grain boundaries (Fig. 6.5).

Both components were considered to have a low carbide phase proportion. For the cup, this was estimated to be in the region of 2%, whereas for the head there was generally an absence of carbides apart from in areas where the casting runners would have been. Chemical analysis showed the material to be high-carbon alloy (C > 0.22%).

Linear wear on both head and cup were found to be $53.5\,\mu m$ and $5.5\,\mu m$, respectively, giving a wear rate of $10.5\,\mu m$ per annum for the head and $1.1\,\mu m$ per annum for the cup. For the cup, the rate was comparable with that of a well-positioned BHR; however, the rate for the head was an order of magnitude higher than would be expected.

From Fig. 6.6 it was seen that wear on the head extended at maximum over an angle of 100 degrees centered at approximately 25 degrees from the pole. Although the values were high, the conformation of the wear patch was unsurprising. For the cup (Fig. 6.7), wear was fully contained within the bearing surface and there was no evidence of wear through contact with the edge of the cup.

This was confirmed by the equatorial trace of the cup (Fig. 6.8), which showed minimal out-of-roundness indicating that the wear area did not extend onto the cup periphery.

Diametral clearances were determined by the methods outlined in Chapter 3. These were as follows. Diametral clear-

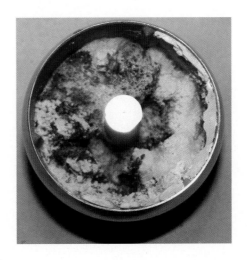

FIG. 6.2.

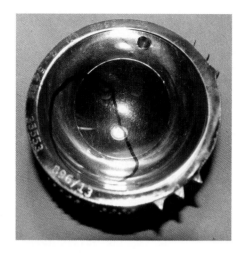

Fig. 6.3.

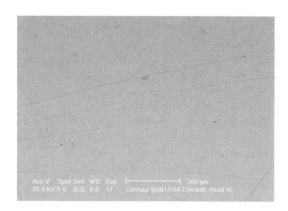

Fig. 6.4.

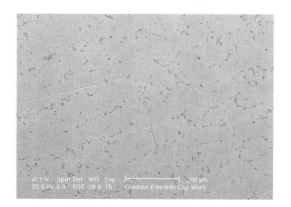

Fig. 6.5.

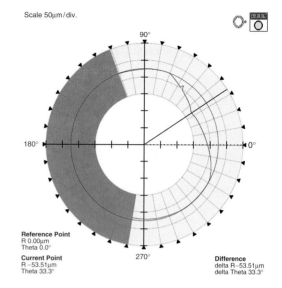

Fig. 6.6.

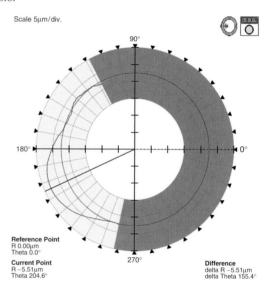

Fig. 6.7.

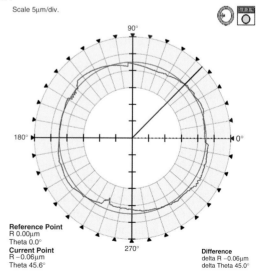

Fig. 6.8.

ance in the noncontact (nonworn) areas was 382 μm. Effective diametral clearance in the contact zone was 87 μm.

Assessment of the anteroposterior (AP) radiograph revealed a cup inclination angle of 45 degrees (radiographic inclination). This would be considered "normal" relative to guideline values.

This device was revised due to osteolysis at 5 years 1 month.

Case 2: S&N Device (BHR); Explanted at 5 Years 10 Months

On visual inspection, the femoral head component still had the resected femoral head remnant on its inner surface (Figs. 6.9 and 6.10). Very fine scratches were observed generally over the bearing surface particularly on the wear zones.

Optical examinations revealed the biphasic structure on both the head and cup, with both components having >5% carbide phase proportion. The chemical analysis confirmed the material to be high carbon alloy (C >0.25%).

Linear wear on both head (Fig. 6.11) and cup (Fig. 6.12) were found to be 5.6 μm and 5.85 μm, respectively, giving a wear rate of 0.96 μm per annum for the head and 1.0 μm per annum for the cup. Both head and cup were wearing at a comparable rate and in line with expectations.

From Fig. 6.11, it is seen that wear on the head extended at maximum over an angle of 60 degrees centered at approximately 35 degrees from the pole. The confirmation of the wear patch was unsurprising. For the cup (Fig. 6.12), wear was fully contained within the bearing surface and there was no evidence of wear through contact with the edge of the cup. This was confirmed by the equatorial trace of the cup (Fig. 6.13), which showed minimal out-of-roundness due to the wear area extending through the equatorial trace.

Diametral clearances were determined by the methods outlined in Chapter 3. These were as follows. Diametral clearance in the noncontact (nonworn) areas was 273 μm. Effective diametral clearance in the contact zone was 270 μm.

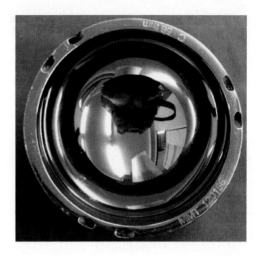

FIG. 6.10.

CAD Assessment of the AP radiograph (Fig. 6.14) revealed a cup inclination angle of 31 degrees (radiographic inclination) and 12 degrees of version (radiographic). The inclination would be considered "low" relative to current guideline values of 40 degrees to 45 degrees.

This device was revised due to pain and suspected cup loosening at 5 years 10 months. This relatively early failure could be attributed to lack of cup stability, although there is no evidence of movement in the wear zones arising from a change in contact position. The linear wear levels are low and, in contrast with the previous case, approximately equal in both head and cup.

It is known that wear rate of metal on metal joints on hip simulators slows down with increasing numbers of cycles. One reason thought to be responsible for this slowdown is that effective clearance in the contact zone reaches a point where fluid film lubrication is sustained, at least in the simulator

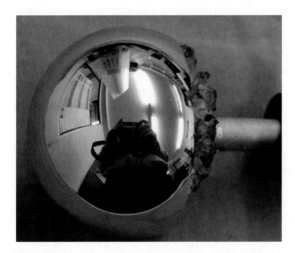

FIG. 6.9.

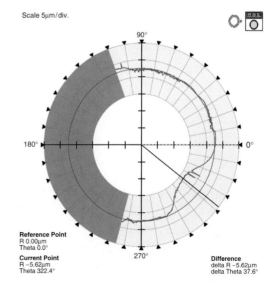

Scale 5μm/div.

90°

180° ——————+—+—+——+—+—+—————— 0°

270°

Reference Point
R 0.00μm
Theta 0.0°

Current Point
R −5.62μm
Theta 322.4°

Difference
delta R −5.62μm
delta Theta 37.6°

FIG. 6.11.

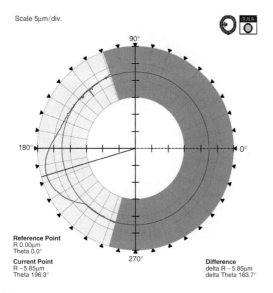

Scale 5µm/div.

Reference Point
R 0.00µm
Theta 0.0°

Current Point
R −5.85µm
Theta 196.3°

Difference
delta R −5.85µm
delta Theta 163.7°

FIG. 6.12.

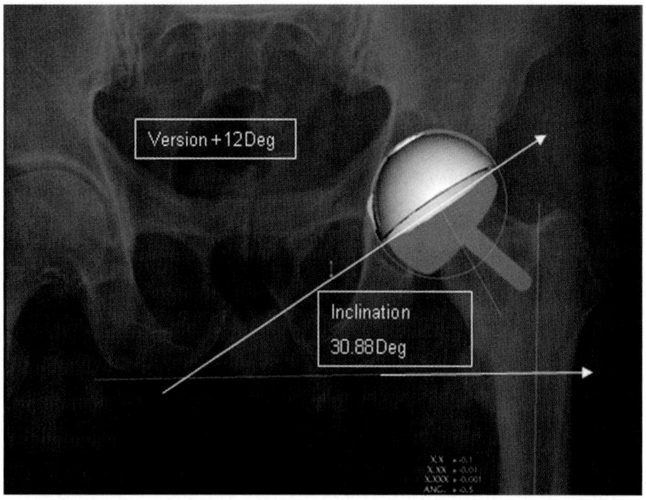

FIG. 6.14.

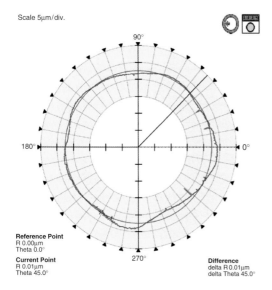

Scale 5µm/div.

Reference Point
R 0.00µm
Theta 0.0°

Current Point
R 0.01µm
Theta 45.0°

Difference
delta R 0.01µm
delta Theta 45.0°

FIG. 6.13.

environment. When this period is reached in the simulator, the wear falls to extremely low steady-state wear rate values. When metal on metal joints of differing clearances are tested on hip simulators, the run-in wear rate of the higher clearance joints is greater than that of lower clearance joints. However, the steady-state wear rates of both high- and low-clearance metal on metal joints are similar. Cases 1 and 2 are interesting examples of *in vivo* wear performance of two different resurfacing systems. In the BHR, the effective clearance at implantation started relatively high (273 µm) and after more than 5 years of use, the effective clearance in the contact zone ended relatively high (270 µm). In the Corin resurfacing (case 1), the effective clearance at implantation started rather higher (382 µm) than the BHR, but after more than 5 years of

use, the effective clearance in the contact zone was relatively low (87 µm). As can be seen in previous chapters, it has been shown that wear as assessed on hip simulators is no different with double heat treated metal on metal devices (an example is Corin) compared with wear of as-cast, metal on metal devices (an example is BHR). Why have these two devices behaved so differently in the examples shown, in clinical use?

Neither of these devices had any suggestion of edge loading due to suboptimal implantation angles.

It could be argued that starting clearance could be the important difference. However, in view of what is known from hip simulator experiments, starting clearance is known to only affect run-in wear. If clearance was the only defining difference between these two joints, we would have expected slightly higher run-in wear in the Corin device, to the point where the effective clearances in the contact zones were equal in the two devices. After that point, we would have expected the steady-state wear to be similar in the two devices, assuming a broadly similar activity profile in the two patients. What has happened, however, is that the wear has continued in the Corin device, beyond the stage when its effective clearance was identical to the BHR, and at the time of revision the Corin device had a much lower effective clearance than the starting value, and much lower than the BHR.

It could be argued that perhaps the patient who had the Corin device had a much higher activity level responsible for his high-wearing resurfacing. Interestingly, this patient had his contralateral hip treated 1 year before with a Corin device, and this hip has remained clinically and radiographically perfect 12 years postoperatively. Why should the patient's high activity level result in very high wear with osteolysis and failure of one hip yet the contralateral side remain clinically and radiographically perfect? It may be further argued that the wear in the patient with the BHR (case 2) was unusually low because of a low activity level. However, the wear rates of this implant are broadly in line with the wear rates of many other BHR explants.

If activity level was the problem in case 1 with harsh conditions in the contact zone resulting, why is the wear rate on one side of the articulation (head) 10 times higher than the cup side of the articulation. As has already been pointed out, the material characteristics are different in this patient's head and cup. The carbide phase proportion is higher in the cup compared with the head, where the numbers of carbides present in the matrix metal are very low. This is the case despite both implants having the same heat treatment regime (double heat treatment; see Chapter 2).

We draw some general conclusions from these two illustrative cases, which fit into the broader picture painted by our experience:

1. The wear of heat-treated components of metal on metal devices *in vivo* is much higher than expected from hip simulator studies.
2. The clinical conditions that these metal on metal bearings are subjected to *in vivo* are harsher from a lubrication standpoint than conditions encountered in hip simulators.
3. The microstructure of metal on metal bearings is profoundly altered by heat treatment regimes.
4. There is great variability in the amount of microstructural damage caused by apparently similar heat-treatment regimes.
5. The wear rates of heat-treated components is component specific and is inversely proportional to the carbide phase proportion in the individual component.
6. High wear rates of metal on metal bearings can lead to metallosis, osteolysis. and clinical failure.

Case 3: DePuy ASR Device; Reported as Explanted at Approximately 2 Years

On visual inspection, the femoral head component still had the resected femoral head remnant on its inner surface with evidence of metallosis (dark staining) (Figs. 6.15 and 6.16).

Both head and cup showed evidence of fine scratches on the wear zone indicative of abrasive wear (Figs. 6.17 and 6.18). Unworn areas of both components showed the original "as-manufactured" surface, with both head and cup showing signs of relief polishing. Examinations of the edge of the bearing surface of the cup showed signs of considerable wear, as part of the manufactured edge radius blend to the introducer feature around the internal periphery of the cup had been worn away.

The head exhibited an as-cast microstructure with a phase proportion greater than 5% (Fig. 6.19), and structure of the cup indicated that it had been through a number of thermal treatments giving rise to smaller more dispersed carbides (Fig. 6.20). These treatments were presumably carried out after application of the sintered bead in-growth surface.

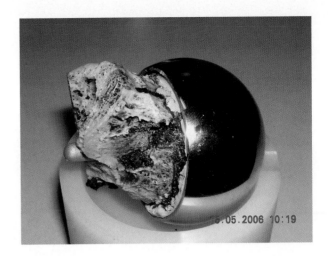

FIG. 6.15.

From Fig. 6.21, linear wear of the head was found to be 70 μm, giving a wear rate of 35 μm per annum, this rate being one order of magnitude higher than would be expected for a well positioned BHR device. From Fig. 6.22, linear wear of the cup was found to be 494 μm, giving a rate per annum of 247 μm, this rate being two orders of magnitude higher than would be expected on a well-positioned device.

Wear on the cup was generally localized to the rim area decreasing linearly to zero approximately 30 degrees from the pole of the cup. Wear on the head was localized to the superior portion of the head from the pole to 50 degrees away from the pole laterally.

As radiographs were available for this device (Fig. 6.23), attention was paid to cup positioning. Cup inclination was found to be 67 degrees (radiographic), and version (assumed anteversion) was 19 degrees (radiographic) (Fig. 6.24). It was also noted that this device had a reduced cup bearing area due to the internal undercut feature; presumably

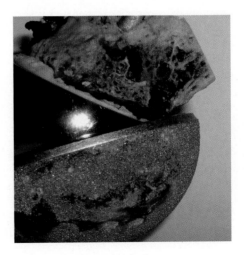

FIG. 6.16.

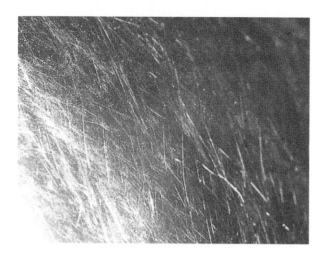

FIG. 6.17.

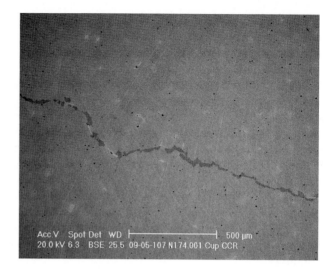

FIG. 6.20.

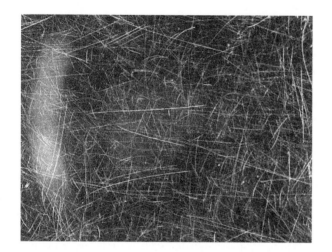

FIG. 6.18.

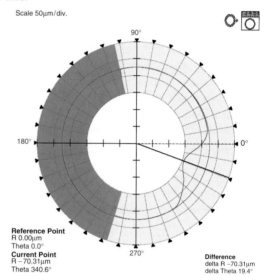

FIG. 6.21.

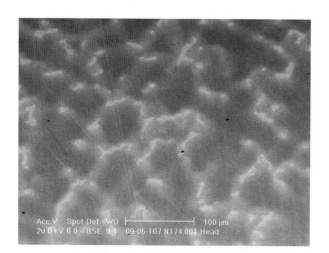

FIG. 6.19.

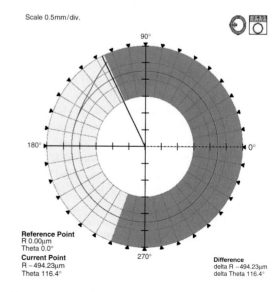

FIG. 6.22.

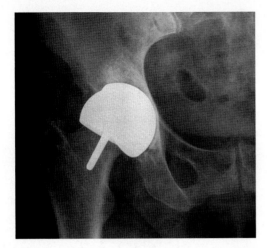

FIG. 6.23.

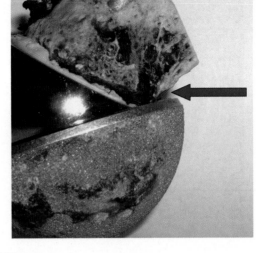

FIG. 6.25.

designed to accept the cup introducer. It was found that by reducing available superior bearing surface, this feature increased the effective inclination by a further 6 degrees. For comparison purposes, the inclination should therefore be reported as 73 degrees.

The high cup inclination found in the positioning study indicated that there was a possibility of impingement between the medial neck at the head neck junction and the rim of the cup (Fig. 6.25). Indeed, a slight recess probably arising from this was identified on the remaining bone that was explanted with the head.

The early failure of this device was attributed to cup position causing impingement followed by subluxation of the head on the edge of the cup. This failure mode was exacerbated by the reduction in bearing area due to the undercut feature. These circumstances led to total loss of lubrication and high contact

pressures finally leading to excessive debris production. The high wear was probably further compounded by the mixed metallurgy of the bearing; with the head exhibiting a higher carbide phase proportion compared with the cup, and the head exhibiting a comparatively lower linear wear value.

Case 4: S&N Device (BHR); Explanted at 11 Months

On visual inspection, the femoral head component still had the resected femoral head remnant at its inner surface (Figs. 6.26 and 6.27). Very fine scratches were observed generally over the bearing surface particularly on the wear zones.

Optical examinations revealed the normal biphasic structure on both the head and cup, with both components having >5%

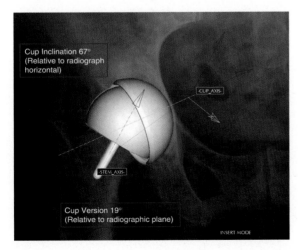

FIG. 6.24.

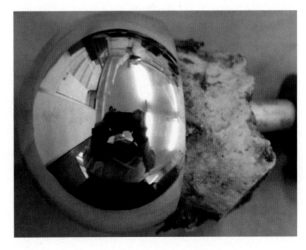

FIG. 6.26.

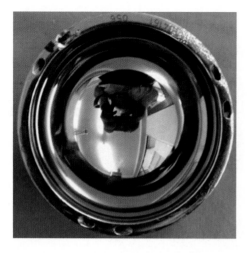

FIG. 6.27

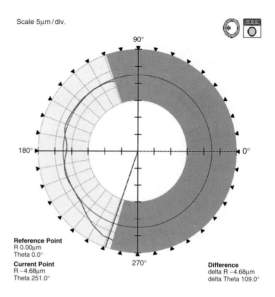

Scale 5μm/div.

Reference Point
R 0.00μm
Theta 0.0°

Current Point
R −4.68μm
Theta 251.0°

Difference
delta R −4.68μm
delta Theta 109.0°

FIG. 6.29.

carbide phase proportion. The chemical analysis confirmed the material to be high carbon alloy (C >0.25%).

Linear wear on both head (Fig. 6.28) and cup (Fig. 6.29) were found to be 29 μm and 5 μm, respectively, giving a wear rate of 31 μm per annum for the head and 5.5 μm per annum for the cup. The head wear was an order of magnitude higher than would be expected, and the cup was wearing at a rate 3 times that of an optimal device

From Fig. 6.28, it is seen that wear on the head extended at maximum over an angle of 60 degrees centered at approximately 30 degrees from the pole. The conformation of the wear patch was unsurprising but high in value. For the cup (Fig. 6.29), wear was not contained within the bearing surface, and

there was evidence of wear through contact with the edge of the cup. This could not easily be confirmed by the equatorial trace of the cup (Fig. 6.30), which showed extreme out-of-roundness due to deformation of the cup, presumably occurring during removal as the position of the deformation corresponds with visible mechanical damage on the edge of the cup.

CAD Assessment of the AP radiograph (Fig. 6.31) revealed a cup inclination angle of 55 degrees (radiographic inclination) and 17 degrees of version (radiographic). The inclination would be considered "high" relative to current guideline values of 40 degrees to 45 degrees.

This device was revised because of issues arising from metallosis at 11 months with pain and a joint effusion. This

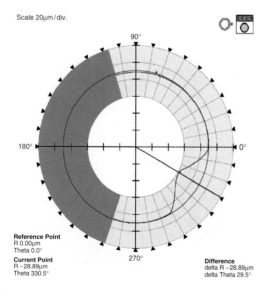

Scale 20μm/div.

Reference Point
R 0.00μm
Theta 0.0°

Current Point
R −28.89μm
Theta 330.5°

Difference
delta R −28.89μm
delta Theta 29.5°

FIG. 6.28.

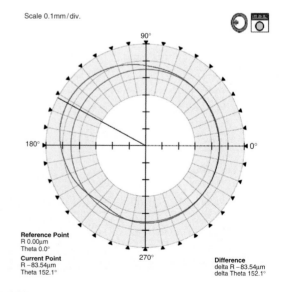

Scale 0.1mm/div.

Reference Point
R 0.00μm
Theta 0.0°

Current Point
R −83.54μm
Theta 152.1°

Difference
delta R −83.54μm
delta Theta 152.1°

FIG. 6.30.

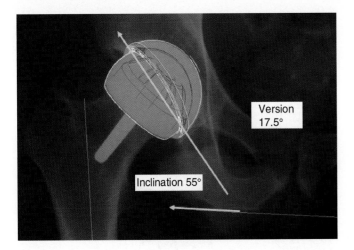

Fig. 6.31.

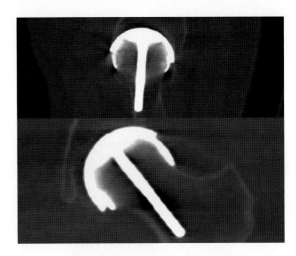

Fig. 6.33.

early failure appears to be largely attributable to issues of cup placement. It would appear that, subject to individual variation, these positioning values mark the boundary where the contact point progresses to the edge of the cup, and high wear ensues. Although it may not be relevant in this case, the compounding effect of bony impingement on subluxation and hence edge wear is hard to ascertain and would require detailed range of motion study for each case.

Case 5: Zimmer Device (Durom); Explanted at 7 Months

The patient was a 63-year-old man who had a left Durom hip resurfacing performed 7 months before revision surgery. During those postoperative 7 months, the patient had unremitting severe groin pain. The clinical features were of psoas irritation. X-ray showed good alignment of com-

ponents, but the acetabular component had not been fully seated (Fig. 6.32).

Multislice computed tomography (CT) scan confirmed incomplete seating of the acetabular component. It further confirmed that the anterior edge of the prosthetic cup protruded 1.1 cm beyond the bony anterior margin of the acetabulum (Fig. 6.33).

At revision surgery, both components were securely fixed. It was confirmed that the acetabular component was indeed protruding beyond the anterior bony acetabular wall. The acetabular component was removed, and a little ongrowth of bone can be seen on the porous surface. Note the sharp edge to the acetabular component. The femoral component was also removed (Fig. 6.34).

The patient had a BHR inserted; his groin pain disappeared immediately, and he has had a good clinical outcome (Fig. 6.35).

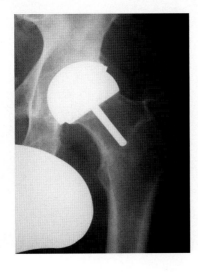

Fig. 6.32.

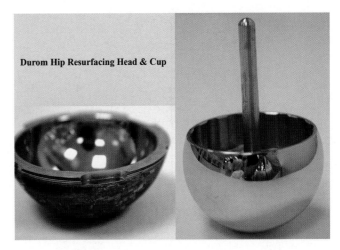

Fig. 6.34.

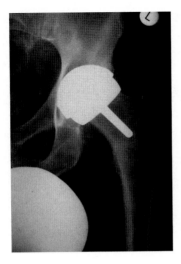

Fig. 6.35.

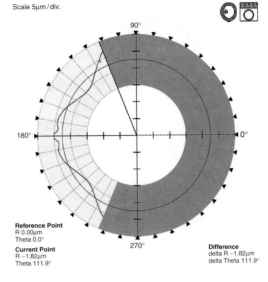

Fig. 6.37.

The retrieved Durom implants were sent to our retrieval analysis laboratory. It is known that the blood titanium concentration is increased after insertion of the Durom resurfacing. The specific question posed was, can you please examine these components for evidence of titanium plasma spray shedding and look for evidence of third-body titanium on the articulating surfaces?

As the head is a forged cobalt chrome device with composite stem and internally machined antirotation features, the manufactured polar form error is relatively large (5–10 μm). When this is combined with very low patient mobility and cup positioning that was optimal in terms of bearing contact position, it was not possible to resolve the anticipated low levels of wear (Figs. 6.36 and 6.37).

Optical examination of the head and cup contact surfaces revealed scratches associated with abrasive wear. Further SEM analysis of the contact surface of the head indicated the presence of patches of extraneous wear debris (Fig. 6.38). The debris possessed characteristic features of adhesion.

Energy Dispersive X-Ray (EDX) spectroscopy analysis (Fig. 6.39), as well as confirming the composition of the CoCr alloy base material, also showed that the adhered debris contained predominately titanium. It was assumed that this originated from the titanium ingrowth surface of the cup.

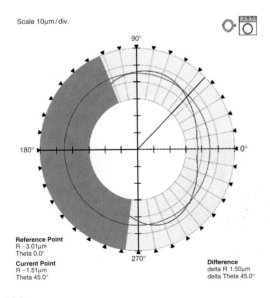

Fig. 6.36.

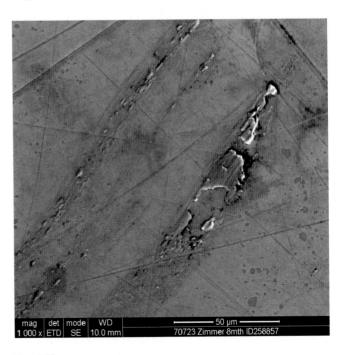

Fig. 6.38.

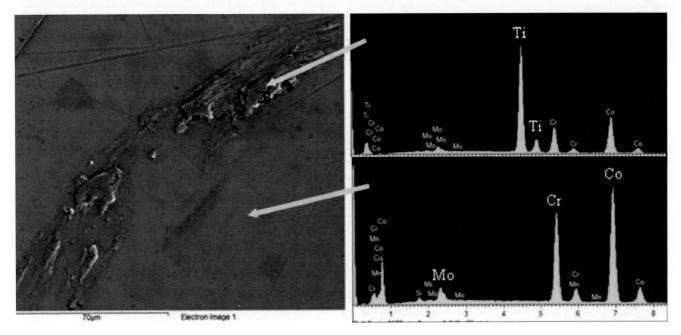

FIG. 6.39.

It has been shown that the entrainment of titanium particles can increase the wear rate of certain metal on metal bearing couples, although, as described above, no wear patch could be detected at 7 months. Failure of this device is attributable to a combination of the design of the acetabular component with a sharp edge and a failure to fully seat the acetabular component at surgery giving rise to tissue irritation and pain.

Discussion

The above case studies serve as indications as to how design, material, and surgical precision (implant position) can contribute to the need for early revision. Whereas engineers who design and manufacture these devices consider the components in optimal positions, any variation to the "ideal" configuration, exposed to physiologic conditions, can exacerbate any inherent weaknesses in the design. This may also provide an explanation as to why hip simulators struggle to reproduce the reality of clinical experience.

It is a truism that this population of retrieved devices, some of which are detailed above, only represents the small percentage of special cases that have required revision.

Hence, conclusions on overall device performance can be misleading.

In the larger group of retrieved devices, the bearing performance is largely in line with expectations, but where it is not, as demonstrated by some of the above cases, the anomalies can largely be attributed to implant positioning and bearing microstructure.

References

1. Kishida Y, Sugano N, Nishii T et al. Preservation of the bone mineral density of the femur after surface replacement of the hip, J Bone Joint Surg Br 2004;86:185–189.
2. Seedhom BB, Dowson D, Wright V. Wear of solid phase formed high density polyethylene in relation to the life of artificial hips and knees. Wear 1973;24:35–51.
3. Schmalzried TP, Szuszczewicz ES, Northfield MR, Akizuki KH, Frankel RE, Belcher G, Amstutz HC. Quantitative assessment of walking activity after total hip or knee replacement. J Bone Joint Surg Am 1998;80:54–59.
4. Daniel J, Ziaee H, Pradhan C, Pynsent PB, McMinn DJ. Blood and urine metal ion levels in young and active patients after Birmingham hip resurfacing arthroplasty: four-year results of a prospective longitudinal study. J Bone Joint Surg Br 2007;89:169–173.

7
Cementing Technique in Birmingham Hip Resurfacing

Stephen McMahon and Gabrielle Hawdon

Introduction

Femoral neck fracture and aseptic loosening are the most common complications associated with modern hip resurfacing arthroplasty, occurring in 0 to 1.5% of most reported series [1–5].

Femoral neck fractures are known to be associated with the orientation of the femoral component [1,6], as well as intra-operative notching of the femoral neck [1].

The reasons for aseptic loosening of the femoral component and for late femoral neck fractures are incompletely understood. It is possible that these failures may occur in patients whose bone is too weak to support the prosthesis, so that failure occurs by fatigue fracture. Fractures occur twice as commonly in women as in men [1]. Thus, patient selection, possibly including assessment of bone mineral density, may play an important part in ensuring success of the arthroplasty. Compromise of the blood supply to the femoral head resulting in avascular necrosis has also been suggested as a mechanism of these failures [7–9] (see also Chapter 9).

Alternatively, failure of femoral resurfacing implants due to femoral neck fracture or aseptic loosening may be related to the method of fixation of the femoral component.

The bone-cement interface is known to be important for survival of the cemented implant. Depth of penetration of cement into the bone, total cement volume, and completeness of the cement mantle might all potentially influence this survival. Large variations in these characteristics were observed in a study of 55 femoral implants retrieved at revision surgery for failed resurfacing arthroplasties [10]. Cement mantle characteristics might in turn be affected by factors such as cement viscosity, bone mineral density, volume of cement instilled into the femoral component prior to implantation, and technique used during implantation. Amstutz et al. reported increased survival of femoral resurfacing implants after a change in implantation technique [11]. Any damage to the bone as a result of the cementing process may also be relevant to the survival of the implant. This might take the form of physical damage (trauma) to the bone, embolization of intraosseous blood vessels due to pressure exerted by cement penetrating into cancellous bone, or thermal damage secondary to exothermic polymerization of the cement.

In dense or normal bone, trabecular spaces occupy a relatively smaller proportion of the total volume of the bone, whereas in soft bone these spaces occupy an increasingly greater proportion of the bone. In another study of femoral heads retrieved at revision surgeries, higher volumes of cement were observed in those cases where failure was due to loosening of the femoral components compared with other modes of failure. Cement-filled femoral cysts were also associated with femoral loosening [12]. The authors suggested thermal damage of bone as a possible mechanism for failure.

This raises the hypothesis that cement penetration and total cement volume might be increased in osteopenic bone, and this in turn may predispose these hips to a higher risk of failure.

A better understanding of the interrelationships between cementing technique, penetration of the cement into bone, and the density of the bone may form a basis for modifying patient selection criteria and/or cementing technique. The ultimate aim is to reduce the incidence of postoperative femoral neck fracture and loosening. We therefore conducted a study to explore the relationship between cement penetration and bone mineral density in Birmingham Hip Resurfacing (BHR), to examine the geographic distribution of the cement mantle, and to determine whether bone is damaged by the cementing process.

Bone Mineral Density Cement Study

Patients undergoing total hip arthroplasty (THA) for osteoarthritis and assessed as being unsuitable candidates for BHR were identified preoperatively. Dual energy X-ray absorptiometry (DEXA) bone mineral density studies of their arthritic femoral heads were undertaken and patients recruited if their DEXA T scores fell within the ranges desired for study.

Patients were grouped according to bone mineral density (T score), measured by DEXA (Group 1: T>0.5, Group 2: -1.5<T<-0.5, Group 3: T<-1.5).

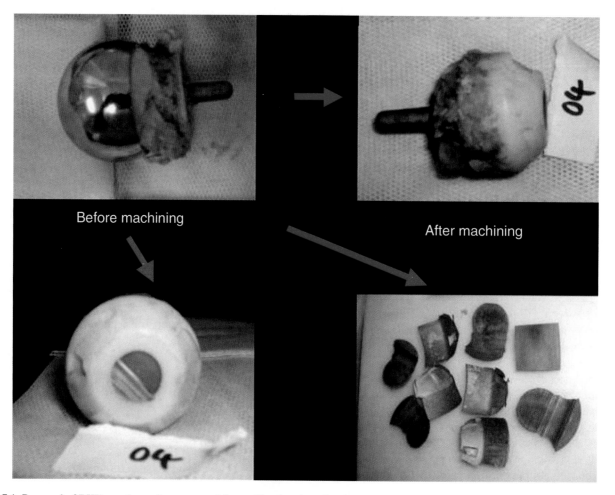

Fig. 7.1. Removal of BHR prostheses from resected femoral heads using electric discharge machining technique.

All procedures were performed by one surgeon, using a standardized posterior surgical approach. The technique used to prepare the femoral head was as follows:

The femoral head was contoured, chamfered, and keyholes made with a burr on the prepared surface in preparation for implantation of the BHR femoral prosthesis. Pulsed lavage was applied to the femoral head, which was then dried using a suction canula inserted via the lesser trochanter. The BHR femoral component was fixed over the prepared native femoral head with low-viscosity cement (Simplex [Howmedica-Limerick, Ireland] with antibiotics [erythromycin and colistin] mixed at 18°C for 1 minute). The volume of cement used was 30% of the internal volume of the femoral prosthesis.

After the cement was polymerized, the femoral head–BHR construct was marked for spatial orientation, removed by femoral neck osteotomy, and sent for analysis. The total hip arthroplasty was then completed.

The BHR femoral prostheses were removed from the retrieved femoral heads (Fig. 7.1), leaving the femoral head and cement mantle intact. The femoral heads were scanned using computed tomography (CT) (Fig. 7.2). They were then sectioned and prepared for histology.

Quantitative Analysis of Cement Penetration

Cement thickness was measured on CT scan images. Measurements were taken at predetermined zones. The geographic extent of the cement mantle was determined and any deficiencies noted. The cement volume for each femoral head was determined from serial CT scans.

Finally, specimens were sectioned and prepared for histology.

Results

On sectioning, all of the femoral prostheses were found to be completely seated.

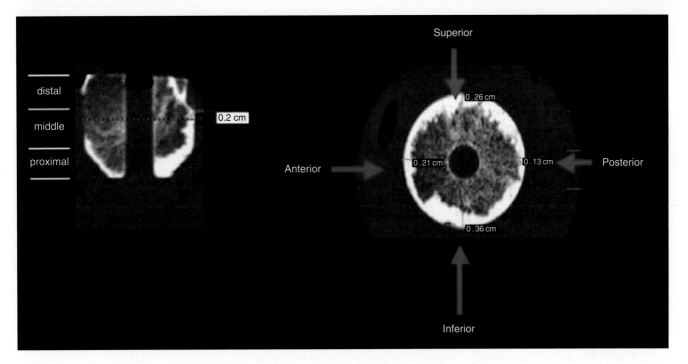

FIG. 7.2. Analysis of cement characteristics of femoral heads using CT and eFilmLite imaging software.

Cement penetration and total cement thickness were greatest at the proximal (polar) end of the femoral heads, tapering toward the distal portion of the head. Cement penetration was not observed to vary with bone mineral density (Fig. 7.3).

Cement mantle thickness (i.e., cement outside the bone) was generally greatest at the distal end of the femoral head and did not vary with bone mineral density (Fig. 7.4).

A posterosuperior deficiency in the cement mantle was noted across all patient groups. This is illustrated in a three-dimensional reconstruction of the cement mantle (Fig. 7.5).

There was no significant difference in cement mantle thickness, cement penetration, total cement thickness, or cement volume between the three bone mineral density groups ($p > 0.05$).

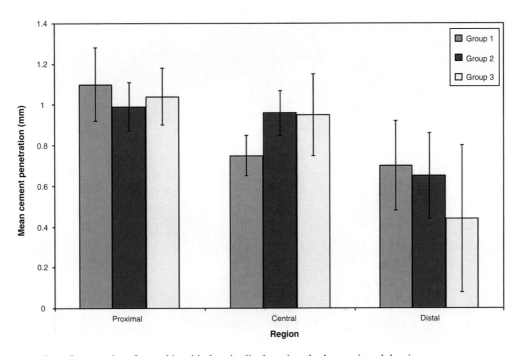

FIG. 7.3. Mean penetration of cement into femoral head in longitudinal sections by bone mineral density.

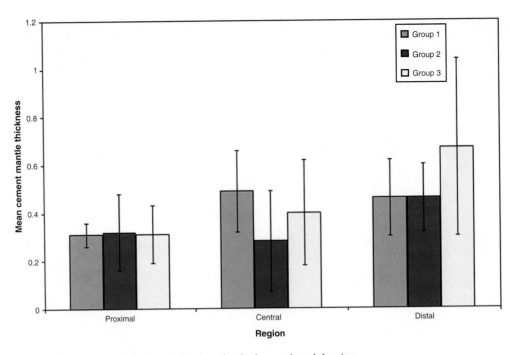

FIG. 7.4. Mean thickness of cement mantle in longitudinal section by bone mineral density.

Microscopy was performed using hematoxylin and eosin staining to examine the bone-cement interface. Most of the sections displayed clean demarcation at the interface with living bone cells adjacent to cement (Fig. 7.6). Some other sections showed bone debris mixed into cement at the interface. One specimen displayed hemorrhage at the bone-cement interface with macrophages and monocytes present. It may be concluded that little if any significant traumatic bone injury

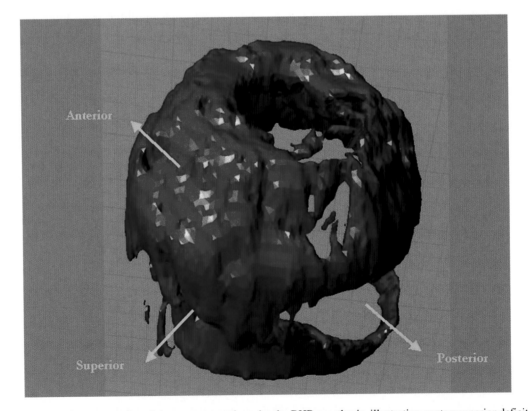

FIG. 7.5. Three-dimensional reconstruction of the cement mantle under the BHR prosthesis, illustrating posterosuperior deficit.

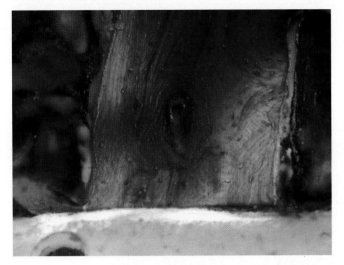

FIG. 7.6. Histology of sectioned femoral head at the bone-cement interface. Little damage to the bone microstructure is evident.

occurs to the femoral head as a result of BHR prosthesis implantation using this cementing technique.

Discussion

This study revealed no significant differences in cement characteristics related to bone mineral density. It may be, therefore, that differences observed in these characteristics in failed femoral implants relate more to implantation technique than to bone mineral density. A study of cementing techniques using simulated femoral heads suggested that considerable variation in cement volume and penetration resulted from differing cementing techniques [13].

It has been suggested that the use of low-viscosity cement in the femoral head may lead to excessive cement penetration and increased risk of thermal necrosis [14]. Our investigation, however, did not reveal excessive volumes or penetration of cement, even into osteopenic bone. In a related study, using the same cementing technique to avoid cement overfilling of the femoral head (including the use of pulsed lavage and a femoral trochanteric suction catheter), the authors have measured temperatures at the bone-cement interface during cement polymerization after implantation of Birmingham femoral prostheses. Maximum temperatures recorded using this technique were insufficient to cause bone necrosis (submitted for publication). Gill et al. reported similar findings after a modification of surgical technique in line with that described above [15].

In our study, all the femoral heads were seen to be fully seated, and no structural or thermal damage was observed on histology.

The mechanism of failure in osteopenic patients may simply be that the soft bone of the femoral head and neck is too weak to support the prosthesis and that it fails by fatigue fracture.

It was observed that the cement mantle was consistently deficient posteriorly. As a result of this observation, we have now modified our cementing technique to include deposition of a small amount of cement directly onto the posterior (i.e., uppermost) surface of the prepared femoral head prior to implantation of the prosthesis. Further work is in progress to examine the cement characteristics resulting from this modification.

This study used a standard cementing technique, including a constant proportional volume (30%) of cement for each femoral prosthesis, a standard mixing time (1 minute), and cement (Simplex with antibiotics) and a single experienced operator. It is likely, therefore, that the resulting cement mantle would be regular and reproducible. Surgical inexperience or variations in cementing technique may lead to greater variability in cement characteristics, which might compromise the success of the procedure. This "learning curve" effect was alluded to by Morlock et al. [10] in a discussion of the heterogeneity observed in retrieved femoral heads from failed resurfacing procedures.

Suggested Cementing Technique

This pilot study has given us some insight into the behavior of low-viscosity cement when used with the BHR femoral component. The suggested technique at this stage is to use low-viscosity cement mixed at 18°C and to implant the prosthesis at 1 to 1.5 minutes. A tapered drill is routinely used to slightly widen the central stem hole in the femoral head prior to implantation (see Chapter 22). At this time, it would be prudent to fill the heads with cement to 30% of their total volume until further results come to hand.

Ongoing research is under way to determine how intraoperative conditions might lead to the massive cement overfilling that is seen in some femoral heads on retrieval. Also under investigation are methods for improving the completeness of the cement mantle; in particular, how the posterosuperior cement mantle defects observed in this study might be prevented.

References

1. Shimmin AJ, Back, D. Femoral neck fractures following Birmingham hip resurfacing: A national review of 50 cases. J Bone Joint Surg Br 2005;87:463–464.
2. Daniel J, Pynsent PB, McMinn DJ. Metal-on-metal resurfacing of the hip in patients under the age of 55 years with osteoarthritis. J Bone Joint Surg Br 2004;86:177–184.
3. Amstutz HC, Campbell PA, Le Duff MJ. Fracture of the neck of the femur after surface arthroplasty of the hip. J Bone Joint Surg Am 2004;86:1874–1877.
4. Treacy RB, McBryde CW, Pynsent PB. Birmingham hip resurfacing arthroplasty. A minimum follow-up of five years. J Bone Joint Surg Br 2005;87:167–170.
5. Back DL, Dalziel R, Young D, Shimmin A. Early results of primary Birmingham hip resurfacings: an independent prospective study of the first 230 hips. J Bone Joint Surg Br 2005;87:324–329.
6. Beaulé PE, Lee JL, LeDuff MJ, et al. Orientation of the femoral component in surface arthroplasty of the hip. A biomechanical and clinical analysis. J Bone Joint Surg Am 2004;86:2015–2021.
7. Beaulé P, Campbell P, Hoke R, et al. Notching of the femoral neck during surface arthroplasty of the hip. J Bone Joint Surg Br 2006;1:35–39.

8. Beaulé PE, Campbell P, Leunig-Ganz K, et al. Vascularity of the arthritic femoral head and hip resurfacing. J Bone Joint Surg Am 2006;88:85–96.

9. Nork SE, Schar M, Pfander G, et al. Anatomic considerations for the choice of surgical approach for hip resurfacing arthroplasty. Orthop Clin North Am 2005;36:163–170.

10. Morlock MM, Bishop N, Rüther W, et al. Biomechanical, morphological, and histological analysis of early failures in hip resurfacing arthroplasty. Proc Inst Mech Eng [H] 2006;220: 333–344.

11. Amstutz HC, Le Duff MJ, Campbell PA, et al The effects of technique changes on aseptic loosening of the femoral component in hip resurfacing. Results of 600 Conserve Plus with a 3 to 9 year follow-up. J Arthroplasty 2007;22:481–489.

12. Campbell P, Beaule PE, Ebramzadeh E, et al. A study of implant failure in metal-on-metal surface arthroplasties. Clin Orthop Relat Res 2006;453:35–46.

13. Bitsch RG, Heisel C, Silva M, et al. Femoral cementing technique for hip resurfacing arthroplasty. J Orthop Res 2007;25: 423–431.

14. Chandler M, Kowalski RS, Watkins ND, et al. Cementing techniques in hip resurfacing, Proc Inst Mech Eng [H] 2006;220:321–331.

15. Gill HS, Campbell PA, Murray DW, et al. Reduction of the potential for thermal damage during hip resurfacing. J Bone Joint Surg Br 2007;89:16–20.

8
Migration Studies

Arne Lundberg and Raed Itayem

Radiostereometric analysis (RSA) is a technique by which very small displacements between segments depicted in radiographs may be measured. There are three fundamental requirements:

1. At least two x-ray exposures must be made, closely enough in time so that the risk of patient movement between the two exposures is minimized. The exposure should cover and include a calibration device (usually a Plexiglas cage with radiopaque markers in known positions).
2. At least a second set of exposures must be made at a user-defined time point (2 years postoperatively, on the same day after maximum internal rotation, etc.). In migration studies, examinations are commonly performed at 6- to 12-month intervals.
3. Before the examination, at least three radiopaque markers have to be established in each segment. In the bone segments (the pelvis and the femur for a hip study), these are usually spherical and in the form of small tantalum beads (0.5–2.0 mm in diameter). On the implant, other features of hemispherical/spherical shape, such as a 28-mm head or a hemispherical uncemented cup backside, are also commonly used. In theory, extremely well-defined other features of an implant could be considered, but this is uncommon in RSA practice. More common in recent times has been to trace the whole outline of the implant and use this in the analysis.

Conventional photogrammetric methods for calculating three-dimensional coordinates from two sets of two-dimensional coordinates are used, as well as standard kinematic software to calculate the displacements between segments. These displacements are—when implant migration is studied—often given as either Euler/Cardan rotations or segment center translations. One alternative description is helical axis component rotations. Methods commonly used in joint kinematics, such as the Grood-Suntay–type coordinate system with floating axes, are very seldom used in implant migration studies.

The accuracy achieved with RSA varies between different study conditions. Notably the size and shape of the segments are important, with a poorer accuracy resulting from segments where the smallest diameter is small (in most instances, a smallest diameter of less than 10 mm will limit the accuracy of rotation assessment). In most precision studies of hip implants, the error for translational migration is 0.1 mm or less, and for rotational migration it will usually not exceed 0.5 degree [1]. In comparison with the precision usually found in assessment of plain radiography (approximately 5 mm), this means that in an implant with a linear migration pattern, RSA will yield relevant stability information in less than one tenth of the time that it will take to collect corresponding information from clinical radiographs. In reality, this difference will be slightly smaller, due to the fact that most implants migrate more in the early postoperative period than subsequently.

The main strength of RSA is its accuracy, whereas its most notable shortcoming is the need for marker insertion into patient and implant. In recent years, methods for RSA with markerless implants have been developed. Although this seems to often give a good accuracy [2], it is dependent on a very good three-dimensional model of the implant, and for symmetric implants, such as press-fit cups without liner markings, and resurfacing heads, a true 6 degrees of freedom analysis cannot be achieved as rotation of the implant about its own axis cannot be assessed.

The Role of RSA in Assessment of New Implants

RSA is one of several methods that are considered indispensable in a controlled introduction of new implant technology [3]. Other methods range from mechanical tests and computer simulations to careful clinical follow-up of early patient cohorts. RSA has its main importance when not only the individual implant type but the whole design concept is new.

Previous RSA information in the literature deals with migration patterns (in conventional cemented femoral stems, >1.2-mm migration at 2 years predicts early revision, whereas in polished tapered stems such as the Exeter it does not) [4–6], but RSA has also been used to completely remove an implant from the market before adverse events had been noticed in clinical groups [7].

RSA and Resurfacing

The major challenge when performing RSA analysis of resurfacing implants is to achieve adequate determination of the cup position. In more conventional implants, the cup is either made entirely from polyethylene or combines a titanium shell with a polyethylene liner. In both cases, it is comparatively easy to detect markers embedded in the liner on radiographs. This possibility is not available in resurfacing, where there is a thin, but very radiopaque monoblock cup, which may easily obscure small tantalum markers. The head also has its challenges, as its outline can be very difficult to accurately trace in order to determine its center, as the cup usually covers a large portion of the head circumference and the "stem" lacks natural positions for markers (such as conventional stems have at the shoulder and at the tip).

The procedure chosen in our studies has been to place markers on titanium towers, protruding from the implant surface at the implant/bone interface; three on the cup (one craniolateral, one caudomedial, and one polar) and three on the "stem" (one at the tip and one each on the craniolateral and caudomedial aspects, about 15 mm from the tip). This gives a segment definition that lacks the redundancy normally sought to improve the analysis, but the shape of the segments is close to ideal. Particularly on the femoral side, the absence of a large metal stem in the metaphysis means that it is comparatively easy to establish a large and well-dispersed marker segment in the greater and lesser trochanter regions. On the pelvic side, optimal segment visualization demands that bone markers are deposited well away from the vicinity of the cup. Placing four markers as high as possible in the ileum plus two in the pubis and two in the ischium has been found to yield optimal segment configuration (Fig. 8.1).

Specific RSA Studies of Resurfacing Implants

To date, there have been at least two RSA studies of resurfacing implants published [8,9]. Several additional studies are under way.

In 1999, a set of BHR implants with RSA markers placed in accordance with the description above were manufactured. The choice of implant combinations was restricted to 50/58 and 54/62 in order to combine enough metal to avoid risk of implant deformation by marker insertion while still providing implants to cover at least a large part of the male patient group.

The study consisted of 20 hips in 19 men, who were all physically active before being limited by osteoarthrosis, and who all returned to their previous high activity level. The age range was from 42 to 63, with an average of 51.

The patients were examined postoperatively (within 48 hours after surgery) and at 2, 6, 12, 24, and 60 months. All examinations were performed in a supine position, with one lab-fixed and one mobile x-ray tube. Synchronization was not exact, but the patients were examined in a relaxed position, which normally means that no motion artifact should occur (such an artifact is identified by the software as an increased distance between the rays from each x-ray tube at their intersection at each marker). Repeat examinations of 26 extra film pairs for the cup side and 47 for the femoral side were analyzed to assess the precision and zero movement error of the specific setup. The repeat cup examinations showed a mean error of approximately 0.2 degrees of rotation and 0.04 to 0.09 mm of translation. The corresponding values for the repeat femoral component examinations were approximately 0.5 degrees and 0.1 to 0.3 mm [8]. These errors are within the range usually encountered in RSA hip studies, indicating that the segment configurations were adequate to offset the disadvantage posed by the lack of redundancy.

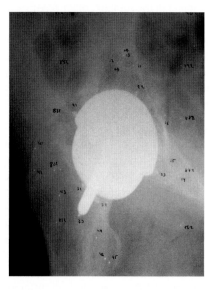

A   B

FIG. 8.1. The two x-ray views of an RSA examination. Note towers protruding from cup and "stem"

In the main study, the rotations and translations encountered were uniformly of very low magnitude. There was no discernible migration pattern, except a possible early proximal implant migration on the acetabular side. This pattern is common for uncemented implants and is seen as a "settling in" phenomenon when migration does not continue after the initial postoperative phase.

In a study of 22 markerless BHR femoral implants followed for 2 years, Glyn-Jones et al. have shown similar results with very little migration and no consistent migration pattern [9]. The results relating to proximal-distal and anterior-posterior migration of the femoral component from the two RSA studies of the BHR are shown in Figs. 8.2 and 8.3.

Proximal-distal migration values for some conventional femoral stems are included for reference; it should be noted that the graphs are not intended to indicate a direct comparison as the implants have not been included in a single study. Also, comparing distal migration of resurfacing versus conventional stems may not be appropriate as their migration pattern may differ. However, the values are provided to give an impression of the magnitudes of migration commonly seen in RSA studies. Femoral component anteversion/retroversion and cup proximal/distal translation are presented in Figs. 8.4 and 8.5; in these only the study with marked implants is included, as such data cannot be provided in a study of markerless implants.

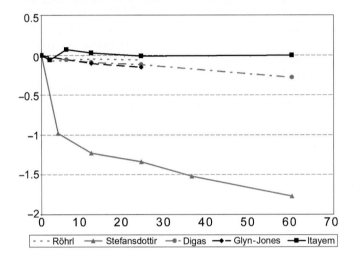

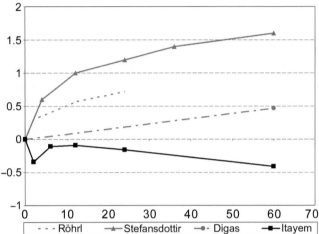

FIG. 8.2. Proximal/distal migration of BHR femoral components over 5 years (solid black line) and over 2 years (Glyn Jones et al. [9], black dash line). Corresponding values for vertical stem migration in conventional THR included as reference (Stefansdottir et al. [4], Exeter stem, gray solid line; Digas et al. [5], Spectron stem, gray dot-dash line; Röhrl et al. [6], CFP cementless short stem, gray dot line)

FIG. 8.4. Anteversion/retroversion of BHR femoral component over 5 years (solid black line). Corresponding values for stem anteversion/retroversion in conventional THR included as reference (Stefansdottir et al. [4], Exeter stem, gray solid line; Digas et al. [5], Spectron stem, gray dot-dash line; Röhrl et al. [6], CFP cementless short stem, gray dot line)

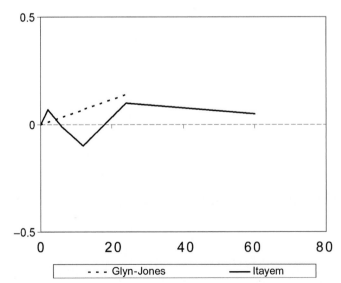

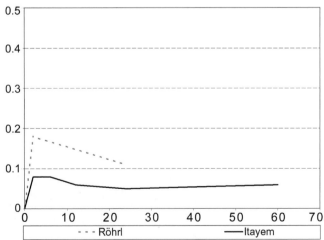

FIG. 8.3. Anteroposterior migration of BHR femoral components over 5 years (solid black line) and over 2 years (Glyn Jones et al. [9], black dash line)

FIG. 8.5. Proximal/distal migration of BHR cups over 5 years (solid black line). Corresponding values for a conventional modular uncemented THR cup (Röhrl et al. [6], HA-coated titanium cup, gray dot line) included as reference. Note in both cases, tendency toward early proximal migration ("settling in") followed by absence of further migration

Whereas results so far have been consistent in showing very low migration values, it has to be remembered that continuous migration is only one possible failure mode in hip implants in general. However, it is equally true that in all instances hitherto analyzed (with the possible exception of polished, tapered, cemented stems), it has been a general finding that the absence of migration is preferable to the presence of migration.

Acknowledgments. We gratefully acknowledge the contributions by our study collaborators: Dr. Anton Arndt, Dr. Joseph Daniel, Mr. Derek J.W. McMinn, and Dr. Lars Nistor.

References

1. Börlin N, Thien T, Kärrholm J. The precision of radiostereometric measurements manual vs digital measurements. J Biomechanics 2002;35:69–79.
2. Alfaro-Adrian J, Gill HS, Murray DW. Cement migration after THR: a comparison of Charnley Elite and Exeter femoral stems using RSA. J Bone Joint Surg Br 1999;81:130–134.
3. Malchau H. On the importance of stepwise introduction of new hip implant technology: assessment of total hip replacement using clinical evaluation, radiostereometry, digitized radiography and a national hip registry. Thesis. Götebory, Sweden: Götebory University, 1995.
4. Stefansdottir A, Franzen H, Johansson R, et al. Movement pattern of the Exeter femoral stem. A radiostereometric analysis of 22 primary hip arthroplasties followed for 5 years. Acta Orthop Scand 2004;75:408–414.
5. Digas G, Kärrholm J, Thanner J. Addition of fluoride to acrylic bone cement does not improve fixation of a total hip arthroplasty stem. Clin Orthop Relat Res 2006;448:58–66.
6. Röhrl SM, Pedersen E, Ullmark G, et al. Migration pattern of a short femoral neck preserving stem. Clin Orthop Relat Res 2006;448:73–78.
7. Nistor L, Lundberg A, Ackerholm P. Rotation and subsidence of a composite femoral component analyzed by Roentgen stereophotogrammetry. Proceedings of the Orthopaedic Research Society, Washington, DC, 1992.
8. Itayem R, Arndt A, Nistor L, McMinn D, Lundberg A. Stability of the Birmingham hip resurfacing arthroplasty at two years. J Bone Joint Surg Br 2005;87:158–162.
9. Glyn-Jones S, Gill HS, McLardy-Smith P, et al. Roentgen stereophotogrammetric analysis of the Birmingham hip resurfacing arthroplasty. J Bone Joint Surg Br 2004;86:172–176.

9

Vascularity of the Femoral Head in Hip Resurfacing

Stephen McMahon and Gabrielle Hawdon

Introduction

Resurfacing arthroplasty was first practiced as early as the 1950s as a treatment for arthritis of the hip. Unfortunately, early resurfacing arthroplasties were associated with a high failure rate. Avascular necrosis of the femoral head (AVN) was thought to play a major role in these failures. It later became evident that these problems were due to polyethylene wear particle–induced osteolysis [1,2]. As a result of these early failures, and the concerns they raised about the vascularity of the femoral head, resurfacing arthroplasty of the hip fell out of favor.

Similarly, early metal on metal hip prostheses showed promise in the form of low wear rates [3] but were also associated with high failure rates secondary to aseptic loosening. This was thought to be related to poor tolerances between prosthetic components or other unfavorable biomechanics [4–7].

In the early 1990s, renewed interest in metal on metal bearing surfaces, stimulated and facilitated by advances in metallurgy and machining technology, coincided with increasing demand from younger patients for a hip replacement that would allow better functional performance and higher levels of activity than were possible with traditional total hip arthroplasty. Resurfacing offered advantages including increased stability, reduced stress shielding in the proximal femur, preservation of femoral bone stock, and easier revision to a conventional stemmed femoral prosthesis if required [8]. Hard metal on metal bearing surfaces offered excellent wear characteristics, an additional advantage in the younger, more active patient population.

Early to mid-term clinical follow-up of hip resurfacing is promising, with 97% to 99% survival at 4 to 6 years [9–11].

By far, the most common mode of failure has been femoral neck fracture. AVN is infrequently reported as a cause of failure. Fracture rates vary from 0 to 2% [12,13].

In a series of 3497 resurfacings performed by Australian surgeons, Shimmin and Back reported 50 failures (1.4%)

as a result of femoral neck fractures but no revisions for AVN of the femoral head [14]. Daniel et al. [9] reported one failure (0.2%), secondary to avascular necrosis, in 446 resurfacing arthroplasties. Amstutz et al. [15] reported a survival of 94.4% of 400 metal on metal hybrid resurfacing arthroplasties at an average follow-up of 3.5 years. Twelve (3%) hips were revised; 7 (1.75%) for femoral loosening, 3 (0.75%) for femoral neck fracture. Treacy et al. [10] followed 144 consecutive Birmingham Hip Resurfacing (BHR) hips for 5 years. They described 98% overall survival. Three (2.1%) femoral components were revised, 2 for infection and 1 (0.7%) for fracture. Back et al. [11] followed 230 BHR patients for a mean of 3 years, reporting 1 failure (acetabular loosening).

McMinn et al. [4] describes the results of 4 different designs used in 235 patients over a period of 5 years. No femoral neck fractures were observed. Little et al. [16] studied 15 revision surgeries from a total of 377 patients from 1998 to 2005: 358 BHRs and 19 Cormet 2000 prostheses were included. Eight (2%) cases involved femoral neck fracture, 5 were revised for component loosening, 1 for inflammation, and 1 for persistent pain.

There is some controversy regarding the etiology of these fractures. Known risk factors include varus position of the femoral component and intraoperative notching of the femoral neck [17–19]. It has also been suggested that interruption to the femoral head's blood supply could contribute to the development of some fractures [16,20].

Hip resurfacing is most commonly performed via a posterior approach, which typically involves posterior capsulotomy, incision of obturator externus, and anterosuperior translocation of the hip. Theoretically, such an approach has the potential to compromise the femoral head's viability by disruption of its extraosseous blood supply. The concept of hip resurfacing, however, depends upon preservation of a significant proportion of the femoral head, so any potential compromise of its blood supply is of genuine concern.

Anatomy of the Femoral Head Blood Supply

It is essential to have a thorough understanding of the anatomy of the blood supply of the proximal femur in order to assess and understand the ramifications of different surgical approaches on the blood supply to the femoral head during resurfacing arthroplasty. Concerns have been raised about the potential for avascular necrosis of the femoral head, particularly when the posterior approach is employed [20–26].

In the normal, nonarthritic adult hip, blood is supplied to the femoral head predominately via the deep branch of the medial circumflex femoral artery (MCFA) [27–29] (Fig. 9.1). The contribution via the ligamentum teres is probably insignificant. Intraosseous blood vessels also contribute to the femoral head blood supply. The MCFA usually arises from the profunda femoris artery and less commonly from the common femoral artery [26]. The deep branch passes posteriorly between pectineus medially and the iliopsoas tendon laterally when it then runs along the inferior border of obturator externus heading toward the intertrochanteric crest. The deep branch gives off a trochanteric branch at the superior border of the quadratus femoris. The trochanteric vessel passes over the intertrochanteric crest and continues on to the lateral aspect of the greater trochanter. The deep branch continues on (as the ascending branch) passing posterior to the tendon of obturator externus and anterior to the tendons of the inferior gemellus, obturator internus, and superior gemellus. At the level of the interval between tendons of the superior gemellus and piriformis, it perforates the capsule and divides into terminal branches. These vessels run a subsynovial course up the posterosuperior neck of the femur to perforate the cortex 2 to 4 mm shy of the articular cartilage of the femoral head [26]. The majority of the vascular foraminae are located in the anterosuperior and posterosuperior quadrants of the femoral head [30]. Therefore, to protect the ascending branch from injury during surgery, the tendon of obturator externus must be preserved [23,26,31,32]. In addition, to protect the retinacular vessels after they have perforated the cortex, notching of the superior neck of the femur with the barrel reamer must be avoided.

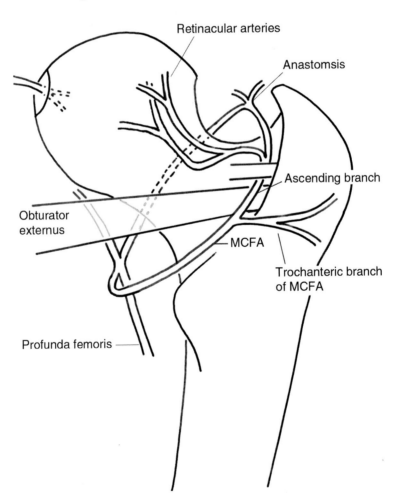

FIG. 9.1. Blood supply to the femoral head.

There is no doubt that the posterior approach can damage the extraosseous blood supply to the femoral head. This circulation is known to be important to the viability of the nonarthritic femoral head. For example, damage to the extraosseous circulation in traumatic dislocation of the hip may lead to AVN of the femoral head in 5% to 50% of cases [33–37]. Intuitively then, one might expect a high rate of femoral component failure secondary to AVN of the femoral head in resurfacing arthroplasties, especially those performed via a posterior approach. However, clinical outcome studies do not support such a high failure rate. Medium-term clinical follow-up of BHR patients has revealed a low incidence of revision for avascular necrosis (<1%) or aseptic loosening (0 to 2%) of the femoral head [4,9,10,11,15,16].

More information on the femoral head circulation is needed to explain this apparent discrepancy.

Femoral Head Perfusion Studies

Given that the extraosseus blood supply to the femoral head is at risk during resurfacing surgery, several studies have been undertaken to examine intraoperative blood flow or tissue perfusion to the femoral head during the surgical approach, reaming of the femoral head, and simulated notching of the femoral neck.

Beaulé et al. used laser Doppler flowmetry to measure blood flow in osteoarthritic femoral heads during total hip arthroplasty, before and after deliberately notching the superior neck of the femur. Ten of 14 hips exhibited reduced flow of greater than 50% after notching. The authors concluded that "vascularity in the osteoarthritic state is similar to the non-arthritic state, where damage to the extraosseous vessels can predispose to avascular necrosis" and suggested that "Surgeons who perform resurfacing arthroplasty of the hip should pay careful attention to these vessels by avoiding excessive dissection around the femoral neck and/or notching" [20].

In a related study, Beaulé, using a vascular-sparing approach [25,38], assessed the effect of femoral reaming on the femoral head blood flow in osteoarthritic heads [39]. He noted a mean decrease in blood flow of 70% in 9 of 10 hips, which he attributed to damage to the retinacular vessels. Thus it would seem that even if the extracapsular blood vessels are preserved by modification of the operative approach, they are still at significant risk of being damaged by the barrel reamer during preparation of the femoral head.

By contrast, Whiteside measured blood flow (using a hydrogen washout method and ink angiography) in normal and arthritic hips in dogs during reaming of the femoral head after stripping of the retinacular vessels. In the normal hips, reaming under these conditions resulted in cessation or severe reduction in blood flow to the femoral head, although hips of arthritic dogs fared better (see later) [40].

Khan et al. used cefuroxime concentration in bone sampled from the femoral head during resurfacing procedures as a proxy measure of bone tissue perfusion. They found that concentration of cefuroxime was significantly lower in hips resurfaced via a posterolateral approach than via a transgluteal approach [24].

Steffen et al. measured oxygen using an electrode in the femoral head during resurfacing procedures performed via a posterior approach. Oxygen concentration was variably reduced in all patients (mean 60% reduction, during approach, and a further 20% reduction with component insertion) and was not significantly improved on wound closure [22].

Retrieval Studies

Several retrieval series exist confirming the vascularity of femoral heads after resurfacing procedures.

Studies performed in 1992–1996 on femoral heads retrieved from early McMinn resurfacing patients undergoing revision surgery for aseptic loosening of cemented acetabular cups revealed well-fixed femoral prostheses. These patients were treated preoperatively with tetracyline, and the retrieved femoral heads were examined with fluorescent light microscopy. Tetracycline uptake observed on the trabecular surfaces of the femoral heads confirmed their vascularity. Histologic examination demonstrated normal hematopoietic marrow and bone structure [4].

Retrieval studies that examined femoral heads obtained at revision surgeries involving other resurfacing prostheses reported incidences of avascular necrosis ranging from 0 to 92%.

Bradley et al. examined retrieved femoral heads from 25 failed femoral resurfacing components. On histologic examination, bone was "substantially alive" in 23 of the 25 cases. [41].

Amstutz [42] describes a pathologic study of femoral heads from 120 surface replacement failures, in which his group "could not identify osteonecrosis as a mode of failure."

Nasser et al. undertook extensive pathologic studies on 21 femoral heads retrieved an average of 32 months after porous surface replacement (PSR) procedures performed between 1983 and 1998. Although the femoral heads showed extensive "cavitation" or lytic lesions of the femoral necks related to polyethylene wear particles, the authors describe "ample viable bone present in the femoral heads proximal to the areas of 'cystic' degeneration" and state that "evidence of avascularity or coagulative necrosis was not identified in any of the retrieved specimens" [43].

Campbell et al. histologically analyzed 25 resurfaced femoral heads (THARIES and PSR) up to 12 years postoperatively and found that osteonecrosis was not induced by the procedure [44].

Howie et al. examined 72 femoral heads retrieved at revision for femoral loosening. Six (8.3%) of the 72 femoral heads showed evidence of osteonecrosis, including one case for whom the indication for initial surgery was AVN. Interestingly, the authors correlated osteonecrosis with the degree of femoral loosening and postulated that some of the necrotic changes observed in femoral heads retrieved for femoral loosening might be secondary to movement of the prosthesis on the bone, rather than to avascularity of the femoral head [45].

In a study of 98 retrieved femoral heads, Campbell et al. reported 7 (7.1%) failures due to osteonecrosis among 28 cases of femoral neck fracture and 23 cases of aseptic femoral loosening [46].

Little et al. studied 13 femoral retrievals from 377 patients. (8 for femoral neck fractures, 3 for aseptic loosening, 1 for inflammation, 1 for persistent pain.) Twelve of the 13 femoral heads showed histologic evidence of osteonecrosis, although the overall postoperative fracture rate was only 1.9% [16].

In another case study of revision surgery after resurfacing arthroplasty, Capello et al. reviewed 24 cases, including 23 Indiana Conservative Hip Arthroplasties and 1 Wagner resurfacing. Three (12.5%) cases were revised for postoperative AVN, diagnosed on bone scan. Perhaps significantly, one of these primary procedures had been performed for AVN, and the other two for inflammatory arthritis, rather than for osteoarthritis [8].

Postoperative Imaging of the Femoral Head

The presence of metallic femoral resurfacing prostheses precludes the use of plain x-ray imaging to detect postoperative changes associated with osteonecrosis of the femoral head. Magnetic resonance imaging (MRI) cannot be used for the same reasons. However, nuclear medicine offers a window into the state of the femoral head inside the resurfacing prosthesis.

Evidence for preservation of vascularity of the femoral head after resurfacing surgery was provided by bone scanning studies performed on 32 patients (36 hips) between 12 and 47 months (average 26 months) after BHR surgery using a posterior approach. Bone scans were performed with technetium-99 m (Tc-99 m) HDP (hydropymethylene diphosphate), using planar and single photon emission computed tomography (SPECT) images, and examined for abnormal patterns of tracer uptake. None of the scans displayed photopenic defects consistent with avascular necrosis. Nor was there any evidence of increased uptake, which might be consistent with femoral fracture or revascularization/remodeling of bone affected by AVN [47] (Figs. 9.2 and 9.3).

A similar study, involving [18F] fluoride positron emission tomography (PET) of resurfaced hips in 10 patients, was reported by Forrest et al. in 2006 [48].

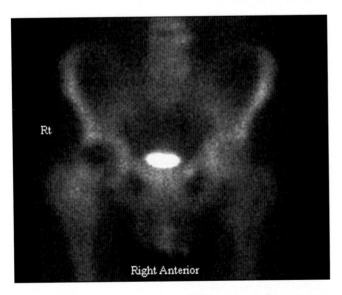

FIG. 9.2. Planar bone scan image of BHR at 32 months postoperatively. Right anterior view. Signal is attenuated by the BHR prosthesis. Preserved bone scan activity under the cap within the residual femoral head.

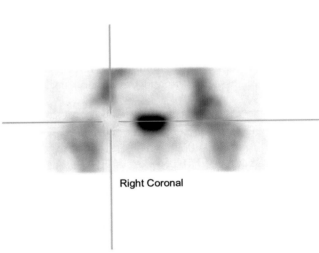

FIG. 9.3. Single photon emission computed tomography (SPECT) image using iterative reconstruction. BHR at 30 months. Coronal view.

BHR resurfacing was performed via a modified anterolateral approach, including circumferential capsulotomy next to the acetabular margin. PET scans were performed an average of 20 months postoperatively, using the nonoperated side as a reference. No areas of osteonecrosis were identifiable in any of the hips studied.

The Case for Preserved Viability of the Femoral Head

These observations, together with the low reported rates of AVN, femoral fracture, and aseptic femoral component loosening, suggest that viability of the femoral head is usually preserved after resurfacing surgery, despite compromise of the extraosseous blood supply intraoperatively. It may be that the intraoperative hypoperfusion insult is transient or insufficient to cause osteonecrosis in most cases, and/or that a collateral circulation (intraosseous blood supply) adequately maintains the viability of the femoral head in these circumstances [49].

To try and explain this apparent discrepancy between the predicted incidence of AVN and what is seen in clinical follow-up, various authors have offered opinions and/or devised studies in an attempt to unravel this conundrum.

Freeman opined that the major blood supply to the arthritic femoral head was from intraosseous blood vessels [50,51]. He described this increased vascularity intraoperatively, postulating that pressure from osteophytes on the retinacular vessels might stimulate the development of an increased intraosseous circulation. Whiteside's study [40] comparing blood flow in femoral heads of normal and arthritic dogs during reaming of the femoral head after stripping of the retinacular vessels showed better blood flow in the arthritic hips than in those of normal dogs. In arthritic hips, "vascular anastomoses between the epiphysis and the metaphysis were abundant," and "all of the femoral heads had detectable blood flow after retinacular stripping and epiphyseal reaming" (the femoral heads were "reamed by hand to a cylindrical shape"). There was still, however, a significant reduction in blood flow to the femoral head, and the authors advised caution in dealing with the retinacular vessels, particularly in cases of early or inflammatory arthritis, when vascular anastomoses may not be fully developed.

Thus it may be that the intraosseous circulation helps to sustain the femoral head, via metaphyseal arteries supplying blood to the femoral head through the epiphyseal scar [40,49–51].

Duncan and Shim conducted an experimental angiographic and histologic study to examine the blood supply to the femoral head after traumatic posterior dislocation of the hip in adult rabbits. They concluded that "the intraosseous epiphyseo-metaphyseal anastomoses across the obliterated growth plate minimize the effects of damage to the extraosseous epiphyseal nutrient system," and that "recovery was not dependent on a parallel return of an extraosseous route of blood supply to the femoral epiphysis" [52].

Yue et al. performed a cadaveric angiographic study, also involving posterior dislocation of the hip, to investigate its effects on the extraosseous and intraosseous blood supply to the femoral head and neck. It was found that changes in extraosseous blood flow did occur as a result of dislocation, and that the vessels most consistently affected were the common femoral and circumflex vessels. Significantly, however, changes in the extraosseous circulation did not consistently lead to changes in intraosseous blood flow. They postulated that this might be explained by the presence of collateral circulation [53].

In 1977, Arnoldi and Lempberg examined arterial blood supply to the femoral head after femoral neck fracture by measuring the intraosseous pressure in the bone marrow intraoperatively, after open reduction of the fracture. They postulated that "damage to the retinacular arteries might not be the single decisive factor" associated with AVN of the femoral head and concluded that "proper fracture reduction with extensive contact between the cancellous bone surfaces and stable fixation seemed to be more important, probably because they offer the best possibilities for re-establishment of transosseous blood flow across the fracture site." This again highlights the potential significance of the intraosseous circulation in helping to preserve femoral head viability when the extraosseous circulation is compromised [54].

Magnetic Resonance Angiographic Studies

The authors are currently undertaking a study using dynamic contrast enhanced magnetic resonance angiography (MRA) to look for any differences in extraosseous and intraosseous blood supply between patients with osteoarthritis and normal controls. Subjects ranged from normal or close to normal through moderate to severe osteoarthrosis. Using Gadovist contrast enhanced imaging, the hip is scanned to visualize the deep branch of the medial circumflex femoral artery (MCFA) posterior to the intertrochanteric neck region of the femur, with particular reference to the presence or absence of the trochanteric anastomosis at the posterior and superolateral aspect of the femoral neck. An initial study of 12 patients suggested that the extraosseous blood supply to the femoral head, as represented by the deep branch of the MCFA and the trochanteric anastomosis, might be reduced in severe osteoarthrosis compared with that of normal subjects (Figs. 9.4 and 9.5). A larger, observer-blinded study is in preparation to further explore this observation.

Discussion

The majority of resurfacing arthroplasties are performed using the posterior approach. This dissection would typically sacrifice the ascending branch of the MCFA. Reaming the femoral head also potentially disrupts the retinacular vessels, especially so if the superior neck is notched [20,39]. Thus, osteonecrosis of the femoral head should occur commonly, and as a consequence, failures due to femoral neck fracture and femoral loosening should be more prevalent. But the clinical outcome studies demonstrate femoral failure rates much less than predicted. How do we explain this?

Let's look at the evidence available.

The intraoperative flow studies tell us that the surgical dissection and femoral head preparation can significantly reduce the femoral head blood flow, at least for the duration of the operation.

The retrieval studies show that AVN may be associated with failures that were caused by femoral neck fractures and femoral loosening [16]. On the other hand, in retrievals of well-functioning femoral components that were revised *en passant*, evidence of AVN is uncommon [4,41–45]. The corollary of this is that, at worst, only about 1% to 2% of resurfacings develop AVN of sufficient severity to precipitate femoral component failure, given that the clinical outcome studies report femoral failure rates of up to 2%. The actual rate of AVN is almost certainly less than this because a number of fractures have a mechanical cause [14,17,51].

In a similar vein, nuclear imaging studies of well-functioning, asymptomatic femoral components demonstrate viability 1 to 2 years after surgery [47,48].

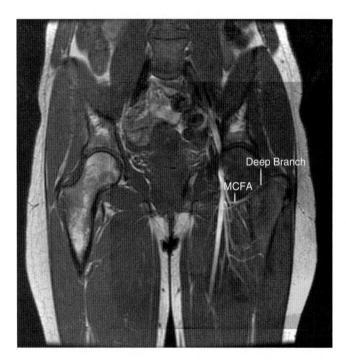

FIG. 9.4. Magnetic resonance angiography (MRA) reconstructed composite image, produced by fusing contrast (Gadovist) enhanced MRA series with coronal high-resolution proton density (PD) view of the hip, to illustrate the presence and position of blood vessels visualized on MRA in relation to the anatomy of the hip. Normal hip. The medical circumflex femoral artery (MCFA) is well demonstrated. (Note: CE-MRA series acquired in coronal plane after 25-second delay after bolus 7.5 mg Gadovist (Bayer Schering Pharma Ag, Germany). In normal MRA studies, the vessels are demonstrated by following them sequentially through the coronal plane images. For illustrative purposes only, the single-plane coronal PD image has been fused with a composite of the coronal angiography images to provide a representation of the vascular anatomy, as seen on MRA, relative to the hip joint).

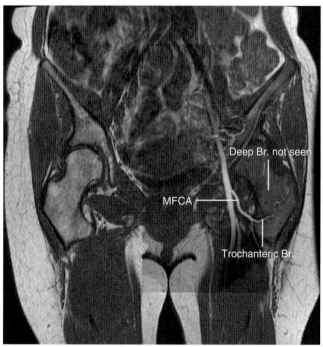

FIG. 9.5. Magnetic resonance angiography (MRA) reconstructed composite image as in Fig. 9.4. Severely osteoarthritic hip. The medial circumflex femoral artery (MCFA) and the trochanteric branch are demonstrated, but the deep branch of the MCFA is not seen.

One possible explanation for these observations is the presence of an additional blood supply to the femoral head. There is good evidence for the existence of an intraosseous blood supply. After resurfacing, the blood supply to the femoral head must improve to, or be maintained at, a level such that any consequent AVN is insufficient to compromise the durability of the femoral implant in all but a small percentage of patients.

This raises the possibility of an injury threshold for AVN. As the degree of compromise to the total femoral head blood supply increases, the risk of developing AVN increases and the possible extent of the AVN also increases. It may be that minor degrees of necrosis do not compromise implant stability, but as the extent of necrosis increases, eventually a point is reached where implant stability is compromised.

Freeman believed that the arthritic process stimulates the intraosseous blood supply [51]. Our MRA studies suggest a diminution of the extraosseous blood vessels in arthritic heads, although our numbers are too small as yet to draw definite conclusions. If Freeman is correct, then this process must occur over some time. Thus it could follow that if the resurfacing is carried out too early in the arthritic process, then the intraosseous blood supply may not have had time to fully develop, and these femoral heads might be at greater risk of developing critical AVN.

It seems that preservation of the extraosseous blood supply may be important in preventing those AVN-related femoral failures that comprise some of the 1% to 2% of resurfacings that fail at 4 to 6 years. The long-term clinical implications of sacrificing the extraosseous blood supply are unknown. Choice of surgical approach has not been shown to have a significant effect on clinical outcomes. The potential advantages of the vascular-sparing trochanteric osteotomy approach described by Beaulé [38] may only be fully realized when the problems of trochanteric nonunion are resolved. Even this approach, however, may not avoid damage to the retinacular vessels during reaming of the femoral head.

Thus if we are to improve our results by avoiding AVN-related failures, we must preserve the extraosseous blood supply, including the retinacular vessels; or somehow identify those patients in whom the intraosseous blood supply would be inadequate to maintain viability of the femoral head if the extraosseous blood supply were to be damaged. Once identified, these patients could be appraised preoperatively of the potentially increased risk of failure and counseled appropriately. At present, there is no reliable imaging or other technique to identify high-risk patients preoperatively. MRA holds some promise, but further investigation is required.

In conclusion, there is a theoretical concern about the femoral head blood supply in resurfacing procedures, and there is some experimental evidence that blood flow or tissue perfusion is decreased intraoperatively. However, we do not know what happens to the blood supply after the procedure. There is evidence from postoperative imaging and from some retrieval studies that significant AVN is not present in postoperative femoral heads. Clearly, more research is required to improve our understanding of the vascularity of femoral heads after resurfacing. Ultimately, however, in clinical practice, the rate of femoral failure in resurfacing procedures is low.

References

1. Howie DW, Cornish BL, Vernon-Roberts B. Resurfacing hip arthroplasty. Classification of loosening and the role of prosthetic wear particles. Clin Orthop Relat Res 1990;255:144–59.
2. Amstutz, HC. History of hip resurfacing. Joint Replacement Institute at Orthopaedic Hospital. Available at http://www.jri-oh.com/hipsurgery/Surface.asp.
3. Clarke Clarke IC, et al. Ultra-low wear rates for rigid-on-rigid bearings in total hip replacements. Proc Inst Mech Eng [H] 2000;214:331.
4. McMinn D, et al. Metal on metal surface replacement of the hip. Clin Orthop 1996;329S:S89.
5. Amstutz HC, Grigoris P. Metal on metal bearings in hip arthroplasty. Clin Orthop 1996;329S:S11.
6. Brown SR, et al. Long-term survival of McKee-Farrar total hip prostheses. Clin Orthop 2002;402:157.
7. Zahiri CA, et al. Lessons learned from loosening of the McKee-Farrar metal-on-metal total hip replacement. J Arthroplasty 1999;14:326.
8. Capello WN, et al. Analysis of revision surgery of resurfacing hip arthroplasty. Clin Orthop 1982;170:50.
9. Daniel J, Pynsent PB, McMinn DJ. Metal-on-metal resurfacing of the hip in patients under the age of 55 years with osteoarthritis. J Bone Joint Surg Br 2004;86:177–84.
10. Treacy RB, McBryde CW, Pynsent PB. Birmingham hip resurfacing arthroplasty. A minimum follow-up of five years. J Bone Joint Surg Br 2005;87:167–70.
11. Back DL, Dalziel R, Young D, Shimmin A. Early results of primary Birmingham hip resurfacings. An independent prospective study of the first 230 hips. J Bone Joint Surg Br 2005;87:324–9.
12. Shimmin AJ, Bare J, Back DL. Complications associated with hip resurfacing arthroplasty. Orthop Clin N Am 2005;36:187–93.
13. Cossey AJ, et al. The nonoperative management of periprosthetic fractures associated with the Birmingham hip resurfacing procedure. J Arthroplasty 2005;20:358–61.
14. Shimmin AJ, Back D. Femoral neck fractures following Birmingham hip resurfacing: a national review of 50 cases. J Bone Joint Surg Br 2005;87:463–4.
15. Amstutz HC, et al. Metal-on-metal hybrid surface arthroplasty: two to six-year follow-up study. J Bone Joint Surg Am 2004;86:28–39.
16. Little CP, et al. Osteonecrosis in retrieved femoral heads after failed resurfacing arthroplasty of the hip. J Bone Joint Surg Br 2005;87:320–3.
17. Markolf KL, Amstutz HC. Mechanical strength of the femur following resurfacing and conventional total hip replacement procedures. Clin Orthop 1980;147:170–80.
18. Jolley MN, Salvati EA, Brown GC. Early results and complications of surface replacement of the hip. J Bone Joint Surg Am 1982;64A:366–77.
19. Amstutz HC, Le Duff MJ, Campbell PA. Fracture of the neck of the femur after surface arthroplasty of the hip. J Bone Joint Surg Am 2004;86:1874–7.
20. Beaulé PE, Campbell PA, Hoke R, Dorey F. Notching of femoral neck during resurfacing arthroplasty of the hip a vascular study. J Bone Joint Surg Br 2006,88:35–9.

21. Beaulé PE, et al. Vascularity of the arthritic femoral head and hip resurfacing. J Bone Joint Surg Am 2006;88:85–96.

22. Steffen RT, et al. The effect of hip resurfacing on oxygen concentration m the femoral head. J Bone Joint Surg Br 2005;87:1468–74.

23. Nork SE, et al. Anatomic considerations for the choice of surgical approach for hip resurfacing arthroplasty. Orthop Clin North Am 2005;36:163–70, viii.

24. Khan A, et al. The effect of surgical approach on blood flow to the femoral head during resurfacing. J Bone Joint Surg Br 2007;89:21–4.

25. Ganz R, et al. Surgical dislocation of the adult hip: a technique with full access to the femoral head and acetabulum without the risk of avascular necrosis. J Bone Joint Surg Br 2001;83:1119.

26. Gautier E, et al. Anatomy of the medial femoral circumflex artery and its surgical implications. J Bone Joint Surg Br 2000;82:679–83.

27. Trueta J, Harrison MHM. The normal vascular anatomy of the femoral head in adult man. J Bone Joint Surg Br 1953;35:442.

28. Crock HV. The Blood Supply of the Lower Limb Bones in Man (Descriptive and Applied). E&S Livingstone, Edinburgh, 1967.

29. Sevitt S, Thompson RG. The distribution of arteries supplying the head and neck of the femur. J Bone Joint Surg Br 1965;47:560.

30. Lavigne M, et al. Distribution of vascular foramina around the femoral head and neck junction: relevance for conservative intracapsular procedures of the hip. Orthop Clin North Am 2005;36:171–6, viii.

31. Stulberg D. Surgical approaches for the performance of surface replacement arthroplasties. Orthop Clin N Am 1982;13:13–14.

32. Hedley AK. Technical considerations with surface replacement. Orthop Clin N Am 1982;13:747–60.

33. Hougaard K, Thomsen PB. Traumatic posterior dislocation of the hip-prognostic factors influencing the incidence of avascular necrosis of the femoral head. Arch Orthop Trauma Surg 1986;106:32–5.

34. Rodriguez-Merchan EC. Osteonecrosis of the femoral head after traumatic hip dislocation in the adult. Clin Orthop 2000;377:68.

35. Epstein HC. Traumatic dislocations of the hip. Clin Orthop 1973;92:116.

36. Brav EA. Traumatic dislocation of the hip. J Bone Joint Surg Am 1962;44:1115.

37. Yang RS, et al. Traumatic dislocation of the hip. Clin Orthop 1991;265:218–27.

38. Beaulé PE. A soft tissue sparing approach to surface arthroplasty of the hip. Oper Tech Orthop 2004;14:75–84.

39. Beaulé PE, Campbell P, Shim P. Femoral head blood flow during hip resurfacing. Clin Orthop Relat Res 2007;456:148–52.

40. Whiteside LA, Lange DR, Capello WN, Fraser B. The effects of surgical procedures on the blood supply to the femoral head. J Bone Joint Surg Am1983;65:1127–33.

41. Bradley GW, et al. Resurfacing arthroplasty. Femoral head viability. Clin Orthop 1987;220:137.

42. Amstutz HC. Letter to the editor. J Bone Joint Surg Am 1986;68:1464.

43. Nasser S, et al: Cementless total joint arthroplasty prostheses with titanium-alloy articular surfaces: a human retrieval analysis. Clin Orthop 1990;261:171.

44. Campbell P, Mirra J, Amstutz HC. Viability of femoral heads treated with resurfacing arthroplasty. J Arthroplasty 2000;15:120–2.

45. Howie DW, et al. The viability of the femoral head after resurfacing hip arthroplasty in humans. Clin Orthop 1993;291:171.

46. Campbell P, et al. A study of implant failure in metal-on-metal surface arthroplasties. Clin Orthop Relat Res 2006;453:35–46.

47. McMahon SJ, et al. Vascularity of the femoral head after Birmingham hip resurfacing. A technetium Tc 99 m bone scan/single photon emission computed tomography study. J Arthroplasty 2006;21:514–21.

48. Forrest N, et al Femoral head viability after birmingham resurfacing hip arthroplasty: assessment with use of [^{18}F] fluoride positron emission tomography. J Bone Joint Surg Am 2006;88:84–9.

49. Harrison MHM, Schajowicz F, Trueta J. Osteoarthritis of the hip: a study of the nature and evolution of the disease. J Bone Joint Surg Br 1953;35:598.

50. Freeman MAR. The complication of double-cup replacement of the hip. In: Ling RSM, ed. Complications of Total Hip Replacement. Churchill Livingstone, Edinburgh, 1994, p. 172.

51. Freeman MAR. Some Anatomical and mechanical considerations relevant to the surface replacement of the femoral head. Clin Orthop 1978;134:19.

52. Duncan CP, Shim SS. Blood supply of the head of the femur in traumatic hip dislocation: Surg Gynaecol Obstet 1977;144:185.

53. Yue JJ, et al. Posterior hip dislocations: a cadaveric angiographic study. J Orthop Trauma 1996;10:447.

54. Arnoldi CC, Lemperg RK. Fracture of the femoral neck. II. Relative importance of primary vascular damage and surgical procedure for the development of necrosis of the femoral head. Clin Orthop 1977;129:217.

10
Femoral Head Blood Supply Studies

Nobuhiko Sugano, Takashi Nishii, and Takehito Hananouchi

Metal on metal resurfacing hip arthroplasty (RHA) has been gaining in popularity due to its concept of bone conservation, stability, and expected longevity [1,2]. There are several papers describing good midterm results of metal on metal RHA, however, 0 to 2.4% of postoperative femoral neck fractures are reported to occur as a unique complication of RHA [1,3–7]. The cause of postoperative femoral neck fracture is controversial, and some literature indicates that mechanical factors such as varus alignment of the stem, notch formation at the supero-lateral femoral neck, and uncoverage of the cancellous bone are related to fractures [3,8]. Others suspect vascular impairment leading to osteonecrosis of the femoral head after resurfacing hip procedures as a causative factor [6,9,10] because it is well-known that osteonecrosis of the femoral head is a complication of traumatic hip dislocation, and RHA requires surgical dislocation that may sacrifice the extraosseous blood supply to the femoral head, including the deep branch of the medial femoral circumflex artery, especially through a posterior approach. In addition, some studies showed that the blood flow in the femoral head was significantly decreased to 20% to 50% of the baseline level by the femoral preparation or notch formation at the femoral neck [9–11]. These levels of decreased oxygen concentration measured with an electrode or decrease in blood flow measured with a laser Doppler flowmeter, however, may not be sufficient to induce large-area osteonecrosis because the incidence of osteonecrosis after RHA is extremely low in clinical studies. A study that measured the blood flow of the greater trochanter after total hip arthroplasty with a laser Doppler flowmeter also showed a 48% decrease in blood flow without inducing osteonecrosis of the greater trochanter [12].

Moreover, a technetium-99 m (Tc-99 m) bone scan/single photon emission computed tomography study proved the preserved femoral head vascularity after Birmingham Hip resurfacing (BHR) [13] and this suggests a substantial blood supply to the femoral head from the intraosseous vascular network. To monitor the blood flow in the femoral head during RHA through a posterior approach, we used a laser Doppler flowmeter in 12 cases that underwent RHA. A laser probe was inserted along a drill hole made from the vastus ridge into the femoral head under guidance of CT-based navigation (Fig. 10.1).

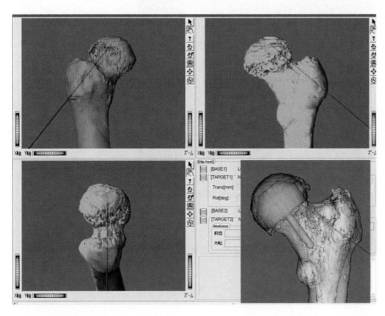

FIG. 10.1. A picture showing the location of a laser Doppler probe in the femoral head on the navigation screen.

The blood flow was measured before cutting the external rotators (T1), after cutting the external rotators (T2), after capsulotomy and dislocation (T3), after femoral head reaming (T4), and after cement fixation of the femoral component (T5). To calculate the blood flow ratio, each measured value at T2 to T5 was divided by the baseline value at T1. The average blood flow ratio decreased significantly after cutting the external rotators, and the average ratio at each timing was 0.74 (T2), 0.60 (T3), 0.46 (T4), and 0.41 (T5). No case showed, however, a zero level even after division of external rotators. In five cases, the laser probe could not be inserted after cementing. In the remaining seven cases, the blood flow was maintained even after cementing (T5) (Fig. 10.2).

It has been our further observation that after a posterior surgical approach, a ligature placed around the femoral neck thus compressing the retinacular vessels markedly diminishes the femoral head blood flow. (Data not shown, work in progress.)

To investigate further the effect of femoral head preparation and cementing on damage to the vascular network in the femoral head, we performed microangiography with micro–computed tomography (microCT) using 20 arthritic femoral head specimens resected at conventional total hip arthroplasty. A 24-gauge intravenous catheter was inserted into the blood vessels in the lateral or medial retinaculum of the femoral neck. Femoral head preparation for RHA was performed in a fashion similar to the clinical setting including cylindrical side reaming, cutting of the femoral head dome, and chamfer reaming. Eight

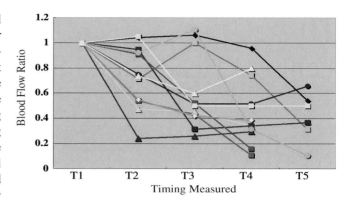

Fig. 10.2. A graph showing the blood flow ratio during the RHA procedure through a posterior approach. T1 to T5 represent the timing of the blood flow measurements; before cutting the external rotators (T1), after cutting the external rotators (T2), after capsulotomy and dislocation (T3), after femoral head reaming (T4), and after cement fixation of the femoral component (T5).

3.5-mm cement anchoring holes with a depth of 20mm were drilled in the femoral head. Bone cement was injected into a plastic replica of the BHR, and the implant was impacted into the prepared femoral head. After the bone cement cured, 50% barium sulfate suspension was infused into the lateral or medial retinacular artery.

Finally, all femoral heads were scanned using microCT (Fig. 10.3).

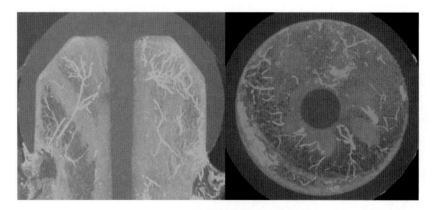

Fig. 10.3. Maximum intensity projection (MIP) images of the resurfaced femoral head with microangiography. A coronal MIP view (left) and an axial MIP view (right) through the center of the femoral head. Vascularity seemed to be maintained in the area without cement.

There was no significant difference in the number of arteries depicted in the femoral heads between the specimens with RHA and those without RHA.

Based on these observations, we think that the intraosseous vascular network blood supply to the femoral head is maintained after RHA even if division of the deep branch of the medial femoral circumflex artery occurs during a posterior approach. Based on our finding, we believe that femoral head preparation and cementing for RHA causes little damage to the vascular network of the femoral head.

References

1. Daniel J, Pynsent PB, McMinn DJ. Metal-on-metal resurfacing of the hip in patients under the age of 55 years with osteoarthritis. J Bone Joint Surg Br 2004;86:177–84.
2. Amstutz HC, Beaule PE, Dorey FJ, Le Duff MJ, Campbell PA, Gruen TA. Metal-on-metal hybrid surface arthroplasty: two to six-year follow-up study. J Bone Joint Surg Am 2004;86:28–39.
3. Amstutz HC, Campbell PA, Le Duff MJ. Fracture of the neck of the femur after surface arthroplasty of the hip. J Bone Joint Surg Am 2004;86:1874–7.
4. Beaule PE, Le Duff M, Campbell P, et al. Metal-on-metal surface arthroplasty with a cemented femoral component: a 7–10 year follow-up study. J Arthroplasty 2004;19(Suppl 3):17–22.
5. Shimmin AJ, Back D. Femoral neck fractures following Birmingham hip resurfacing: a national review of 50 cases. J Bone Joint Surg Br 2005;87:463–4.
6. Little CP, Ruiz AL, Harding IJ, McLardy-Smith P, Gundle R, Murray DW, Athanasou NA. Osteonecrosis in retrieved femoral heads after failed resurfacing arthroplasty of the hip. J Bone Joint Surg Br 2005;87:320–3.
7. Treacy RB, McBryde CW, Pynsent PB. Birmingham hip resurfacing arthroplasty: a minimum follow-up of five years. J Bone Joint Surg Br 2005;87:167–70.
8. Freeman MA. Some anatomical and mechanical considerations relevant to the surface replacement of the femoral head. Clin Orthop Relat Res 1978;134:19–24.
9. Steffen RT, Smith SR, Urban JP, McLardy-Smith P, Beard DJ, Gill HS, Murray DW. The effect of hip resurfacing on oxygen concentration in the femoral head. J Bone Joint Surg Br 2005;87:1468–74.
10. Beaule PE, Campbell PA, Hoke R, Dorey F. Notching of the femoral neck during resurfacing arthroplasty of the hip: a vascular study. J Bone Joint Surg Br 2006;88:35–9.
11. Beaulé PE, Campbell P, Shim P. Femoral head blood flow during hip resurfacing. Clin Orthop Relat Res. 2007;456:148–52.
12. ElMaraghy AW, Schemitsch EH, Waddell JP. Greater trochanteric blood flow during total hip arthroplasty using a posterior approach. Clin Orthop Relat Res 1999;363:151–7.
13. McMahon SJ, Young D, Ballok Z, Badaruddin BS, Larbpaiboonpong V, Hawdon G. Vascularity of the femoral head after Birmingham hip resurfacing. A technetium Tc 99 m bone scan/single photon emission computed tomography study. J Arthroplasty 2006;21:514–21.

11
Acetabular Bone Conservation

Joseph Daniel, Hena Ziaee, and Derek J.W. McMinn

It is an established fact that hip resurfacing is bone conserving on the femoral side. Dual energy X-ray absorptiometry (DEXA) studies discussed in Chapter 12 establish the fact that the conserved bone is also better preserved. Does this however come at the cost of excess acetabular bone loss?

The first publication [1] on this subject was based on a study in which hip resurfacings and hip replacements performed by a surgeon during the same time period were retrospectively studied in two cohorts of patients. The two groups were different in terms of their age groups and sex ratios, which makes the comparison unequal. The authors used the contralateral "normal" hip as a normalizing measure, which is also not an ideal solution. They found that the resurfacing needed greater bone resection, but their claims have been contested by other studies [2] and independent responses [3]. In the interests of safety in order to avoid notching, it is possible that an individual surgeon may err on the side of caution and upsize the femoral component resulting in greater bone removal from the acetabulum.

With resurfacing having been established as a successful procedure, it would be considered unethical to carry out a prospective randomized trial comparing resurfacing with a total hip replacement (THR) in young patients who are otherwise suitable for a resurfacing, although some centers have indeed conducted such a trial. Our patients would never enter such a trial. That leaves us with limited options to test the reality of whether a resurfacing procedure involves a greater or lesser acetabular bone loss.

The very nature of the osteoarthritic process makes patients with this condition an extremely heterogeneous group in terms of the pathoanatomy around the hip. The most rigorous matching of patient demographics, diagnoses, and other variables may not be sufficient to fully account for the variability in hip morphology between patients in one group undergoing hip replacement and patients in another group undergoing hip resurfacing.

Method

We have used a very simple practical technique to overcome this variability. We use the morphology of the hip being operated upon as a measure to calculate acetabular bone loss. We measure the existing femoral head and neck sizes during the Birmingham Hip Resurfacing (BHR) procedure. Because the femoral head has been located within that socket before the operation, these measurements give us an indication of the exact preoperative acetabular dimensions. Comparing that data with the cup size used in each individual case gives an estimate of the acetabular bone removed in order to implant the resurfacing.

We have been performing these measurements since 2001, and we present the results from 1606 BHRs performed with a regular socket. Out of a consecutive series of 1707 BHRs, 79 who needed a dysplasia BHR and 22 in whom it was impossible to get accurate measurements have been excluded.

After the hip is dislocated, the neck osteophytes are cleared to expose the true neck. The maximum and minimum head diameters and the maximum and minimum neck diameters are then measured with a Vernier caliper before proceeding with the rest of the operation. We have made these measurements a routine in every BHR case at our center. The rest of the operation proceeds as usual. The sizing of the femoral and acetabular components is made according to the existing dimensions and needs of the individual case irrespective of the measurements taken.

Observations

The shape of an arthritic femoral head is not spherical. It is generally expanded more in an oblique coronal plane than in the sagittal plane. An arthritic acetabulum also assumes this nonspherical shape to accommodate the femoral head.

Our measurements show that the mean cup size used almost matches the mean maximum head size measured (mean difference 0.3 mm) (Figs. 11.1–11.3). This is equivalent to a conversion of the nonhemispherical acetabulum into a hemisphere with a diameter that equals its original maximum diameter on average.

It has been our experience that in most patients, we are able to allow the acetabular dimensions to dictate the component size rather than be constrained by the femoral neck diameter.

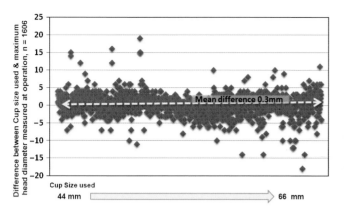

FIG. 11.1. Scattergraph showing the difference between cup size used and maximum femoral head diameter measured. The mean difference is 0.3 mm

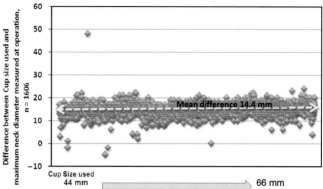

FIG. 11.3. Scattergraph showing the difference between cup size used and maximum neck diameter measured. The mean difference is 14.4 mm

In only the most exceptional cases did we have to overream the acetabulum in order to avoid a component that would notch the neck. It is our current practice that, should significant overreaming of the acetabulum be required in order to perform a BHR, then we would rather perform a total hip replacement than sacrifice valuable acetabular bone stock.

In earlier years, most models of resurfacings came in only 4-mm increments of femoral head sizes and 2-mm increments of cup sizes. This might have necessitated overreaming in a few patients with a large neck diameter and a relatively small acetabulum. With the availability of 2-mm increment head sizes, this difficulty has been overcome with the BHR.

There is also the concern about femoral impingement due to a poor femoral head-neck offset as a result of being too conservative on the acetabular side. It is certainly possible to upsize the femoral and acetabular components in order to give a greater head-neck offset and better range of movement without impingement. It is a delicate balance and a difficult decision, choosing between a marginal reduction in offset and sacrificing too much bone on the acetabular side.

Acetabular design and in particular the sector angle of articulation plays a part in impingement. By reducing the sector angle, the femoral neck is allowed a greater range of motion for a given head-neck ratio. However, too small a sector angle creates another problem. It reduces peripheral cover for the femoral head and is less forgiving of minor surgical error in device implantation. It is well-known that there is always a degree of variability in component placement at operation, and decreasing the sector angle reduces the allowance available for this margin of error. A small increase in the angle of inclination can lead to edge wear and device failure. On the basis of a large number of BHRs performed in young patients with demanding physical activities, it can be said with confidence that the acetabular component of the BHR is well-designed to allow the unavoidable small variability in surgical component placement without causing femoral neck impingement.

The strength of our assessment of acetabular bone loss lies in the large number of patients studied. By using the patient's own dimensions, the problem of individual variability is overcome, and in conclusion it can be said that the BHR does not lead to excess acetabular bone loss, at least as practiced at our center.

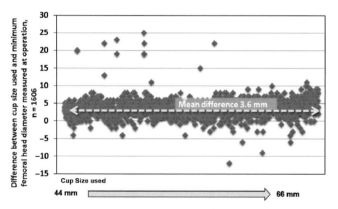

FIG. 11.2. Scattergraph showing the difference between cup size used and minimum femoral head diameter measured. The mean difference is 3.6 mm

References

1. Loughead JM, Starks I, Chesney D, Matthews JN, McCaskie AW, Holland JP. Removal of acetabular bone in resurfacing arthroplasty of the hip: a comparison with hybrid total hip arthroplasty. J Bone Joint Surg Br 2006;88:31–4.
2. Venditioli PA, Lavigne M, Girard J, Roy AG. A randomised study comparing resection of acetabular bone at resurfacing and total hip replacement. J Bone Joint Surg Br 2006;88:997–1002.
3. Muirhead-Allwood SK, Patel C, Mohandas P. Removal of acetabular bone in resurfacing arthroplasty of the hip. J Bone Joint Surg Br 2006;88:1117; author reply 1117.

12
Femoral DEXA Studies in Hip Arthroplasty

Nobuhiko Sugano

Proximal bone resorption around femoral stems is commonly seen after cementless total hip arthroplasty. The reasons for this phenomenon include stress shielding (bone remodeling) and an inflammatory reaction to small particles produced by the various wear modes (bone resorption). The remodeling patterns are thought to be affected by several factors. These include patient-related factors, such as gender, age, initial femoral bone stock, and patient activity, as well as prosthesis-related factors, such as the type of fixation, stem length, stiffness, design, the extent of the coating area, and the method of femoral bone preparation [1–6]. Even though recent improvements in the quality of bearing materials may reduce the influence of bone resorption due to wear particles, femoral bone atrophy under mechanical unloading above the lesser trochanter level is still inevitable in most of the total hip systems. Loss of periprosthetic bone may predispose the site to periprosthetic fracture, reduce prosthetic stability, and make revision difficult. Therefore, minimizing proximal bone loss after hip replacement is desirable.

Maintenance of proximal femoral bone quality requires maintenance of physiologic load transfer to the proximal femur [7,8]. Among the various types of hip prosthesis, hip surface replacement is the most efficient way to maintain physiologic load on the proximal femur. To understand the strain-adaptive bone remodeling after hip replacement, the finite element method (FEM) is often used. Although some FEM studies suggest that proximal femoral stresses and strains after hip resurfacing are nonphysiologic and stress shielding may occur in the femoral head within the component [9–12], the strain energy density in the medial femoral neck area is quite similar to that of the intact femurs [13,14]. To prove these simulation studies, monitoring the femoral bone mineral density (BMD) after total hip arthroplasty using a radiologic method is of primary importance.

Serial plain radiographs can provide useful information on periprosthetic bone remodeling (Fig. 12.1), and grading of stress shielding is possible by using Engh's method [15].

This radiographic evaluation of the periprosthetic BMD by human eyes, however, is not so sensitive to small changes in BMD and is not quantitative. Dual-energy x-ray absorptiometry (DEXA) is a precise method for quantifying bone mass and small changes in BMD around femoral implants after total hip arthroplasty.

We have studied BMD changes in the femur with various types of implants using DEXA [4–6,16,17]. The BMD was measured by DEXA (DPX-L; Lunar, Madison, WI, USA) at 3 weeks and then at 6, 12, and 24 months after surgery. The software (Orthopaedic Software Package; Lunar) used in our study was designed to measure periprosthetic bone mineral content and density in the seven Gruen zones (Fig. 12.2).

We used the BMD at 3 weeks postoperatively for the reference baseline, and the BMD ratio of each zone was calculated as a percentage of the value obtained 3 weeks after the operation. It has been generally recognized that proximal femoral BMD decreases after conventional cementless THA and that considerable bone remodeling occurs in the first postoperative year [4]. One year after cementless THA using a stem made of CoCr alloy, the BMD ratio has been reported to be 73% to 76% in zone 1 and 75% to 80% in zone 7. One year after using a femoral component made of Ti alloy, which has a lower stiffness than CoCr alloy, the BMD ratio has been reported to be 77% to 90% in zone 1 and 75% to 88% in zone 7. Table 12.1 summarizes our DEXA study results of the femoral BMD ratios in the seven Gruen zones at 1 year after surgery using various types of implants. Decrease in the BMD ratio is seen even in the area below the lesser trochanter such as zone 2 and zone 6. On the other hand, our DEXA results of BHR for which a standard stem template was used to create Gruen zones (Fig. 12.3A) showed minimum BMD loss in zone 1, and interestingly, we observed an increased BMD in zone 7, which was never seen in conventional total hip arthroplasty (Table 12.1).

We also looked at the BMD changes in the femoral neck area after BHR more in detail by dividing the femoral neck area around the stem into four zones (Fig. 12.3B). BMD ratio at 1 year after resurfacing was 105% in zone L1, 101% in zone L2, 105% in zone M2, and 110% in zone

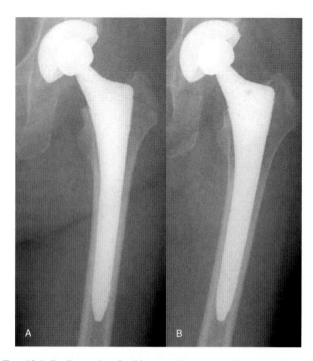

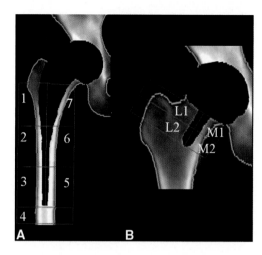

FIG. 12.3 (A) DEXA image showing the template of a standard stem superimposed on the bones treated with the BHR system to allow similar Gruen zones. (B) DEXA image showing the four locations L1, L2, M1, and M2 to evaluate BMD changes around the short stem of the BHR components.

FIG. 12.1. Radiographs of a 66-year-old woman with osteoarthritis at (A) 3 weeks and (B) 1 year after cementless THA using a Versys FM Taper stem. When these two radiographs are compared, it is apparent that the radiodensity of the proximal medial cortex up to 1 cm below the lesser trochanter showed atrophy at 1 year after surgery.

TABLE 12.1. DEXA study results of the femoral BMD ratios in the seven Gruen zones at 1 year after surgery using various types of implants

Type of implant	Number of implants examined	Femoral BMD ratios						
		Zone 1	Zone 2	Zone 3	Zone 4	Zone 5	Zone 6	Zone 7
Lübeck (CoCr)	32	76	87	91	89	88	84	79
Axcel (Ti6Al4V)	13	90	97	102	93	102	99	88
Versys FMT (Ti6Al4V)	58	77	90	101	95	99	96	75
BHR	13	96	100	96	101	103	96	105

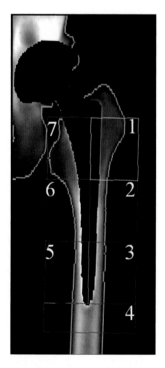

FIG. 12.2. The location of the seven Gruen zones, defined according to the length of the stem.

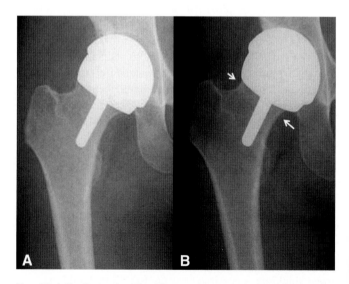

FIG. 12.4. Radiographs of a 45-year-old woman with osteoarthritis at (A) 3 weeks and (B) 1 year after BHR. Cortical thickening of the superolateral and medial femoral neck is seen (arrows).

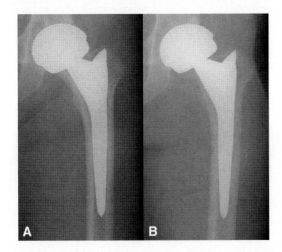

FIG. 12.5. Radiographs of a 76-year-old woman with osteoarthritis at (A) 3 weeks and (B) 1 year after cementless THA using a Freeman HA-coated cementless stem. The femoral neck was preserved by fenestration of the neck saddle and reposition of the fragment after the stem insertion. Resorption of the femoral neck at 1 year after surgery is obvious.

M1, respectively. These mean that BMD of the medial and superolateral femoral neck areas increase after resurfacing (Fig. 12.4). This phenomenon was apparent even on plain radiographs when femoral neck remodeling after Birmingham Hip Resurfacing (BHR) was observed. In contrast, after insertion of the Freeman stem using a femoral neck retention technique, the femoral neck has resorbed 1 year later (Fig. 12.5) [17].

We conclude that the BHR system transfers load to the proximal femur in a more physiologic manner than long-stem devices, and that it prevents stress shielding and preserves the bone stock of the proximal femur.

References

1. Engh CA, Bobyn JD. The influence of stem size and extent of porous coating on femoral bone resorption after primary cementless hip arthroplasty. Clin Orthop Relat Res 1988;231:7.
2. Engh CA Jr, Sychterz C, Engh C Sr. Factors affecting femoral bone remodeling after cementless total hip arthroplasty. J Arthroplasty 1999;14:637.
3. Pritchett JW. Femoral bone loss following hip replacement. A comparative study. Clin Orthop Relat Res 1995;314:156.
4. Nishii T, Sugano N, Masuhara K, Shibuya T, Ochi T, Tamura S. Longitudinal evaluation of time related bone remodeling after cementless total hip arthroplasty. Clin Orthop Relat Res 1997;339:121.
5. Yamaguchi K, Masuhara K, Ohzono K, Sugano N, Nishii T, Ochi T. Evaluation of periprosthetic bone-remodeling after cementless total hip arthroplasty. The influence of the extent of porous coating. J Bone Joint Surg Am 2000;82:1426.
6. Hananouchi T, Sugano N, Nishii T, Nakamura N, Miki H, Kakimoto A, Yamamura M, Yoshikawa H. Effect of robotic milling on periprosthetic bone remodeling. J Orthop Res 2007;25:1062–9.
7. Huiskes R, Weinans H, Grootenboer HJ, Dalstra M, Fudala B, Slooff TJ. Adaptive bone-remodeling theory applied to prosthetic-design analysis. J Biomech 1987;20:1135–50.
8. Huiskes R. The various stress patterns of press-fit, ingrown, and cemented femoral stems. Clin Orthop Relat Res 1990;261:27–38.
9. Huiskes R, Strens PH, van Heck J, Slooff TJ. Interface stresses in the resurfaced hip. Finite element analysis of load transmission in the femoral head. Acta Orthop Scand 1985;56:474–8.
10. Watanabe Y, Shiba N, Matsuo S, Higuchi F, Tagawa Y, Inoue A. Biomechanical study of the resurfacing hip arthroplasty: finite element analysis of the femoral component. J Arthroplasty 2000;15:505–11.
11. Ong KL, Kurtz SM, Manley MT, Rushton N, Mohammed NA, Field RE. Biomechanics of the Birmingham hip resurfacing arthroplasty. J Bone Joint Surg Br 2006;88:1110–5.
12. Long JP, Bartel DL. Surgical variables affect the mechanics of a hip resurfacing system. Clin Orthop Relat Res 2006;453:115–22.
13. Little JP, Taddei F, Viceconti M, Murray DW, Gill HS. Changes in femur stress after hip resurfacing arthroplasty: Response to physiological loads. Clin Biomech (Bristol, Avon) 2007;22:440–8.
14. Radcliffe IA, Taylor M. Investigation into the effect of varus-valgus orientation on load transfer in the resurfaced femoral head: a multi-femur finite element analysis. Clin Biomech (Bristol, Avon) 2007;22:780–6.
15. Engh CA, Bobyn JD, Glassman AH. Porous-coated hip replacement. The factors governing bone ingrowth, stress shielding, and clinical results. J Bone Joint Surg Br 1987;69:45–55.
16. Kishida Y, Sugano N, Nishii T, Miki H, Yamaguchi K, Yoshikawa H. Preservation of the bone mineral density of the femur after surface replacement of the hip. J Bone Joint Surg Br 2004;86:185–9.
17. Hayaishi Y, Miki H, Nishii T, Hananouchi T, Yoshikawa H, Sugano N. Proximal femoral bone mineral density after resurfacing THA and after standard stem-type cementless THA, both having similar neck preservation and the same articulation type. J Arthroplasty (in press).

13
Metal Ions

Joseph Daniel and Hena Ziaee

Cobalt-Chrome Alloy

Cobalt-chrome alloy has been used in hip arthroplasty devices since 1938 when Smith-Petersen started using it as Vitallium in his "mould arthroplasty" [1]. In addition to several other trace elements, the alloy consists of three main constituents—cobalt, chromium, and molybdenum—all of which belong to the transition element (Fig. 13.1) series. Transition elements have several unpaired electrons in their outer shells that can be shared between nuclei to form a lattice structure at room temperature. The greater this electron sharing, the stronger is the metal. They therefore tend to have high density and melting points and excellent strength. These unpaired electrons also mean that they can potentially exist in several oxidation states (valencies) and enter into complex molecular structures (See Table 13.1). In nature, they are found not in their elemental ground state but in the lower-energy oxidized states as ores.

Cobalt is a hard metal, and is used in several corrosion-resistant and wear-resistant applications including superalloys in gas turbines, aircraft engines, high-speed steels, and cutting tools. In industry, cobalt exposure occurs in occupations such as the pottery industry and in hard-metal industries (where tungsten carbide is used along with nickel and cobalt matrices).

Chromium is a steel-gray, lustrous, hard metal. When exposed to the atmosphere, it forms a chromium oxide passivating layer on the surface that prevents corrosion and gives it a shiny surface. Its corrosion-resistance is one of its main uses in the CoCr alloy as in several other applications. For the same reason, it is used in stainless steel and chrome plating. Its compounds are also used in tanning leather.

Metal Ions

Metal on metal (MM) bearings used in arthroplasty devices are subject to wear and corrosion resulting in the release of insoluble particles and soluble metal ions. Conventional replacements have also been shown to release metal from metal stems and socket carriages. Metal ions are soluble and are cleared into the bloodstream subsequently being excreted in the urine. They have the potential to cause systemic effects. Metal particles are insoluble and collect in the joint fluid and periarticular tissues. Some particles are phagocytosed by macrophages and giant cells where intracellular chemicals such as peroxides and chlorides and organelles such as lysosomes have the potential to enzymatically degrade the particles partially into soluble metal ions. Additionally, metal particles are transported through the lymphatic system and are deposited in the regional lymph nodes, liver, and spleen.

Biochemical Role of Cobalt, Chromium, and Molybdenum

Cobalt, chromium, and molybdenum are the main constituents (Figs. 13.2–13.5) of the alloys used in MM bearings. All of these are essential trace elements (Fig. 13.5) for humans and are found in the water supply and food. Measurable metal ion levels are present in the blood and urine of subjects with no artificial metal devices in the body.

Cobalt is the only metallic element in cyanocobalamin (Fig. 13.4) (vitamin B_{12}; $C_{63}H_{88}CoN_{14}O_{14}P$, molecular mass 1355.37 g/mol) and is as critical to its function as iron is to hemoglobin. Methionyl aminopeptidase, an enzyme involved in intracellular functional regulation and protein turnover, also contains cobalt ions. Several other roles of cobalt have been identified in the study of biochemical cofactors in non-human experiments.

Until recently, elemental cobalt was administered as a supplement for patients with anemia. Excessive administration of cobalt is believed to produce goiter. Cobalt-induced cardiomyopathy has been described in the context of the Quebec Beer-Drinkers' Disease. In the 1960s in some parts of North America and Belgium, it was reported that some brewers added cobalt to beer to improve its foaming quality. A percentage of those who consumed large quantities of this beer developed cardiomyopathy 4 to 8 weeks later [2].

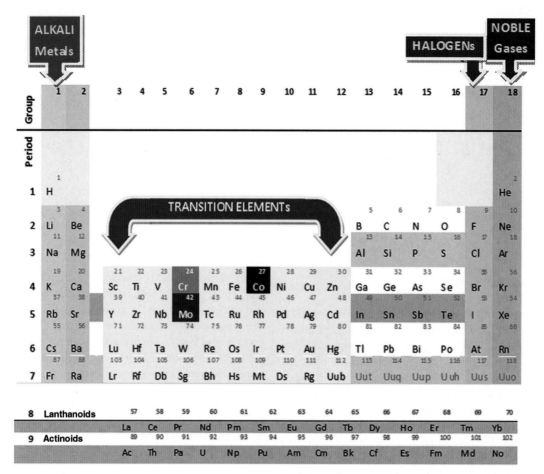

FIG. 13.1. Cobalt (Co), chromium (Cr), and molybdenum (Mo), and, in fact, most elements we commonly call metals, belong to the broad group called transition elements. "What are transition elements?" The chemical nature of elements and their physical properties depend on their electron configurations and especially whether there are any unfilled electron slots in their orbits. For instance, the noble gases on the right-hand side of the Periodic Table have their electron shells completely filled and are therefore not in a hurry to react with any element. The halogens to their left are short of just one electron and are therefore highly reactive. Likewise the alkali metals on the extreme left-hand side have just one excess electron and are therefore trying to get rid of that all the time and are quick to react. Each successive cell to the right along each row has another electron added to it. The transition elements therefore have several unpaired (free) electrons and therefore can react in different ways (different valencies) and form complex structures. They can also share these free electrons in a lattice and therefore form strong, dense structures. We exploit these characteristics to produce strong structural materials and use them in different applications including artificial joints.

TABLE 13.1. Conversion factors and a few key properties of cobalt and chromium

	Chromium	Cobalt
Atomic number	24	27
Atomic mass number	52	59
Density at room temp (g/cm³)	7.15	8.9
Unpaired electrons in the outer shells	6	3
Oxidation states (valencies)	2, 3, 6 (3 is most stable)	2, 3
Conversion factor for units of concentration in blood, urine, etc.		
1 mole	51.9961 g	58.9332 g
1 nmol/L =	0.052 ppb or µg/L or ng/mL	0.059 ppb or µg/L or ng/mL

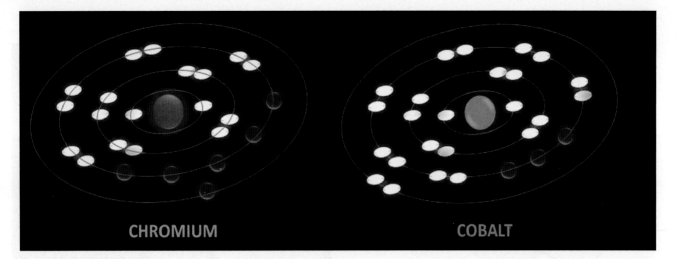

CHROMIUM COBALT

Fig. 13.2. Chromium has six unpaired electrons (shown in red) with which it can form compounds in several oxidation states, the most common being the trivalent and hexavalent states. Hexavalent chromium compounds are formed under high-energy situations such as welding and chrome plating. Strong chemicals, such as chromic acid used in tanning, also release hexavalent chromium. The relatively low-energy reactions involved during *in vivo* metal release from arthroplasty devices generate predominately trivalent chromium. The small amounts of hexavalent chromium released in the body are also believed to be subsequently reduced to trivalent chromium. Trivalent chromium is nontoxic and noncarcinogenic. Hexavalent chromium is classed as a potential carcinogen with a threshold effect. Cobalt has three unpaired electrons and has valencies of 2 and 3. Cobalt is noncarcinogenic in humans.

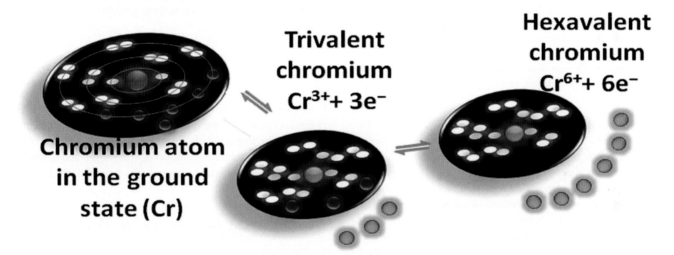

Trivalent chromium $Cr^{3+} + 3e^-$

Hexavalent chromium $Cr^{6+} + 6e^-$

Chromium atom in the ground state (Cr)

Fig. 13.3. "What are ions?" "When we speak of cobalt and chromium in blood, serum, or urine, do they exist as atoms, ions, or particles?" These are some questions that are frequently asked by many budding orthopedic surgeons.

Metal particles are not soluble and therefore stay suspended in the joint fluid and become deposited in the tissues around or are transported through the lymphatic system. They are also subject to corrosion and ionization. As a rule, only dissolved metal in the form of metal ions gains free entrance into the systemic circulation.

An ion is a charged particle. An atom acquires a positive charge when it loses electrons (oxidation) or a negative charge when it gains extra electrons (reduction) from a neighboring atom. For instance, chromium tends to easily give up some or all of its unpaired electrons and become positively charged. This oxidized state is the lower-energy state for chromium and for many other metals (see also chapter 5).

When metallic atoms are dissolved in solution, they readily find their level (like fluids) and reach the lowest energy level (become oxidized or give up electrons) and therefore become charged. Furthermore, in the body fluids they easily find friendly neighbors that are willing to readily accept these spare electrons. For instance oxygen and water together take up these electrons (e^-) and produce hydroxyl $[OH]^-$ ions:

$$O_2 + 2H_2O + 4e^- \rightarrow 4[OH]^-$$

Therefore, when these metals are in a state of solution, they tend to slide into the ionic state rather than stay at the higher unionized or ground state. That is the reason we speak of metal *ion* levels in blood or serum.

Sometimes, instead of losing or gaining electrons, atoms share electrons to form covalent bonds. These can be single, double, triple, or quadruple bonds depending on the number of electron pairs shared. In fact chromium, and only chromium of all the known elements, has been shown to enter into a quintuple bond (six pairs of electrons shared between two atoms of chromium).

These multiple, unpaired electrons give metals the ability to enter into complex molecular structures and thereby function as excellent catalysts to accelerate reactions of other elements. The cellular biochemical apparatus exploits this ability of metals and utilizes them in various coenzymes that have catalytic roles. That is the reason these metals are essential for metabolic functions.

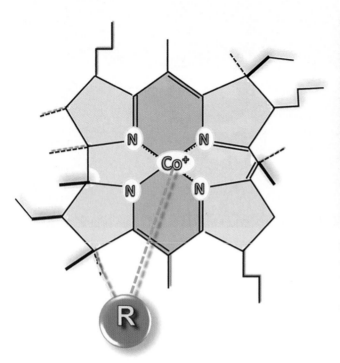

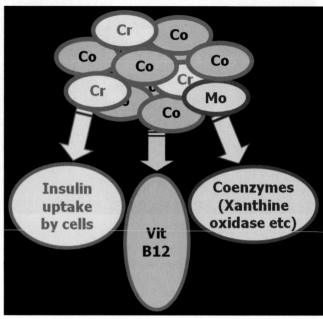

FIG. 13.5. Some of the biological roles of cobalt, chromium, and molybdenum. In addition, all of them participate in several coenzyme systems.

FIG. 13.4. Cobalt (Co) occupies the central position in the corrin ring of cobalamin, which is schematically depicted here. The radical (R, which may be CN, OH, CH_3, or deoxyadenosyl) attached to cobalt decides the type of cobalamin. (i.e., cyano, hydroxyl, methyl, or deoxyadenosyl cobalamin, etc.)

The estimated doses of cobalt in these drinks are many times larger than the exposure risks from MM bearings. However, the cobalt doses in alcohol were low in comparison with the therapeutic doses of cobalt used as a hematinic in the past, and the hematinic use of cobalt has not been implicated as a source of heart disease. Thus it appears that the combination of cobalt and *substantial* amounts of alcohol were needed for the occurrence of this condition [2].

Molybdenum is essential as a cofactor for a number of enzymes involved in amino acid metabolism such as sulfite oxidase, which is necessary for the metabolism of cysteine, and aldehyde oxidase and xanthine oxidase, which process hydroxylation reactions of drugs and toxins and assist in the breakdown of nucleotides to form uric acid. Deficiencies of the above coenzymes occur as part of rare inherited inborn errors of metabolism. The recommended daily allowance of molybdenum in a healthy adult is 45 µg. Dietary deficiency is almost unknown except in those who are on total parenteral nutrition.

Chromium is essential for all the energy functions of the cell. It is part of the cellular structure that facilitates cells to respond to insulin and allows the entry of glucose. Chromium deficiency has been reported in patients on long-term parenteral nutrition. They develop impaired cellular glucose uptake and do not respond even to very high doses of insulin but respond well to chromium supplementation. Because chromium appears to potentiate the action of insulin and because chromium deficiency results in disturbed glucose tolerance, chromium insufficiency has been hypothesized to be a possible contributing factor in the development of type 2 diabetes. The recommended daily allowance in a healthy adult is 25 µg. Its utilization is increased in those who exercise regularly.

In the tissues, chromium exists in mainly two valencies, 3 and 6. The essential cellular functions of chromium are carried out in its trivalent form. The International Atomic Energy Agency (IAEA) classifies trivalent chromium as a human noncarcinogen and hexavalent chromium as a potential carcinogen with a threshold effect.

Bearing Wear *In Vitro* and *In Vivo*

In Vitro Wear Measurements

Hip function simulators described in Chapter 4 are useful for preclinical testing of an arthroplasty device. Although much effort is made to make the loads and lubricants in some ways similar to *in vivo* conditions, the wide variation of real-life loads in young and active patients are unlikely to be fully replicated in any simulator. Therefore, it is possible that a device that may eventually prove wear-prone in real life may not be detected by the predictable regimens of the simulators. However, they do provide an accelerated means of bench-testing device wear in a relatively short time frame. Hip simulator studies of MM bearings show that these bearings go through a phase of increased wear (5 to 10 µm linear wear) during the first 500,000 to 1 million cycles (Mcyc). During this running-in phase, the bearing surfaces tend to become modified (Fig. 13.6) resulting in an improvement in their lubrication regime as seen from the reduced friction factors in Fig. 13.7.

Subsequently, they enter into a reduced steady-state wear rate of around a micrometer per million cycles linear wear (more than an order of magnitude lower compared with the run-in wear) and

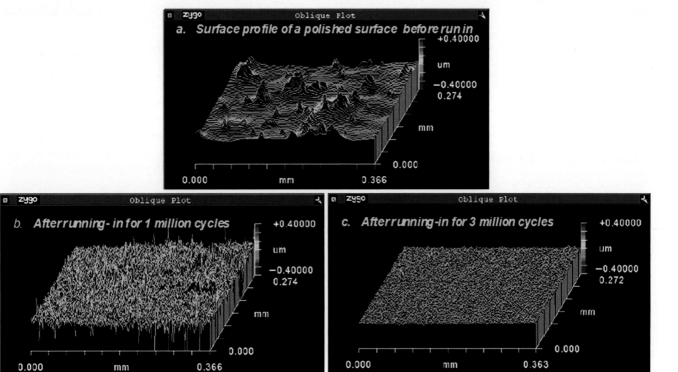

FIG. 13.6. Surface profiles of a Birmingham Hip Resurfacing before and after running-in, measured using the Zygo NewView 100 noncontacting interference profilometer. Ten measurements were taken on the contact area of each component. Representative measurements are shown here. The asperities seen protruding beyond the surface before run-in are removed through wear, making the surface progressively smoother. The surface also assumes a negative profile with troughs, known to fill with lubricant and assist lubrication. Figures 13.6 to 13.8 relate to the different results (surface profiles, friction, and linear wear) during a single wear simulator experiment. (Figure modified from Vassiliou K, Elfick A, Scholes S, Unsworth A. The effect of 'running-in' on the tribology and surface morphology of metal-on-metal BHR device in simulator studies. Proc I Mech E Part H J Eng Med 2006;220:269–77, with kind permission of Peter Williams, Academic Director, Professional Engineering Publishing.)

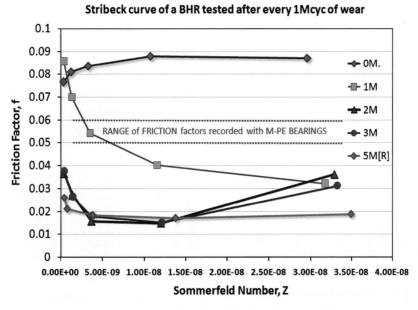

FIG. 13.7. Friction measurements made on a Durham Hip Function Friction Simulator. The Stribeck curves pertain to one of the BHRs after successive million cycle runs on the Durham Wear Simulator in the experiment mentioned earlier. They show that bearing friction progressively decreases and reaches levels below those recorded for metal-polyethylene bearings in the same laboratory using the same equipment and lubricants. After 2 million cycles, the friction plots are in the region that would apply to fluid film lubrication and demonstrate that large-diameter MM bearings can be shown to enter into this mode after the initial running-in period. (Figure modified from Vassiliou K, Elfick A, Scholes S, Unsworth A. The effect of 'running-in' on the tribology and surface morphology of metal-on-metal BHR device in simulator studies. Proc I Mech E Part H J Eng Med 2006;220:269–77, with kind permission of Peter Williams, Academic Director, Professional Engineering Publishing.)

around 2 mg/Mcyc (Figs. 13.8 and 13.9). It is estimated that an average individual logs around 1 to 2 million walking cycles a year. Therefore, it can be safely assumed that 1 million cycles in a hip simulator corresponds with 6 months to 1 year of normal hip use. Young and active patients log many more walking cycles per year. Wear measurements performed on metal components retrieved from revisions or postmortem specimens also confirm this extremely low long-term wear rate.

In Vivo Wear Measurement

Hip simulator data provides a good estimate of *in vitro* bearing wear, but how can we measure *in vivo* bearing wear? Do we have a good surrogate measure of this process? In end-stage renal failure, serum cobalt levels increase 100-fold compared with the levels in patients with normal renal competence [3]. The fact that such high levels are not seen in renal-competent patients leads us to the conclusion that there is no cumulative buildup of

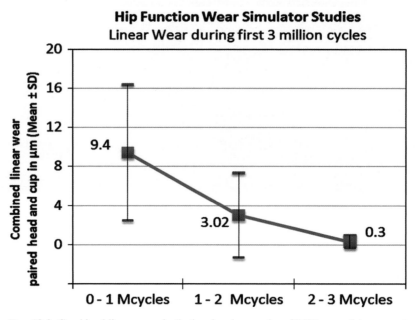

FIG. 13.8. Combined linear wear in the head and cup pairs of BHRs, n = 5 (measured using a coordinate measuring machine and roundness assessment; see Chapter 3) after each 10⁶ cycles on the Durham Mark I wear simulator. Linear wear rate starts higher but progressively decreases thereafter.

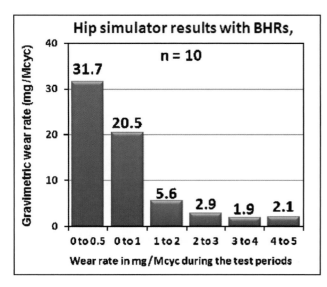

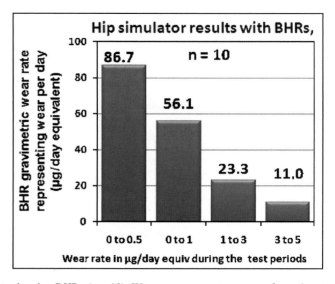

FIG. 13.9. Gravimetric wear rates (mg per Mcyc) with 50-mm-diameter bearing BHRs (n = 10). Wear measurements were performed up to 5 million cycles on a Prosim Wear Simulator using diluted calf serum as the lubricant. (Data provided by courtesy of Kamali et al., S & N Implant Development Centre, UK). The total wear between 0 and 0.5 Mcyc was doubled to obtain the (per Mcyc) wear rate up to that point. The wear rates at subsequent points are the actual readings at the respective stages of the experiment. The results show that the wear in a simulator falls by more than an order of magnitude in the later wear cycles compared with the earlier cycles. The wear per day equivalent is calculated by dividing the total wear during the respective time interval by 365.

metal in the system and that an equilibrium is established between metal release from the bearing and metal clearance in urine. Hence the daily urinary output of metal ions is almost equal to the metal generated from the device. This allows urinary metal output to be used as a measure of *in vivo* bearing wear.

There is an increase in the urinary metal output in patients with a MM bearing in the early months as predicted by hip simulator results. After the first year, there is a relative fall in the output as seen from Fig. 13.10. However, the reduction of metal ion output in subsequent years is not as dramatic as would be expected given the reduction of wear rates seen in hip simulators (Fig. 13.9).

Source of Metal Ions *In Vivo*

How do we reconcile the simulator finding of negligible wear after early run-in phase and the clinical observation that metal ion levels do not drop down to nearly normal after the running-in period? In real life, does metal wear continue to occur throughout the life of the bearing as depicted in the model in Fig. 13.11A or do the bearings enter into fluid film lubrication after the initial run-in leading to negligible wear thereafter as predicted by hip simulators? In order to explain the discrepancy between *in vitro* simulator tests and *in vivo* observations, it has been hypothesized by some authors that the total metal

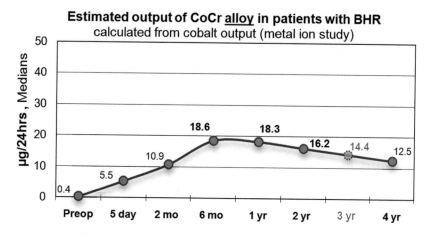

Fig. 13.10. The *in vivo* alloy output is calculated from the daily output of cobalt (cobalt content of alloy is ~65%) in the longitudinal study (ref. Fig. 13.22). The three-year output shown above is an average of the 2 and 4-year outputs. since we obtained 1, 2 and 4-year collections only. All other readings shown are actual measurements.

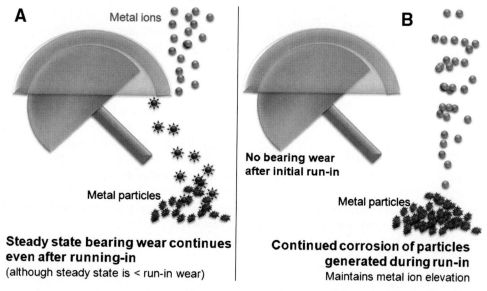

Fig. 13.11. Two models have been described for *in vivo* metal ion generation during the life of a MM bearing. In model A, the bearing continues to wear throughout its life, and real-time bearing wear is responsible for elevated metal ions. In model B, wear occurs only during initial run-in, and subsequent metal ion elevation is from passive corrosion of accumulated run-in wear particles.

wear burden that a patient is going to receive from a MM bearing is generated within the early run-in period and that continued elevation of metal levels in later years occurs due to the slow degradation/corrosion of the particles released during run-in as shown in Fig. 13.11B.

In order to test this hypothesis, we measured metal ion release in patients who have had MM bearings that were subsequently revised to a non-MM bearing. We know that particle dissemination and accumulation occur in the periarticular tissues and also in distant sites such as paraaortic lymph nodes as well as liver and spleen. If corrosion of accumulated wear particles were to be the main source of metal ions *in vivo*, then corrosion of disseminated particles should have continued even after removal of the MM joint, resulting in persistent elevation of metal levels after revision. However, contrary to that expectation, in our small cohort of patients, metal release in these patients fell sharply after removal of the MM bearing. This strongly suggests that continued metal ion elevation in patients with well-functioning implants is maintained by release from continued wear from the bearing, even after the initial run-in period, and not from corrosion of accumulated wear particles released during run-in.

This has important implications. If run-in wear is the only factor to be reckoned with, then the wear properties of the bearing do not matter at all. Once self-polishing has occurred and running-in has created the correct environment for the establishment of fluid film lubrication, all bearings would behave in the same way. However, if bearing wear truly occurs throughout the period of usage of the bearing, then low-wear bearings are likely to perform better in the long-run and therefore there is a need to continue research to improve bearing wear performance.

How then do we reconcile this discrepancy—the markedly different trends of metal loss in simulator studies and daily metal ion release in clinical studies? As mentioned in Chapter 4, it is possible for a high-wear bearing to be protected from wear in a simulator through the influence of several factors including the loading regime, amplitude of oscillation, lubricant used, and so forth. Do hip simulators then really not reflect clinical wear rates? We look at the answers to these questions in the following section.

Metal Particle Versus Metal Ion Release *In Vivo*

In an attempt to understand the dynamics of metal release from MM bearings, we drew up a balance sheet of metal release from the hip simulator work on the BHRs (Fig. 13.9) and compared them with clinical metal ion studies (Fig. 13.10). In any such calculation, we have some data and we need to make a few assumptions. The strength of our final conclusions will depend on the validity of the assumptions we make, and it is for the reader to judge their validity.

The data we have are

(a) Hip simulator gravimetric and volumetric loss measurements;
(b) Clinical metal ion studies;
(c) Step activity monitor measurements of device usage in young patients which show average activity levels of 2 million cycles a year, and
(d) Mean residual cobalt release after MM bearing revision to a metal-on-polyethylene (MPE) bearing, which is 0.9 μg/24 h (equivalent to 1.4 μg/day of CoCr alloy).

The assumptions we made are

(a) *In vivo* device wear rate is roughly equivalent to *in vitro* (hip simulator) wear rate;
(b) Activity in young patients during the first year is approximately 1 Mcyc per year. Thereafter it reaches the steady-state usage of 2 Mcyc per year, and
(c) Residual metal release after MM bearing removal is produced from corrosion of disseminated metal particles. Metal particles in the proximity of the hip (capsule, joint fluid, etc) that would have been removed at the time of revision have the potential to contribute at least as much metal from corrosion as the disseminated particles.

In order to compare the simulator and clinical data, all the readings were first converted into common units (μg/day or equivalent). The simulator gravimetric wear rates (per Mcyc or per 2 Mcyc depending on whether it is run-in or steady-state wear period) are converted into equivalent daily wear by dividing it by 365. The proportion of cobalt in the alloy is ~65% and correcting for that gives us the estimated alloy wear *in vivo* (Fig. 13.10). If hip simulator data is correct and all the metal released from the device *in vivo* is excreted in urine, then we would expect to see the simulator wear loss and the daily metal output approximating each other closely. We then plotted the obtained values on a graph (Fig. 13.12). Contrary to our expectation, we found that during the first 6 months, the clinical readings account for only a fifth of the wear seen in simulators. From there on, the two plots begin to converge and actually almost coincide at the 3-year stage

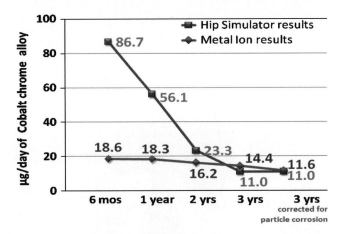

FIG. 13.12. Comparison between (*in vivo*) gravimetric wear rate in a hip simulator and (*in vivo*) alloy wear calculated from cobalt output in a metal ion study.

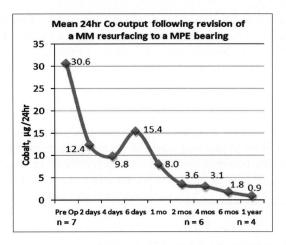

FIG. 13.13. Cobalt output after revision of a MM bearing resurfacing to a MPE bearing THR showing a steep fall in output after the revision.

Reviewing our data, we realize that we have omitted an important factor (i.e., metal release in the form of particles). We know, from simulator studies, that the particulate debris is greatest during early run-in and that the particle sizes are greatest during this phase. Can we attribute this initial difference to particulate debris shed from the bearing, which, being insoluble, is not excreted in the urine? If that is true, it gives us a clue that in the first 6 months more than four fifths of the wear debris is particulate and only a fifth is in the form of soluble metal ions (Fig. 13.12). The ratio of metal ions to particles is around 1:4.7. Closer to a year the ratio is around 1:3 and at 2 years it is 1:1.4. At 3 years, simulator wear is actually lower than daily metal ion output, 1:0.8.

How do we account for this lower estimate with simulators at the 3-year stage? Should we conclude that the simulator is now protecting the bearing when it has reached a self-polished state?

We reviewed the data for other missing factors and realized that we had not considered metal release from corrosion of deposited particles. From the study of metal levels after revision of a MM bearing to an MPE bearing, we know that at 1 year the cobalt output is around 0.9 µg/24 h (alloy equivalent 1.4 µg/day) (Table 13.2 and Fig. 13.13 to 13.14). This is metal release from disseminated wear particles. It is reasonable to

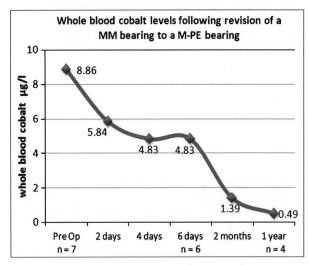

FIG. 13.14. Cobalt levels in blood also show a steady fall over a period after MM bearing removal, reaching almost normal levels at around 1 year.

assume that at least an equivalent amount of corrosion would have occurred from metal particles in the proximity of the joint that have been removed in these revision cases but that would be active in patients with functioning BHRs such as those in our clinical study. It is therefore not unreasonable to assume that in the steady state, in patients with well-functioning devices, metal release from shed wear particles would amount to at least twice the levels released in the post-revision cases. When we factor this into our calculation, it emerges that at 3 years the simulator prediction of metal release perfectly coincides with the clinical data, and the ratio is 1:0.95. This suggests that at this 3-year stage, most of the wear that is occurring is in the form of soluble metal which is effectively cleared by the renal mechanisms. That is probably one reason why we do not see black debris staining the tissues in patients undergoing revision of well-functioning MM bearing hips even if they have been

TABLE 13.2. Metal output in patients after revision of a MM bearing to a MPE bearing

Metal output after revision of a MM to a MPE bearing	Cobalt (µg/day)	Alloy equivalent (µg/day)
Pre-revision	30.6	47.1
2 days post-revision	12.4	19.0
4 days	9.8	15.0
6 days	15.4	23.7
1 month	8.0	12.3
2 months	3.6	5.5
4 months	3.1	4.7
6 months	1.8	2.7
1 year	0.9	1.4

in situ for several years. It also shows that nearly a fifth of the metal release in the steady-state phase actually comes from corrosion of metal components or wear debris particles.

In conclusion, if our assumptions are correct, then during the run-in period (i.e., the first 6 months after implantation), four fifths of bearing wear is in the form of insoluble particulate debris and a fifth is soluble metal ions. This relationship changes as the bearing progresses through the steady-state phase. At around the 3-year stage, even if we assume that most of the real-time bearing wear releases soluble metal ions, around 20% of it can only be accounted for through passive corrosion of the components or the accumulated wear particles.

Transport of Metal Particles

Metal particles are insoluble and collect in the synovial fluid and are deposited in the periarticular tissues. They are also phagocytosed by macrophages and giant cells and are transported to the regional lymph nodes and reticuloendothelial organs like liver and spleen (Fig. 13.15 to 13.16).

In a postmortem and biopsy study of cases with MPE replacements, Urban et al. [4] found that metal particles were found in the paraaortic lymph nodes in two thirds of cases and in the liver and spleen in a third of patients. Disseminated metal particles were detectable in more than 80% of specimens among those who had mechanically failed replacements. This does strongly indicate that metal particles are indeed transported along lymphatic channels.

"Are particles transported hematogenously as well?" is a frequently asked question. Urban et al. [4] reported that in exceptional cases with extensive wear, particles were found in the fixed macrophages or Kupffer cells lining the hepatic sinusoids, suggesting the possibility of hematogenous dissemination. However, if hematogenous dissemination of particles is the rule rather than the exception, then the first bed of deposition of these particles would be the pulmonary capillary system.

Unfortunately, Urban et al. did not examine the lungs in their cases. Case et al. [5] studied cadaveric specimens of patients with metal devices and found metal particles in the regional lymph nodes, liver, and spleen; and structural changes in the

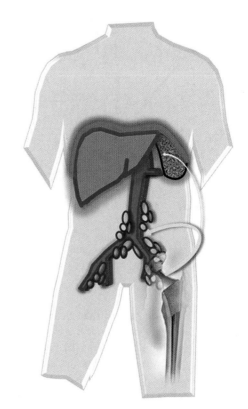

Fig. 13.16. Metal particles are insoluble and do not enter the circulation freely. To an extent, they undergo dissolution and oxidation to release metal ions. The remainder collects in the joint fluid and in the periarticular tissues. If in excess, they have the potential to cause osteolysis and implant loosening. Some are taken up by macrophages and giant cells and are subjected to further dissolution. They can be transported in the lymphatic channels and reach the regional and paraaortic lymph nodes. In a few they even spread to the liver or spleen, where they are found in small aggregates of macrophages apparently "without apparent pathological importance" (Urban et al. [4]).

lymph nodes. However, they found neither metal particles nor distinct changes in the lungs on light microscopy and no metal concentration in lung tissue on mass spectrometry. It is therefore unlikely that the hematogenous route is a major mode of metal particle transport.

Transport of Metal Ions

Metal ions are soluble and freely enter the bloodstream. Cobalt is more soluble than chromium and therefore tends to clear from the local site faster than chromium. Both cobalt and chromium are transported in serum, both in the free ionic form and in the protein-bound form. Being the most abundant protein, albumin is believed to be an important transport medium for these ions. Transferrin has also been identified as a carrier for chromium. The binding is reversible and allows transport to a site such as the kidney where they can be released and excreted. Hexavalent chromium is more soluble and is able to pass through cell membranes. Intracellularly, it is reduced to its trivalent form, which, unable to traverse the cell membrane, becomes sequestered within cells.

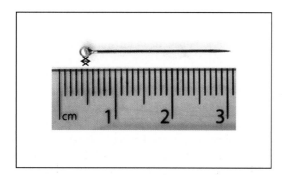

Fig. 13.15. It has been estimated that the total volume of metal wear that occurs over 15 years of usage of a MM bearing hip device is equivalent to the volume of a pin head.

Clearance of Metal Ions

Renal excretion is the predominant route of clearance of excess metal ions from the system (Fig. 13.17). Animal experiments wherein metal injected intravenously is recovered from urine suggest that 85% of injected cobalt is recoverable within 24 hours [6,7] and 95% within 3 days. Molybdenum is also excreted in urine rapidly within 24 hours. The content of molybdenum is low in the alloy and it is rapidly eliminated in urine, and therefore it is not believed to produce any adverse toxic effects in the body. In comparison, chromium tends to take longer to be eliminated, and only 44% of chromium is recoverable within 3 days.

"Are metal ion levels after MM arthroplasty breaching renal threshold and leading to systemic metal buildup?" is another frequently asked question. In order to study the concentrating efficacy of kidneys, we studied more than 250 unselected concurrent specimens of urine and whole blood from unilateral and bilateral arthroplasty patients before their operation and those with different well-functioning and failing resurfacings at various stages. We found that among preoperative controls, the ratio between urine and whole blood levels of cobalt is 0.7, indicating that there is renal conservation of cobalt (Fig. 13.18).

In patients with a MM bearing, the ratio goes up to between 4 and 5, indicating the ability of kidneys to concentrate cobalt in urine against a concentration gradient when there is an excess. If we assume that patients with high levels of metal output begin to breach the renal threshold, then the ratio of urine to blood levels should be lower in such patients. On the contrary, we find that in patients with the greatest *in vivo* metal generation as evidenced by high daily output of cobalt (to the right side of plot in Fig. 13.18), the ratio is between 6 and 9, demonstrating that renal clearance

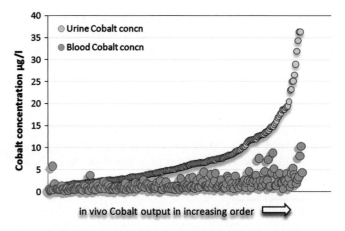

FIG. 13.18. Cobalt levels in concurrent urine and whole blood specimens from patients with different well-functioning and failing resurfacings arranged in increasing order of cobalt output in urine. The ratio of urine to whole blood concentrations increases toward the right side of the plot.

efficiency holds up even against this steep gradient and that the threshold is not breached within clinically relevant levels. Brodner et al. [8] reported on the serum metal levels in two patients with MM total hip replacements who had developed chronic renal failure. They found 100-fold elevation in their cobalt levels compared with those with similar prostheses, but normal renal function. In the absence of effective renal clearance, the cumulative buildup of metal has the potential to raise metal levels enormously. The fact that such a buildup does not occur in renal-competent patients suggests that a dynamic equilibrium is estabilished between metal release from the device and metal ion output in urine. Therefore timed output of metal in urine is a good surrogate measure of in vivo bearing wear.

Therefore, MM arthroplasty is not advisable in patients with chronic renal failure. It has been suggested that modern dialysis machines have the ability to clear excess cobalt and chromium, but we have been unable to confirm this from published literature or from experience. A successful renal transplant, however, is able to reestablish dynamic metal equilibrium as we have found in one of our patients. She developed renal failure unrelated to her MM hip resurfacing a few years after the procedure. She has since undergone a renal transplant and her cobalt, chromium, and molybdenum levels are within the expected range.

Do cobalt and chromium cause renal damage? Case et al. [5] studied postmortem specimens of kidneys in patients with metal implants including those with metal staining and evidence of wear in joints. They did not find any adverse tissue changes in the kidneys. Metal particles in the kidneys were only found in one case where there was extensive debris elsewhere and "minimal metal particles" in renal tubular epithelial cells.

Urban et al. [9] studied renal tubular deposition in patients with failed or long-term replacements. One patient who had received gold injections for rheumatoid arthritis had deposition of gold particles in the glomeruli. Two patients (one with multiple revision hips and unintended cobalt-chrome on

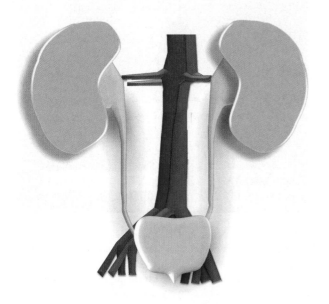

FIG. 13.17. Metal ions are soluble and enter the circulation. There is a renal clearance mechanism for their elimination that is effective across the clinically relevant range of systemic metal elevations seen in patients with arthroplasty.

stainless steel corrosion and another with a knee replacement with evidence of femoral component scratching) showed submicrometer deposits of chromium-orthophosphate in the renal tubules. They found no alloy particles in the kidneys of any of the patients although these could be detected in the lymph nodes, livers, and spleens in all of them.

Chromate-induced tubular necrosis has been extensively studied in experimental animals after parenteral administration of large doses (15 mg/kg body weight) of (hexavalent) potassium chromate [10]. Such high levels of chromate are not clinically relevant in arthroplasty patients.

There have been reports [10] of low-molecular-weight (LMW) proteinuria in factory workers who handle chromium. However, even among those who are exposed to metals at levels close to the limits of safety, no reports of metal-induced chronic renal failure have been reported [10]. Furthermore, LMW proteinuria occurs after a variety of physiologic stresses, is usually reversible, and cannot by itself be considered evidence of chronic renal disease [10]. Studies performed in cobalt workers who were exposed to levels close to the limits of safety also did not show any adverse renal effects in these workers [11].

The absence of nephrotoxicity among factory workers exposed to high levels of cobalt and chromium for prolonged periods suggests that it is highly unlikely that there exists a causal relationship between MM arthroplasty and chronic renal failure.

Measurement of Systemic Metal Exposure

The long-term effects of systemic metal ion exposure are not fully understood, and there is a need for continued monitoring of systemic metal exposure in patients with metal devices. In the earlier section we considered the reason why daily urinary output of metal is a good measure of *in vivo* bearing wear. Systemic monitoring has been done in the past using one of several blood specimens including whole blood, plasma, serum, or erythrocytes. In the bloodstream, metal ions are transported both in the plasma and within the blood cells. In the case of chromium, it has been shown that the chromium trapped in the blood cells is not in dynamic equilibrium with extracellular chromium and that the ratio of metal in the intra- and extracellular compartments is widely variable [12]. Serum metal ion concentrations correspond only with the extracellular component and do not take into account intracellular metal ions. Therefore, whole blood metal concentrations are a better measure of systemic metal ion load.

Confusion is created due to the fact that different specimens and different techniques of analysis are used in different studies. A panel of experts conceded this inadequacy through the statement that "to date, no study has reported a comparison of whole blood, serum, and erythrocyte levels on the same specimens in patients with metal-on-metal bearings" [13] and that serum analysis is recommended only due to the relative ease of analysis rather than on the basis of a scientific comparison of concurrent specimens.

Analytical Techniques

Two techniques are commonly used in metal analysis. Atomic absorption spectrometry (AAS) is used frequently to perform serum metal ion analysis (Fig. 13.19). For a variety of reasons,

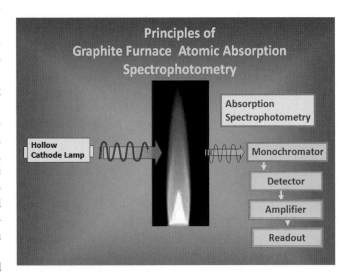

FIG. 13.19. Atomic absorption spectrometry works on the principle of spectral absorption. Metals emit and absorb light at specified wavelengths. The specimen is first allowed to burn in a flame. A powerful beam of light is then passed through it, and the pattern and intensity of light absorbed as it passes through the flame can be measured against a standard to estimate the concentration.

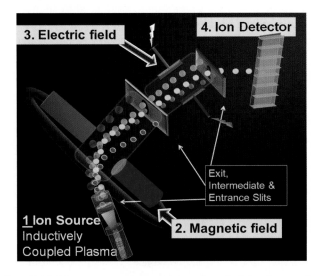

FIG. 13.20. Mass spectrometry works on the principle of separation of particles according to their mass-charge (m/z) ratio. When charged particles (ions) are passed through an electric and/or magnetic field, they deflect toward the opposite electrode or pole depending on their m/z ratio. Lighter particles with a greater charge deflect more and vice versa. A detector at the other end determines the concentrations of the sorted particles. The entrance and exit slits filter in the particles of interest. Adjusting slit width controls resolving power, which typically extends up to 10,000. The typical detection limits vary between 1 ppb and 1 ppt (part per trillion) depending on the element and matrix.

it is not easy to analyze whole blood with AAS. High-resolution inductively coupled plasma mass spectrometry (HRICPMS) is a more advanced and sensitive technique (Fig. 13.20).

HRICPMS is able to effectively overcome the interference caused by the complex matrix in whole blood. Multielement analysis can be performed on a single run reducing sample handling and hence the risk of contamination. Furthermore, multiple specimens can also be analyzed in a batch without the need for recalibration, making the measurements more uniform [14].

Specimen Selection

Using concurrent specimens of whole blood and serum, we found that the disagreement between the readings obtained with the two specimens was greater than ±67% for cobalt and greater than ±85% for chromium [15] (Fig. 13.21). This calls into question the appropriateness of continuing to use serum specimens for measurement.

to assess these through a longitudinal study in patients with Birmingham Hip Resurfacing (BHR) devices. Cross-sectional studies are subject to individual variability in metal transport and excretion. However, they are useful in planning a longitudinal study.

We therefore first performed a retrospective cross-sectional study in order to determine the critical time points at which patients need to be assessed and specimen collection organized. We obtained 12-hour urine collections at two monthly intervals up to 1 year followed by annual intervals thereafter. The cross-sectional study showed peak levels at the 1-year follow-up period.

Accordingly, we planned our longitudinal study with whole blood collections preoperatively and at the 1-year and 4-year time periods and urine collections at more frequent intervals (i.e., preoperative, 5-day, and 2, 6, 12, 24, and 48 months). Based on power analysis, we included 26 consecutive patients who received unilateral BHRs, with one of two bearing diameters (50 and 54 mm).

Metal Ion Levels in Arthroplasty

We therefore decided to use whole blood analysis as a measure of systemic metal burden and daily output of metal ions in urine as a good measure of *in vivo* bearing wear. We proceeded

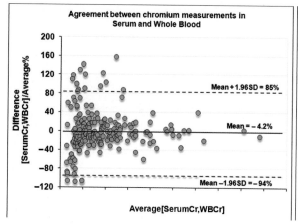
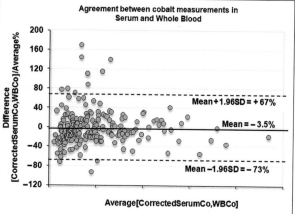

FIG. 13.21. Bland and Altman comparison shows that the disagreement between the readings obtained with serum and whole blood was greater than ±67% for cobalt and greater than ±85% for chromium. (Reproduced from Daniel J, Ziaee H, Pynsent PB, McMinn DJ. The validity of serum levels as a surrogate measure of systemic exposure to metal ions in hip replacement. J Bone Joint Surg Br 2007;89:736–41, with permission and copyright © of the British Editorial Society of Bone and Joint Surgery.)

We recently reported their 4-year results [16] and are currently at the 6-year stage (Figs. 13.22 and 13.23). All patients were found to have well-functioning hips at their 4-year follow-up with an average step activity rate of 2.1 million cycles per year. Their activities included participating in heavy occupational work and pursuing impact-loading leisure activities like running, mountain hiking, playing hockey, tennis, and squash.

Cobalt output in these patients showed a steady increase up to the 6-month stage (Fig. 13.22). After this, there is a steady decline in the output until the 4-year stage. Preliminary results indicate that the decreasing trend continues at their 6-year follow-up as well. Chromium output shows a similar but less pronounced increasing trend up to the 1- and 2-year postoperative stage, followed by a decrease at the 4- and 6-year stages. Blood levels also show an early rise followed by a reducing trend (Fig. 13.23).

A review of past literature found only one longitudinal study of daily metal ion output in urine employing HRICPMS analysis in patients with MM hips. In that study, in addition to daily urine output of metal, erythrocyte metal levels were assessed rather than whole blood levels. The metal output with the MM device used in that study was found to be so great (cobalt output 50 µg/24 h) that further recruitment into the study was reportedly discontinued at that center after 2 years [17].

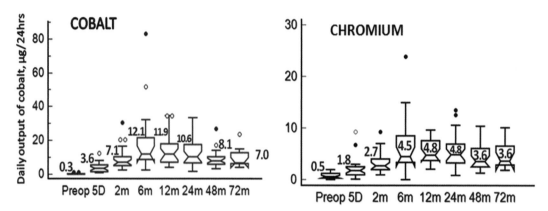

Fig. 13.22. Daily output of cobalt and chromium. Values in figures are medians (horizontal lines). The boxes are interquartile ranges, 95% confidence intervals of medians are notches, and the whiskers extend to values within 1.5 times the box length. Outliers beyond are shown as data points. Only 11 specimens have been analyzed at the 72-month follow-up to date.

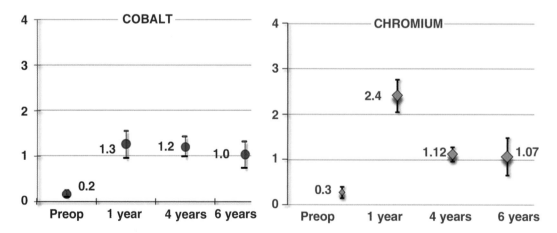

Fig. 13.23. Whole blood levels of cobalt and chromium (means and 95% confidence intervals). Only 11 specimens have been analyzed at the 72 month follow-up to date.

The steady increase of metal ion output in the first 6 months appears to fit in with the 1 million cycles of run-in wear predicted by simulator and retrieval studies. If the wear regimen *in vivo* were to continue to follow the predicted laboratory results (such as those from hip simulators), one would expect the output to enter a phase of dramatically reduced output, reaching a level close to the preoperative levels. Metal ion levels do not show such a reduction. The reducing trend in metal release with the BHR, however, allays the fear that all MM bearings lead to a cumulative buildup of metal in the system with progressively increasing blood levels.

We compared the 2-year output and 1-year blood levels in the above group with patients who underwent a unilateral 28-mm Metasul MM total hip replacement (THR) [18] and with another group of patients who underwent a large-diameter MM THR (with diameters in the range of modern MM resurfacings). We found no significant difference between the metal levels in BHRs and either the 28-mm THRs or the large-diameter MM THRs (Fig. 13.24).

The metal levels from several other studies are quoted in Table 13.3. The specimens and analytical techniques are different in the various studies as shown in the table, and therefore they do not provide a direct comparison. It may be noted that the highest cobalt levels (>3 μg/L) are found in two studies. One of these is RBC cobalt level in 28-mm mixed bearing (low carbon–high carbon) THRs reported by MacDonald et al., and another is whole blood cobalt level in low-carbon 28-mm THRs reported by Pfister et al. In addition to the data in the table, Hart et al. [19] published blood metal levels in patients with MPE total hip replacements and BHRs. However, Hart admits that there was a measurement error in their cobalt levels

to the tune of 2 μg/L and that the true cobalt level in the BHRs in their study is 2.18 μg/L (4.18 − 2 = 2.18 μg/L).

There were three reports of blood chromium levels >3 μg/L. One of these is the report by MacDonald et al. in mixed bearing 28-mm MM THRs with an erythrocyte chromium level of 3.03 μg/L. Interestingly, the highest chromium levels have been reported by Luetzner et al. [20] in cobalt chrome on polyethylene total knee replacements. The serum chromium levels were 3.28 μg/L in unilateral and 4.28 μg/L in bilateral MPE total knee replacements.

Metal Ion Sequelae Including DNA and Chromosome Damage and Carcinogenesis

Chromosome translocations (or sister chromatid exchanges; SCEs) are structural changes in which part of an arm of a chromosome is exchanged with that of another chromosome. Aneuploidy is a numerical change in the number of chromosomes resulting in a gain or loss compared with the normal diploid (a pair of each) number of chromosomes, resulting in trisomy (three chromosomes with the same number) or monosomy (a single chromatid with its number) (Figs. 13.25–13.29).

Both of these changes occur in normal subjects, too, and accumulate with time. Their frequency reportedly increases with age and factors such as consuming diet drinks, watching television for several hours a day, and high-altitude travel. However, it is also known that there are mechanisms in the body that monitor and repair DNA changes; and there are systems that protect against their effects.

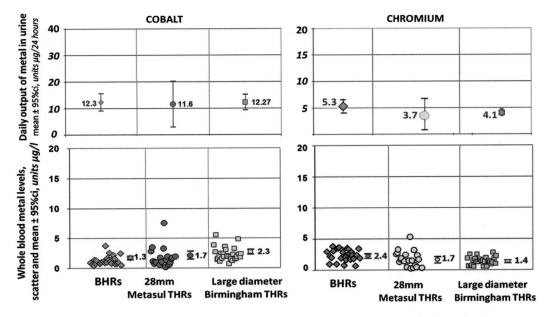

Fig. 13.24. Daily output of metal ions in urine and blood metal levels in patients with 28 mm Metasul THRs, BHRs, and large-diameter MM THRs. The smaller diameter bearings did not show a significant difference from either the BHRs or the large-diameter MM THRs.

TABLE 13.3. Metal ion levels from several studies in patients with different arthroplasties*

Studies on CoCr THRs	n	Alloy	Specimen	Technique	Follow-up	µg/L Co	SD	µg/L Cr	SD
Farvard, 2001 [37]	16	HC	SE	HRICPMS	1 y	1.71	±3.4	1.62	±2.6
Savarino et al., 2002 [38]	26	HC	SE	GFAAS	2.2 y	1.33	±0.25 (se)	1.72	±0.33
Pfister et al., 2002 [39]	113	HC	WB	HRICPMS	4.1 y (1–5.9)	2.6	±7.4		
Pfister et al., 2002 [39]	17	LC	WB	HRICPMS	2.9 y (0.9–4.8)	3.1	±2.4		
Clarke et al., 2003 [40]	22	Mixed	SE	HRICPMS	1.3 y	1.3	0.9–5.1 (range)	1	
MacDonald et al., 2002 [17]	23	Mixed	RBC	HRICPMS	2.9 y	3.46		3.03	
Back et al., 2005 (BHR) [41]	20	HC	SE	ICPMS, GFAAS	3 mo	0.8		1.5	
Back et al., 2005 (BHR) [41]	20	HC	SE	ICPMS, GFAAS	6 mo	1		1.6	
Back et al., 2005 (BHR) [41]	20	HC	SE	ICPMS, GFAAS	9 mo	0.9		1.8	
Back et al., 2005 (BHR) [41]	20	HC	SE	ICPMS, GFAAS	12 mo	0.7		1.5	
Back et al., 2005 (BHR) [41]	20	HC	SE	ICPMS, GFAAS	24 mo	0.5		1.3	
Back et al., 2005 (BHR) [41]	120	HC	SE	ICPMS, GFAAS	3 mo to 24 mo	0.8		1.5	
Heisel et al, 2005 (Low activity) [42]	7	HC	SE	GFAAS	1.5 y	1.4	±0.85	2.08	±0.90
Heisel et al, Jacobs, 2005 (Treadmill) [42]	7	HC	SE	GFAAS	1.5 y	1.41	±0.79	2.11	±0.93
Heisel et al, 2005 (High activity) [42]	7	HC	SE	GFAAS	1.5 y	1.29	±0.63	2.12	±0.87
Dunstan, 2005 (Historic MM) [43]	5		WB	HRICPMS	30y+	0.65	0.3–1.1	2.16	1.9–2.4
Dunstan, 2005 (Historic MM, etc.) [43]	3		WB	HRICPMS	30y+	1.97	1.1–2.4	2.17	1.7–2.5
Daniel et al., 2006 (BHR) [18]	26	HC'	WB	HRICPMS	1 y	1.3	0.76	2.4	0.96
Daniel et al., 2006 (28 mm) [18]	20	HC	WB	HRICPMS	1 y	1.7	±1.6	1.7	±1.3
Daniel et al., 2007 (BHR) [16]	26	HC'	WB	HRICPMS	4 y	1.2		1.1	
Luetzner et al., 2007 [20]	18	MPE TKRs	SE	GFAAS	5 y	0.92		3.28	
Luetzner et al., 2007 [20]	23	MPE TKRs	SE	GFAAS	4 y+	0.98		4.28	

HC, high-carbon cobalt-chrome alloy; LC, low-carbon cobalt-chrome alloy; Mixed, mixed bearing combination wherein one component is HC and another LC; SE, serum; WB, whole blood; RBC, red blood cells or erythrocytes; GFAAS, graphite furnace atomic absorption spectrometry; ICPMS, inductively coupled plasma mass spectrometry; HRICPMS, high-resolution ICPMS; Co, cobalt; Cr, chromium; SD, standard deviation.

* All the studies relate to MM THRs except Luetzner et al. (2007), which relate to metal polyethylene total knee replacements (MPE TKRs).

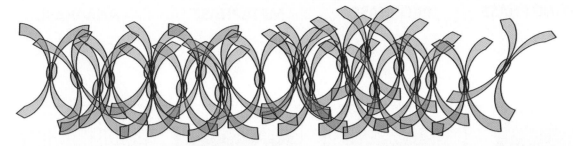

FIG. 13.25. A normal human cell has 23 pairs of chromosomes. Each pair consists of homologous copies of each other and these are attached at a structure called the centromere. They are faithfully copied and replicated during cell division, but the individual chromosomes cannot be identified or stained during the resting phase of the cell when they are hidden in the chromatin material of the nuclei.

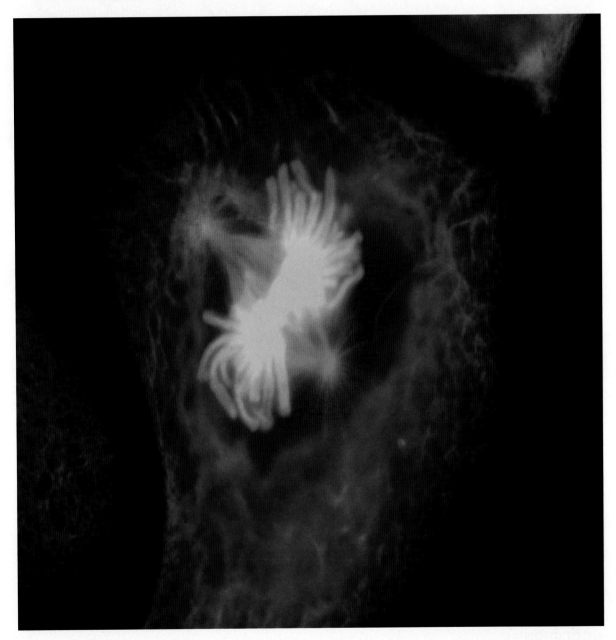

FIG. 13.26. When the cell starts dividing, the chromatin condenses itself into chromosomes. One of these phases of cell division is called *metaphase*, when the chromosomes are arranged along the equator of the cell. We are then presented with an opportunity to study their number and structure and look for abnormalities. Shown is an electron micrograph of a Newt lung cell in the metaphase stage of cell division. (Photograph by Dr. Conly L. Rieder, Wadsworth Center, Albany, NY, USA.)

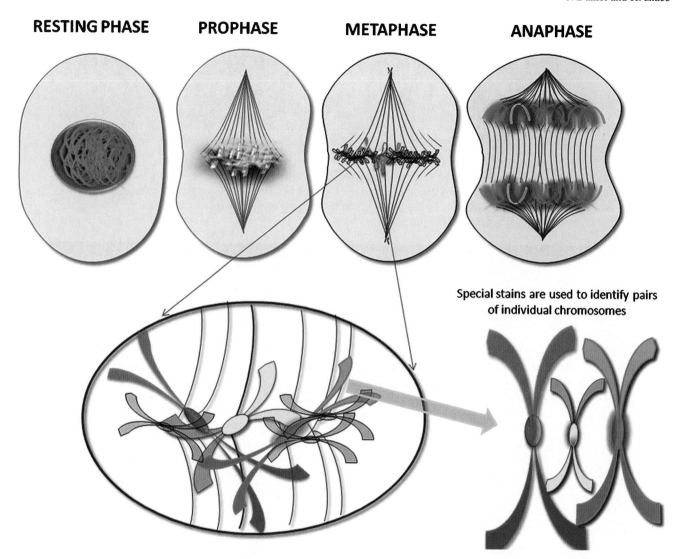

RESTING PHASE **PROPHASE** **METAPHASE** **ANAPHASE**

Special stains are used to identify pairs
of individual chromosomes

FIG. 13.27. During cell division the chromatin condenses into chromosomes and becomes arranged along the equator of the cell. The pairs of chromosomes are then separated and are drawn toward the opposite poles before the cell divides. During metaphase, these pairs can be identified and stained to identify errors. In the work done at Bristol, three pairs of chromosomes of the 23 pairs were studied with the fluorescent *in situ* hybridization technique, and the investigators looked for two types of specific changes.

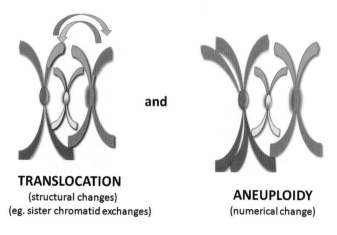

and

TRANSLOCATION
(structural changes)
(eg. sister chromatid exchanges)

ANEUPLOIDY
(numerical change)

FIG. 13.28. In rapidly dividing cells, both physical and chemical influences can lead to copying errors leading to a change in the number of chromosomes (aneuploidy) or a change in their structure including loss of material or exchange of chromatid material between different pairs of chromosomes. These changes are used in cancer cytogenetics as markers of certain cancers when they are above a certain threshold level.

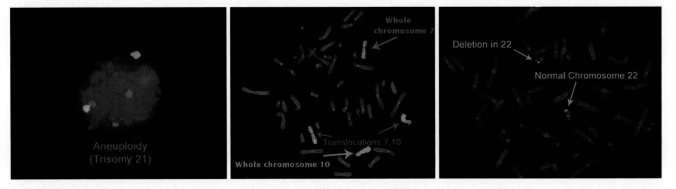

FIG. 13.29. Fluorescent *in situ* staining used on interphase and metaphase cells showing aneuploidy (trisomy 21 of Down syndrome), deletion in chromosome 22 (DiGeorge syndrome), and translocation between chromosomes 7 and 10. (Photomicrographs courtesy Dr. Dominic McMullan, West Midlands Regional Genetics Laboratories, Birmingham, UK.)

A cross-sectional study [21] from the Bristol Implant Research Centre (BIRC) analyzed these changes in the peripheral blood lymphocytes in a group of patients at the time of revision arthroplasty (revision of predominately metal on polyethylene replacements except for two who had MM bearing replacements). They then compared the results with tests from controls presenting for primary arthroplasty.

The BIRC study showed that there was an increase of nonspecific translocations and aneuploidy in the study group, and that there were differences between CoCr- and titanium-containing implants. Patients with titanium prostheses had a nearly fivefold increase in aneuploidy but no change in chromosomal translocations. Those with CoCr prostheses had a 2.5-fold increase in aneuploidy and a 3.5-fold increase in chromosomal translocations.

Another longitudinal study performed at the same center [22] on patients with MM hip replacements showed that the increase in chromosome aberrations in these patients was not as great as that previously reported for the metal on polyethylene prostheses in the cross-sectional study mentioned above. They did, however, state that the postoperative intervals in the MM longitudinal study are shorter, and the devices in these cases were well-functioning replacements rather than failed implants. No significant relationship was found between the chromosome changes and the blood levels of cobalt or chromium. Studies from the same center also demonstrate that ceramic-ceramic bearing replacements also show similar chromosome changes in the peripheral blood [23] (Table 13.4).

TABLE 13.4. Chromosome studies on peripheral blood lymphocytes, reported from Bristol Implant Research Centre*

Bearing	Number of patients	Authors	Type of study	Findings	Comments of Case et al. in the respective publications
Predominately metal on polyethylene THRs	31 study patients and 30 controls	Doherty AT et al., J Bone Joint Surg Br 2001 [21]	Cross-sectional	5× increase in aneuploidy in patients with Ti alloy components; 2.5× aneuploidy and 3.5× translocations in those with CoCr components.	
Metal on metal THRs	95 patients	Ladon D et al., J Arthroplasty 2004 [22]	Prospective longitudinal, 2 years	Increase in translocations and aneuploidy at 2 years are *not* as severe as with MPE hips	Chromosome aberrations are not quite as great as that which were reported with MPE bearings
Ceramic on ceramic THRs	24 patients	Ladon D et al., Transactions 51st Annual Meeting of the Orthopaedic Research Society 2005 [23]	Prospective longitudinal, 1 year	"Pattern and level of chromosomal changes similar to that with metal on metal prostheses"	Chromosome aberrations are caused either by the SS Protasul stem in the bone marrow or by a small particle effect or by some nonspecific effect of surgery

*Case and colleagues from the Bristol Implant Research Centre performed FISH (fluorescent *in situ* hybridization) studies on chromosomes 1, 2, and 3 in peripheral blood lymphocytes in patients before and after hip replacements. They found no difference in the chromosome changes found in association with the three types of bearings.

The possibility of DNA damage has been studied in synovial fluid obtained from replaced joints using the comet assay [24]. This is a nonspecific test of the DNA damage potential of the fluid. The results suggest that DNA damage does occur with synovial fluid obtained from joints with CoCr MM devices. However, the same study reports a similar range of changes in those with CoCr MPE knee replacements (Fig. 13.30). These studies were performed in the same laboratory using the same techniques by the same team and are therefore directly comparable.

There has been concern that these chromosome and DNA changes can lead to carcinogenic effects in the subjects and mutagenic and teratogenic effects in the offspring. However, the changes in patients with MM bearings are no greater than in those with either MPE or ceramic-ceramic bearings. Therefore, on the basis of chromosome changes, the risk of carcino-genesis should be no greater in MM bearings compared with the other bearing combinations.

First-generation MM hip replacements were used during the 1960s and 1970s. Long-term studies of a cohort of 579 Nordic patients (9756 person-years) with these historic (McKee-Farrar) replacements in patients who had osteoarthritis have shown that compared with the general population, there is no increase in the all-site cancer rate or in the site-specific cancer rates in these patients at 28 years follow-up (mean follow-up 16 years) [25]. Significantly, there was no increase in cancer rates in the target organs of liver, kidney, or urinary tract. Temporary increases in hematopoietic cancers at interim follow-up periods were not sustained in the longer-term follow-up. The only site-specific cancer that showed a statistically significant difference between the MM cohort and the general population was that of lung cancer, and the incidence

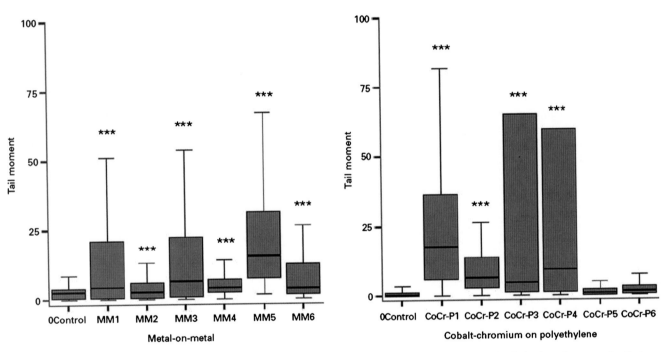

FIG. 13.30. Results of the comet assay of DNA damage for synovial fluids from metal on metal (MM) and cobalt-chromium on polyethylene (CoCr-PE) bearing joints. (Reproduced from Davies AP, Sood A, Lewis AC, Newson R, Learmonth ID, Case CP. Metal-specific differences in levels of DNA damage caused by synovial fluid recovered at revision arthroplasty. J Bone Joint Surg Br 2005;87:1439–44, with permission and copyright © of the British Editorial Society of Bone and Joint Surgery.)

was lower in the MM group compared with the general population (Fig. 13.31).

Around 400,000 MM bearings have been implanted since the late 1980s. No case of local sarcoma has been reported among these patients at the local sites. Several patients among these have reported having had babies in the years after device implantation. There have been no published reports of evidence of mutagenic/teratogenic effects directly attributable to the MM replacements; nor have there been such reports in those treated with the earlier-generation MM hip replacements.

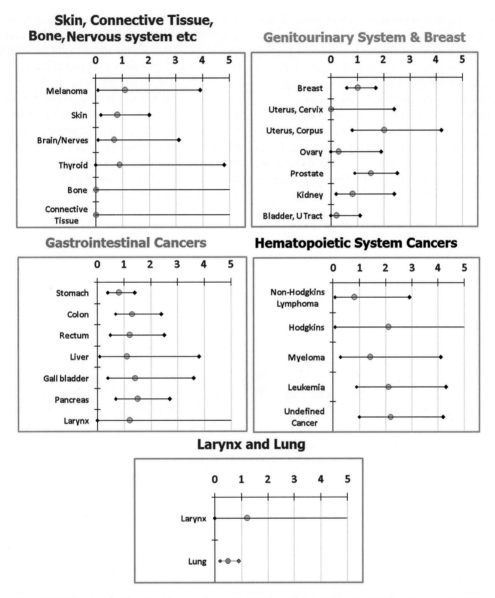

Fig. 13.31. The standardized incidence ratios with 95% confidence intervals of different cancers in 579 patients with McKee-Farrar THRs with primary replacements performed since 1967 and followed up for a maximum period of 30 years. The 95% CIs in all but one cancer straddle 1 implying that there is no significant difference between the observed cancers in this cohort and that expected in the general population. The only cancer whose 95% CI does not cross 1 is lung cancer, which interestingly is less than 1 (0.2 to 0.9) indicating that the observed rate is lower in the MM group compared with the general population. The annual incidence of all-site cancer rates in this cohort tracked the general population closely year on year. (Modified from Visuri T, Pukkala E. Does metal-on-metal hip prosthesis have influence on cancer? A long-term follow-up study. In: Reiker C, Oberholzer S, Wyss U, eds. World Tribology Forum in Arthroplasty. Bern, Toronto, Seattle: Hans Huber, 2001:181–8.)

Placental Transfer

The concern regarding possible teratogenicity could be resolved in part if it was known whether metal ions are transferred across the placenta. One study [26] of the transplacental transfer of metal ions in patients with MM hip devices led to the conclusion that the elevated metal ion levels in maternal blood do not lead to raised levels in the umbilical cord blood and that the placenta acts as an effective barrier to metal ions released from metal devices. This would imply that the rapidly dividing and differentiating tissues in the developing fetus are not exposed to the elevated metal ion levels and are therefore not subject to the potential adverse effects predicted by the laboratory experiments.

That study was based on a study of serum levels in three subjects using graphite furnace atomic absorption spectrometry (GFAAS). In fact, the analysis could not detect metal ions in the sera of two of the three mothers or in that of the three babies at the time of delivery. We found this surprising as these elements are essential for the babies as well.

We felt compelled to perform a controlled study of placental transfer of cobalt and chromium in patients with MM bearings and controls with no metal implants. We reported [27] on this subject earlier, and more subjects have been added to the cohort since then. We found that metal ions were detected in all the maternal and cord blood specimens in the study and control groups (Fig. 13.32). No congenital abnormality was observed at birth in any of the babies in either group.

In the control group, the mean metal levels in the cord blood were 97% to 99% of the mean maternal levels, and the differences between the mean maternal and cord blood levels were statistically not significant (Fig. 13.33). This suggests that, far from acting as a barrier, there is an almost-free passage of these ions across the placental barrier at the levels expected in the normal population. The finding that the placenta does not act as a total barrier to these elements is understandable when we realize that these essential trace elements are also required by the developing fetus for its cellular and metabolic functions.

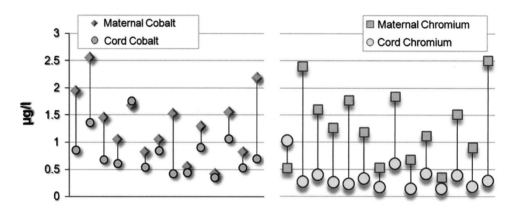

FIG. 13.32. Cobalt and chromium levels in maternal and cord blood in patients with metal-metal bearings, n = 14; whole blood analysis with HRICPMS.

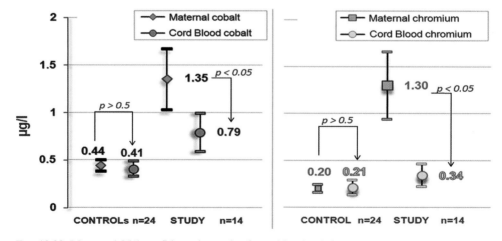

FIG. 13.33. Mean and 95% confidence intervals of metal ion levels in the maternal and cord blood of study patients, with metal-metal bearings and controls with no metallic devices.

The relative levels of metal ions in the maternal and cord blood in patients with MM bearings reveal that the placenta does exert a modulatory effect on metal transfer at the higher metal levels expected in these patients. The mean cord blood levels of cobalt and chromium in the study group are only 60.4% and 29.4% of the maternal blood levels, respectively. The differences between the cord metal levels and maternal levels in the MM group were statistically significant indicating that the placenta was blocking a significant proportion of the maternal chromium from passage into the cord blood. Furthermore, the difference in cord chromium levels between the MM and control groups was not statistically significant (Fig. 13.33) indicating that the chromium milieu in the babies in the MM group was unchanged compared with the general population. Thus, compared with the almost-free passage of metal in those with no metal implants, the placentas in those with MM bearings were preventing a large percentage of maternal chromium and cobalt from entering the fetal circulation.

In the light of the findings that metal ions are elevated in patients with MM bearings, and that these metals do cross the placenta, what advice should be offered to young women at child-bearing age who choose to undergo a conservative hip arthroplasty? Metal on metal bearings are known to go through higher wear rates while they run-in over the first 6 months after implantation. During this period, urine and blood studies show that there is a greater systemic exposure and renal output of metal ions. Our female patients who are planning a resurfacing and a pregnancy in the foreseeable future are offered the advice that they have the baby before the resurfacing, or postpone a pregnancy for at least 2 years after the resurfacing.

Metal Hypersensitivity

It is a well-known fact that all artificial joints generate debris. If the debris generated is above a threshold level, it can trigger off a lysosomal cascade in the periarticular tissues leading to osteolysis, in a manner similar to that seen with polyethylene debris. Therefore, a high-wear bearing is likely to cause osteolysis more frequently than is a wear-resistant bearing. This is an expected and normal response to an (over-the-threshold level of an) abnormal substance and should not be confused with hypersensitivity.

Hypersensitivity is an abnormal exaggerated immune reaction to an innocuous antigen leading to adverse effects on normal tissues. Metal ions or particles by themselves do not initiate a hypersensitivity response. They can however react with an existing organic substance such as a protein or form a metal-protein complex to create an antigen that has the potential to initiate an immune response.

Merritt and Brown describe their adaptation of Koch's postulates as proof of allergic response to a metal device [28]. They suggest that a patient with a suspected immune reaction to a device (1) should undergo a laboratory test, such as one of those described below, to confirm an immune response;

(2) this is followed by device removal with disappearance of symptoms; (3) reinsert the device and observe reappearance of symptoms; and then (4) demonstrate a positive laboratory test response for immunity again. These have been used in dermatological and dental disciplines but they acknowledge that steps 3 and 4 are in fact inadvisable in orthopedic surgery.

Gell and Coombs classified hypersensitivity into four types. Types I, II, and III are antibody-mediated reactions [29]. Type I hypersensitivity (atopic or anaphylactic) is an immediate allergic reaction provoked by exposure to a previously exposed specific antigen mediated by IgE antibodies and results in the release of substances like histamine that can produce local or systemic effects. Symptoms vary from mild irritation to sudden death from anaphylactic shock. Type II hypersensitivity (antibody-dependent hypersensitivity) is when the antibodies produced by the immune response bind to antigens on the patient's cell surfaces and form complexes causing cell lysis and cell death. Autoimmune hemolytic anemia, Hashimoto's thyroiditis, Graves' disease, myasthenia gravis, and hemolytic disease of the newborn are some examples. In type III hypersensitivity (immune complex hypersensitivity), soluble immune complexes (aggregations of antigens and IgG and IgM antibodies) form in the blood and are deposited in various tissues (typically the skin, kidney, and joints) where they may trigger an immune response according to the classic pathway of complement activation. Immune complex glomerulonephritis, serum sickness, and Arthus reaction are some examples.

Metal-induced hypersensitivity is of the type IV variety. Unlike the other types, it is not antibody mediated but rather is a type of cell-mediated response. An antigen-presenting cell (APC) first processes the antigen and presents it along with the major histocompatibility complex (MHC) on its surface to T cells (CD8 [cytotoxic] or CD4 [helper]). The APCs (macrophages, dendritic cells, or B-cells) also release interleukin 1 to stimulate the proliferation of further CD4 cells, which release interleukin 2 and interferon gamma and other cytokines, which are immune-response mediators. Activated CD8 cells destroy target cells on contact, and activated macrophages produce hydrolytic enzymes and can transform into multinucleated giant cells. Some clinical examples are contact dermatitis, temporal arteritis, and transplant rejection.

The prevalence of hypersensitivity to cheap jewelry containing nickel and that of positive skin test to nickel are high in the general population (more than 10%). If all the metals contained in the cobalt chrome alloy are taken into account, the incidence is higher. The prevalence of positive skin tests is higher if patients with a MM device are tested, in particular among those with failing replacements (13% to 70%) [30]. However, metal on metal bearing failure secondary to hypersensitivity is a very rare (around 1 in 1000) phenomenon. An Australian national review of failures in 3497 MM resurfacings [31] reported only one case of presumed hypersensitivity that led to a revision.

In our series of more than 3500 MM bearings, we have had only one patient who reported developing an eczematous rash after a MM resurfacing (Fig. 13.34). This 59-year-old woman, who had no history of skin problems before her operation, developed a skin rash with itching and eczematous change on the operated right leg a few weeks after a BHR in 1998. Her dermatologist diagnosed it as eczema and prescribed her medication that controlled the rash in a few weeks. Since then, every year she continues to develop an eczematous rash for a few weeks during the winter, which responds well to applications of different creams.

Eight years later, she started developing pain in her right hip on severe activity. A multislice CT scan confirmed two small areas of osteolysis in zones 1 and 3 of the acetabulum and fluid in the iliopsoas bursa. A skin patch test showed that she had a weak positive sensitivity to cobalt, but so weak, her dermatologist was not convinced of its significance. We then performed a lymphocyte transformation test on her, which showed no reaction to cobalt, chromium, and molybdenum and a positive reaction to copper. Her hip pain has since subsided and although she has not returned to playing golf, her activity is not otherwise restricted. She knows that there is a problem with her hip, which will need conversion to a THR if symptomatic.

Another patient was found to be allergic to nickel on lymphocyte transformation test and has been revised to a ceramic on polyethylene THR. However, her histology did *not* show any evidence of the typical aseptic lymphocytic vasculitis (ALVAL) described in MM bearings.

There are reports of dermal metal hypersensitivity reported in other orthopedic devices, predominately internal fixation devices such as plates and screws implanted superficially. The discrepancy between the high incidence of dermal metal hypersensitivity and the extremely low incidence of hypersensitivity to arthroplasty devices implanted deep in the tissues has intrigued researchers for a long time. It has been suggested that one reason for this is the fact that the antigen-presenting cells in skin (Langerhans dendritic cells) handle antigens in a different manner compared with systemic antigen-presenting cells (macrophages and monocytes). Therefore, many individuals who have skin reactivity to a metal will never develop any reaction at the site of a prosthesis composed of that metal. Thus, conclusions based on skin patch testing are likely to yield a high prevalence of false positives. The following two histologic studies suggest that hypersensitivity to metal is indeed a distinct possibility.

Willert et al. [32] studied periprosthetic tissues obtained from 19 consecutive revisions of MM hips, a majority of whom had persistence or early recurrence of preoperative pain and/or hip effusion after the original hip replacement. Radiolucent lines were found in five hips and osteolysis in seven hips. At revision, both components were found to be well fixed in nine patients. Fourteen had the MM device revised to a non-MM articulation and five received a second MM THR. Three other groups of patients, two of which were treated primarily with non-MM implants and one with historic MM implants, served as controls.

Histology of the study group specimens revealed an active cellular reaction with diffuse and perivascular infiltrates of T and B lymphocytes and plasma cells, high endothelial venules, massive fibrin exudation, accumulation of macrophages

FIG. 13.34. Eczematous skin rash that developed in a 59-year-old woman after a BHR. Good joint function for 8 years. Pain, iliopsoas fluid collection, and a small area of acetabular osteolysis in two zones suggests the possibility of hypersensitivity to the implant. Although her skin patch test showed weak positive reaction to cobalt, lymphocyte transformation test showed a positive reaction only to copper.

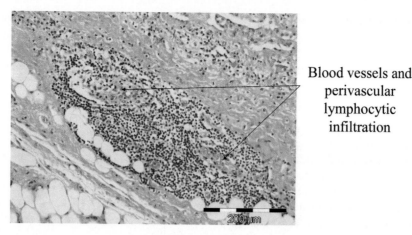

Blood vessels and
perivascular
lymphocytic
infiltration

FIG. 13.35. Perivascular aggregation of lymphocytes in a patient who underwent an excision of an iliopsoas bursa. The histology was described as ALVAL (aseptic lymphocytic vasculitis and associated lesions).

with drop-like inclusions, and infiltrates of eosinophilic granulocytes and necrosis. Only a few metal particles were detected. This histology was different from that expected in a typical type IV (DTH) reaction and was described as aseptic lymphocyte-dominated vasculitis-associated lesion (ALVAL) (Fig. 13.35). In the non-MM control groups, the predominant finding was one of foreign-body reaction. The group with no CoCr components showed no lymphocytes, whereas the historic MM control group showed the presence of lymphocytes but to a lesser extent. Study patients who received another MM articulation at revision had no relief of symptoms, whereas those who were revised to a non-MM device experienced symptom relief.

The persistence or early reappearance of symptoms, joint effusion, and osteolysis after a MM THR procedure in the study suggests the possibility of a metal hypersensitivity reaction. The distinctive histologic pattern found in these patients with MM hips supports this possibility.

Davies et al. [33] studied tissues obtained from revision of 25 MM hips some of which had failed with osteolysis and aseptic loosening, and others with no osteolysis, such as autopsy specimens of hips that had been well functioning, and those retrieved from hips that had failed due to femoral neck fractures. They compared these with 19 MPE THR retrievals. Tissue samples obtained from the MM hips showed features similar to Willert's findings. However, among MM hips, surface changes and lymphocytic infiltration were more pronounced in those that had failed due to aseptic loosening compared with those that had failed from reasons other than aseptic loosening (non–bearing related failures). In fact, the surface changes in these non–bearing failures were equivalent to those seen with M-PE joints.

This raises a fundamental question, whether deep hypersensitivity to these essential metals does exist at all in reality. Dorr [34,35], with his extensive experience in metal on metal bearings, studied failures from unexplained pain in patients with MM bearings and suggests that over-the-threshold wear debris generation is the primary cause of the histopathologic

changes, rather than an inherent genetically determined hypersensitivity to metal.

Tests for Hypersensitivity

Skin testing has been in use for several decades in the assessment of contact dermatitis. As noted above, this test may not have a direct relationship to the incidence of deep hypersensitivity. Furthermore, there is a small but definite incidence of sensitization after skin testing. Therefore, we do not routinely use skin testing in the assessment of metal hypersensitivity. Two other *in vitro* tests that have been used in the assessment of metal hypersensitivity include the lymphocyte transformation test (LTT) and the leukocyte migration inhibition factor (MIF) test.

Lymphocyte Transformation Test

The LTT involves measuring the proliferative response of lymphocytes after activation. A radioactive marker such as [H³]-labeled thymidine is added to lymphocytes along with the desired activating agent. The radioactive [H³]-thymidine gets incorporated into the DNA during cell division and allows quantification of the proliferation response. Measurement of radioactivity at day 6 helps determine the proliferation factor or stimulation index (SI). SI is calculated as a ratio of mean radiation counts per minute (cpm), with and without treatment.

$$SI = \frac{\text{Mean cpm with traeatement}}{\text{Mean cpm without treatment}}$$

The logistical difficulties involved in the transport of blood samples with vital cells to a specialist laboratory within hours of drawing the sample, the technical difficulties involved in the test itself, and the cost of LTT limit its use in clinical testing for metal hypersensitivity. However, there are reports suggesting that LTT is suitable for the assessment of metal-hypersensitivity in arthroplasty.

Leukocyte Migration Inhibition Factor Test

Another *in vitro* test involves the use of MIF. *In vitro*, leukocytes possess a natural tendency to migrate both in a random fashion and toward specific chemoattractants, such as those released by bacteria. In the presence of a sensitizing agent such as a solution of metal ions, their migration is slowed down, and this inhibition of migration can be quantified as a measure of the sensitivity to the agent. The test is positive if there is no migration and negative if the migration continues unchanged indicating that they have not been sensitized to the metal. One of several types of media can be used to allow the migration. It may be a capillary tube, two-cell culture chamber separated by a membrane (Boyden chamber), agarose, or collagen gel [30].

Our understanding of metal hypersensitivity reactions in patients with metallic implants is incomplete. However, case reports and histologic studies suggest that metal on metal bearings initiate a distinctive immune response. Although the prevalence of true hypersensitivity in patients with MM replacements is unknown, metal sensitivity should be borne in mind while investigating a patient with local or systemic signs of hypersensitivity related to device implantation. A high index of suspicion is essential while investigating a patient for persistent unexplained joint pain or swelling after an arthroplasty procedure. Hypersensitivity should be considered in the differential diagnosis if investigations rule out any explicable cause such as infection. In the presence of a positive test result that suggests hypersensitivity, exchange to a non-MM bearing should be considered and performed early.

The ultimate benefit from *in vitro* testing would be the development of a sensitive and reliable screening test that would preoperatively diagnose whether a person has a genetic predisposition to hypersensitivity to a specific metal or group of metals. That would enable a patient and his or her clinician to make an informed decision regarding the choice of bearing material in that individual case. Identification and validation of such a test would involve a large study recruiting thousands of patients undergoing a MM bearing arthroplasty before their operations and following them up longitudinally over several years.

Conclusion

There are many gaps in our understanding of the nature of these essential elements (cobalt, chromium, molybdenum, and other trace elements) and the nature of the threat from their persistent elevation over long periods of time. Several laboratory tests and markers raise the possibility that adverse effects cannot be ruled out. However, epidemiologic studies have not upheld these claims to date. What is becoming abundantly clear with each passing year, however, are the potential benefits from conservative arthroplasty that are made possible through metal on metal bearing devices. Until the development of another class of devices proven to produce equivalent benefits without similar or other risks, the usage of metal on metal bearings will continue. While we continue to use metal on metal bearings, the potential risks serve as an impetus to try and improve materials and bearing design to minimize wear and corrosion and thereby reduce systemic metal exposure risk.

References

1. Smith-Petersen MN. Evolution of mould arthroplasty of the hip joint. J Bone Joint Surg Br 1948;30:59–75.
2. Klatsky AL. Alcohol and cardiovascular diseases: a historical overview. Ann N Y Acad Sci 2002;957:7–15. Review.
3. Brodner W, Grohs JG, Bancher-Todesca D, Dorotka R, Meisinger V, Gottsauner-Wolf F, Kotz R. Does the placenta inhibit the passage of chromium and cobalt after metal-on-metal total hip arthroplasty? J Arthroplasty 2004;19(suppl):S102–106.
4. Urban RM, Jacobs JJ, Tomlinson MJ, Gavrilovic J, Black J, Peoc'h M. Dissemination of wear particles to the liver, spleen, and abdominal lymph nodes of patients with hip or knee replacement. J Bone Joint Surg Am 2000;82:457–76.
5. Case CP, Langkamer VG, James C, Palmer MR, Kemp AJ, Heap PF, Solomon L. Widespread dissemination of metal debris from implants. J Bone Joint Surg Br 1994;76:701–12.
6. Brown SA, Zhang K, Merritt K, Payer JH. *In vivo* transport and excretion of corrosion products from accelerated anodic corrosion of porous coated F75 alloy. J Biomed Mater Res 1993;27:1007–17.
7. Merritt K, Brown SA. Distribution of cobalt chromium wear and corrosion products and biologic reactions. Clin Orthop Relat Res 1996;329(suppl):S233–43. Review.
8. Brodner W, Grohs JG, Bitzan P, Meisinger V, Kovarik J, Kotz R. [Serum cobalt and serum chromium level in 2 patients with chronic renal failure after total hip prosthesis implantation with metal-metal gliding contact]. Z Orthop Ihre Grenzgeb 2000;138:425–9.
9. Urban RM, Jacobs JJ, Tomlinson MJ, Galante JO. Renal tubular chromium deposition in patients with failed or long-term joint replacement. Paper #0165: 47th Annual Meeting, Orthopaedic Research Society, February 25–28, 2001, San Francisco, CA, USA.
10. Wedeen RP, Qian LF. Chromium-induced kidney disease. Environ Health Perspect 1991;92:71–4. Review.
11. Franchini I, Bocchi MC, Giaroli C, Ferdenzi O, Alinovi R, Bergamaschi E. Does occupational cobalt exposure determine early renal changes? Sci Total Environ 1994;150:149–52.
12. Merritt K, Brown SA. Release of hexavalent chromium from corrosion of stainless steel and cobalt-chromium alloys. J Biomed Mater Res 1995;29:627–33.
13. MacDonald SJ, Brodner W, Jacobs JJ. A consensus paper on metal ions in metal-on-metal hip arthroplasties. J Arthroplasty 2004;19(8 Suppl 3):12–6.
14. Case CP, Ellis L, Turner JC, Fairman B. Development of a routine method for the determination of trace metals in whole blood by magnetic sector inductively coupled plasma mass spectrometry with particular relevance to patients with total hip and knee arthroplasty. Clin Chem 2001;47:275–80.
15. Daniel J, Ziaee H, Pynsent PB, McMinn DJ. The validity of serum levels as a surrogate measure of systemic exposure to metal ions in hip replacement. J Bone Joint Surg Br 2007;89:736–41.

16. Daniel J, Ziaee H, Pradhan C, Pynsent PB, McMinn DJ. Blood and urine metal ion levels in young and active patients after Birmingham hip resurfacing arthroplasty: four-year results of a prospective longitudinal study. J Bone Joint Surg Br 2007;89:169–73.

17. MacDonald SJ, McCalden RW, Chess DG, et al. Hip Society Open Scientific Meeting 2002, Dallas, Texas. Available at http://www.hipsoc.org/openmeet02162002.html. Accessed August 24, 2007.

18. Daniel J, Ziaee H, Salama A, Pradhan C, McMinn DJ. The effect of the diameter of metal-on-metal bearings on systemic exposure to cobalt and chromium. J Bone Joint Surg Br 2006;88:443–8.

19. Hart AJ, Hester T, Sinclair K, Powell JJ, Goodship AE, Pele L, Fersht NL, Skinner J. The association between metal ions from hip resurfacing and reduced T-cell counts. J Bone Joint Surg Br 2006;88:449–54.

20. Luetzner J, Krummenauer F, Lengel AM, Ziegler J, Witzleb WC. Serum metal ion exposure after total knee arthroplasty. Clin Orthop Relat Res 2007;461:136–42.

21. Doherty AT, Howell RT, Ellis LA, Bisbinas I, Learmonth ID, Newson R, Case CP. Increased chromosome translocations and aneuploidy in peripheral blood lymphocytes of patients having revision arthroplasty of the hip. J Bone Joint Surg Br 2001;83:1075–81.

22. Ladon D, Doherty A, Newson R, Turner J, Bhamra M, Case CP. Changes in metal levels and chromosome aberrations in the peripheral blood of patients after metal-on-metal hip arthroplasty. J Arthroplasty 2004;19(8 Suppl 3):78–83.

23. Ladon D, Bhamra M, Turner J, Case CP Changes in chromosome aberrations and metal levels in the peripheral blood of patients after ceramic-on- ceramic hip replacement. Poster No. 1145. 51st Annual Meeting of the Orthopaedic Research Society, Washington, DC, 2005.

24. Davies AP, Sood A, Lewis AC, Newson R, Learmonth ID, Case CP. Metal-specific differences in levels of DNA damage caused by synovial fluid recovered at revision arthroplasty. J Bone Joint Surg Br 2005;87:1439–44.

25. Visuri T, Pukkala E. Does metal-on-metal hip prosthesis have influence on cancer? A long-term follow-up study. In: Reiker C, Oberholzer S, Wyss U, eds. World Tribology Forum in Arthroplasty. Bern, Toronto, Seattle: Hans Huber, 2001:181–8.

26. Brodner W, Grohs JG, Bancher-Todesca D, Dorotka R, Meisinger V, Gottsauner-Wolf F, Kotz R. Does the placenta inhibit the passage of chromium and cobalt after metal-on-metal total hip arthroplasty? J Arthroplasty 2004;19(suppl):S102–106.

27. Ziaee H, Daniel J, Datta AK, Blunt S, McMinn DJ. Transplacental transfer of cobalt and chromium in patients with metal-on-metal hip arthroplasty: a controlled study. J Bone Joint Surg Br 2007;89:301–305.

28. Merritt K, Brown SA. Distribution of cobalt chromium wear and corrosion products and biologic reactions. Clin Orthop Relat Res 1996;329(suppl):S233–43. Review.

29. Riedl MA, Casillas AM. Adverse drug reactions: types and treatment options. Am Fam Physician 2003;68:1781–90. Review.

30. Hallab N, Merritt K, Jacobs JJ. Metal sensitivity in patients with orthopaedic implants. J Bone Joint Surg Am 2001;83:428–36. Review.

31. Shimmin AJ, Back D. Femoral neck fractures following Birmingham hip resurfacing: a national review of 50 cases. J Bone Joint Surg Br 2005;87:463–4.

32. Willert HG, Buchhorn GH, Fayyazi A, Flury R, Windler M, Koster G, Lohmann CH. Metal-on-metal bearings and hypersensitivity in patients with artificial hip joints. A clinical and histomorphological study. J Bone Joint Surg Am 2005;87:28–36.

33. Davies AP, Willert HG, Campbell PA, Learmonth ID, Case CP. An unusual lymphocytic perivascular infiltration in tissues around contemporary metal-on-metal joint replacements. J Bone Joint Surg Am 2005;87:18–27.

34. Long WT, Dorr LD, Gendelman V. An American experience with metal-on-metal total hip arthroplasties: a 7-year follow-up study. J Arthroplasty 2004;19(8 Suppl 3):29–34.

35. Shahrdar C, Campbell P, Mirra J, Dorr LD. Painful metal-on-metal total hip arthroplasty. J Arthroplasty 2006;21:289–93.

36. Vassiliou K, Elfick A, Scholes S, Unsworth A. The effect of 'running-in' on the tribology and surface morphology of metal-on-metal BHR device in simulator studies. Proc I Mech E Part H J Eng Med 2006;220:269–77.

37. Farvard L. Damie F. Blood serum levels with metal-metal and metal-on-polyethylene arthroplasties. In: Reiker C, Oberholzer S, Wyss U, eds. World Tribology Forum in Arthroplasty Bern, Toronto, Seattle: Hans Huber, 2001:143–146.

38. Savarino L, Granchi D, Ciapetti G, Cenni E, Nardi Pantoli A, Rotini R, Veronesi CA, Baldini N, Giunti A. Ion release in patients with metal-on-metal hip bearings in total joint replacement: a comparison with metal-on-polyethylene bearings. J Biomed Mater Res. 2002;63(5):467–74.

39. Pfister AJ, Widmer KH, Friedrich NF. Increased whole blood levels of cobalt, chromium and molybdenum in hip arthroplasty with metal metal bearings. Presented at the 7th Swiss Congress de l'Union des Societes Chirurgicales Suisses. 19–22, June 2002. Lausanne, Switzerland. 2002

40. Clarke MT, Lee PT, Arora A, Villar RN. Levels of metal ions after small- and large-diameter metal-on-metal hip arthroplasty. J Bone Joint Surg Br. 2003 Aug;85(6):913–7.

41. Back DL, Young DA, Shimmin AJ. How do serum cobalt and chromium levels change after metal-on-metal hip resurfacing? Clin Orthop Relat Res. 2005 Sep;438:177–81.

42. Heisel C, Silva M, Skipor AK, Jacobs JJ, Schmalzried TP. The relationship between activity and ions in patients with metal-on-metal bearing hip prostheses. J Bone Joint Surg Am. 2005 Apr;87(4):781–7.

43. Dunstan E, Sanghrajka AP, Tilley S, Unwin P, Blunn G, Cannon SR, Briggs TW. Metal ion levels after metal-on-metal proximal femoral replacements: a 30-year follow-up. J Bone Joint Surg Br. 2005 May; 87(5):628–31.

14
Patient Selection and Timing of Operation

Joseph Daniel, Chandra Pradhan, and Hena Ziaee

Indications

Hip resurfacing arthroplasty is an option for people with advanced hip disease who would otherwise receive and are likely to outlive a conventional primary total hip replacement (THR), particularly for younger patients who wish to be reasonably active [1]. That guideline from the National Institute for Clinical Excellence (NICE), a statutory body in the United Kingdom, broadly sums up the indications in which a hip resurfacing device should be used.

A patient who would receive a conventional THR is someone with significant pain and disability arising from severe hip arthritis and in whom nonoperative treatment has failed. Several proven hip arthroplasty devices are available for the management of hip arthritis in elderly inactive patients. These can be used with a reasonable expectation that the device would outlast the patient. The Birmingham Hip Resurfacing (BHR) is neither indicated nor desirable in such patients, in whom progressive osteoporosis is inevitable and constitutes a risk factor for failure through femoral neck fracture or femoral head collapse. Young patients and especially those who are active jeopardize the longevity of any device and may need multiple revision procedures during their lifetime. It is in these young and active patients that there is a need to go conservative and it is for them that the Birmingham Hip Resurfacing (BHR) is really indicated.

By far the most common indication in any Western series is primary osteoarthrosis of the hip. Other indications include any hip disease that can lead to secondary arthritic change. The list of conditions in which we have used the BHR is given in Table 14.1 and Fig. 14.1.

There are some patients in whom a resurfacing is particularly preferable to a replacement in the absence of other adverse factors:

- Young active patients (better revision options retained).
- Young patients with a particularly large femoral offset. In spite of the availability of high offset THR stems, the offset in some patients is too large for an artificial stem to match. This makes a BHR preferable.
- Patients with a wide femoral canal or a femoral shaft deformity are awkward for stem implantation.
- Patients with osteopetrosis (marble bone disease) in whom it is almost impossible to fit a stem in the nonexistent femoral canal.

Contraindications

From the preamble that the indication for a resurfacing is a patient who would otherwise have received a conventional THR, it follows that those patients who would have been excluded from being considered for a THR would be excluded from a resurfacing as well. These include patients with:

- recent active infection in and around the hip;
- current active infection elsewhere;
- severe vascular deficiency in the limb;
- inadequate motor power around the hip;
- and the skeletally immature.

Patients who are unfit for an anesthetic or a major elective operation are also not suitable for a resurfacing. These include the following:

- Patients graded as ASA 4 and 5 (according to the physical status classification system of the American Society of Anesthesiologists); or those with medical conditions that substantially increase the risk of serious perioperative complications or death.
- Short life expectancy or where the expected benefits do not outweigh the risks.
- Recent history of coronary or cerebrovascular episodes.
- Patients with uncontrolled diabetes or other systemic diseases.

The contraindications specific to a metal on metal bearing include:

- Patients in end-stage renal failure or those on dialysis.
- Patients with a known or proven hypersensitivity to metal.

TABLE 14.1. Different indications in which a BHR was performed

Sequelae of childhood hip disorders
  Congenital hip dysplasia
  Developmental dysplasia
  Multiple epiphyseal dysplasia
  Dysplasia with neurofibromatosis
  Post–Perthes disease
  Old septic arthritis
  Old slipped capital femoral epiphysis (SCFE)
  Any of the above with previous surgery

Adult hip disorders
  Primary osteoarthrosis
  Early destructive arthritis
  Posttraumatic arthritis
  Avascular necrosis
  Protrusio acetabulae
  Synovial chondromatosis

Inflammatory disorders
  Rheumatoid arthritis
  Juvenile rheumatoid arthritis
  Psoriatic arthritis
  Other seronegative arthritis
  Idiopathic ankylosis of hip
  Idiopathic chondrolysis
  Ankylosing spondylitis

Women of child-bearing age who are planning to have a baby in the near future should be advised to have the baby before the resurfacing or wait for at least 2 years after the operation before having a baby.

In addition to the above, the specific contraindications to hip resurfacing include:

- Patients with poor quality bone in the femoral head and neck (cystic degeneration or osteopenia).
- Older inactive patients in whom conventional THRs have a proven track record of success. A simple chronological cut-off age (for instance, men >65 years and women >60 years) is not always workable. Other considerations such as patient

activities, comorbidities, and bone quality have to be taken into consideration while using age as a criterion.

- Crowe grade IV dysplasia of the femur in which the socket is too hypotrophic and poorly developed to implant a cup large enough for a resurfacing.
- Malignant tumors in and around the hip are best treated with regular or custom THR.
- Severe femoral head avascular necrosis (AVN) is a relative contraindication due to the higher rate of postresurfacing femoral head collapse. It is better treated with a Birmingham Mid-Head Resection (BMHR) prosthesis or a THR.
- Severe post–Perthes disease or post–slipped capital femoral epiphysis arthritis (SCFE) are relative contraindications especially if the anatomic abnormality cannot be restored with a resurfacing. A BMHR prosthesis is preferable in these young patients.
- Patients with severe leg length discrepancy. Hip resurfacing cannot produce large leg length adjustments.

The Ideal Candidate for a Hip Resurfacing

A symptomatic young active patient in end-stage hip arthritis (i.e., cartilage loss and bone-on-bone articulation) with acceptable femoral head bone quality and a reasonably regular anatomy of the acetabulum and proximal femur would benefit the most from a hip resurfacing.

Timing of Operation

A caveat has to be added to the generalization in the NICE guideline that hip resurfacing is an option for people who would otherwise receive a conventional primary THR. A young patient with an arthritic hip and no other restraining physical disabilities was until recently considered a relative contraindication to hip replacement. Therefore, if a young patient with end-stage arthritis were to find his symptoms manageable with daily long-term anti-inflammatory medications, he would be considered as one who did not need a hip replacement yet, thereby ruling out a hip resurfacing too according to the NICE guideline.

In the era when a conventional hip replacement was the only option, it was wise to delay the procedure by every means possible as suggested by Sir John Charnley. That delay was purported to achieve two purposes: (a) it hopefully allowed the patient to grow older and reach an age at which he would be suitable for a replacement, and (b) the delay would bring his activity level down to a lower state thereby reducing the demands on the prosthesis and favoring longer implant survival.

Hip resurfacing has now been shown to perform best in young active patients, the very group who produce the worst results with a conventional hip replacement. We reported [2] a series of 446 hip resurfacings (79% males) in patients under the age of 55 years with osteoarthritis and there was

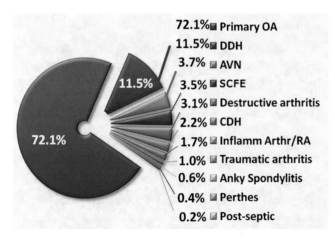

FIG. 14.1. Incidence of different etiologies for which a BHR was performed at our center (1997–2005), n = 2600.

72.1% Primary OA
11.5% DDH
3.7% AVN
3.5% SCFE
3.1% Destructive arthritis
2.2% CDH
1.7% Inflamm Arthr/RA
1.0% Traumatic arthritis
0.6% Anky Spondylitis
0.4% Perthes
0.2% Post-septic

15
Anesthesia, Pain Control, and Thromboprophylaxis

Jonathan W. Freeman

The anesthetic technique currently used for the Birmingham Hip Resurfacing (BHR), and in fact for all of our joint arthroplasty surgery, has evolved over the past 14 years during the evolution of this innovative surgery. As an anesthetic team, we have reviewed the work in other centers, trawled the literature for novel techniques, traveled to see what we think is good practice elsewhere, and have developed our own distillation that we believe works well for us. That birthing process has taken us from normotensive and hypotensive techniques under general anesthesia (GA), through regional techniques and local anesthetic blocks, with and without sedation, to a technique of epidural-induced hypotension under light general anesthesia that we practice today. We have played with both autologous and homologous blood transfusions, predonation transfusions, and intraoperative and postoperative salvage and have ended up with a technique that leads us to transfusing only 1.4% of our primary BHRs and 8.3% of our total hip replacements (THRs), and we no longer routinely cross-match blood for our patients. Postoperative pain relief has gone from intramuscular opiates through prolonged epidural blocks and patient-controlled analgesia (PCA and PCEA) techniques to what is now early mobilization after a short-duration patient-controlled epidural pump (PCEA) technique and local infiltration followed by routine oral analgesia. Thromboprophylaxis has always been a difficult decision—a conflict of increased blood loss but reduction of nonfatal and fatal deep vein thrombosis (DVT) and pulmonary embolism (PE). The world's health care professions are divided on what is best treatment, and we have also struggled with this dilemma. The National Institute of Clinical Excellence (NICE) in the United Kingdom has recently deliberated this issue and has issued guidance on good practice that is at conflict with the mixed views of the U.K. orthopedic fraternity. There is no doubt that thromboembolism is a reality and causes much morbidity and mortality in patients undergoing orthopedic surgery, but as I shall outline later in the chapter, our experience and regimen is different than most and could be construed to be at odds with the treatment prophylaxis recommended both nationally and internationally.

Anesthesia

Preoperative Assessment

We realized quite early in the development of our anesthetic technique that there is no single standard anesthetic for hip arthroplasty. A technique should be developed that takes into account the premorbid state of the patient as well as the type of proposed surgery. Fortunately, the majority of our patients are "relatively young" and fit, wishing to pursue their social and sporting activities into later life. However, as they progress through their middle and late-middle age, there are frequent covert medical conditions that need to be uncovered prior to surgery, as they can cause problems with anesthesia especially if we use a hypotensive technique. All our patients are reviewed in detail in clinic, and if there is any comorbidity of note, they are all referred to the anesthetic team for consideration before surgery is planned. Some of the easier conditions requiring further investigation include symptomatic cardiovascular disease such as poorly treated hypertension and coronary artery disease including those having had coronary artery stenting and cardiac bypass grafting. Asymptomatic but treated insulin-dependent diabetes frequently has associated silent coronary artery disease that needs review, and orthopedic conditions such as ankylosing spondylitis and severe rheumatoid disease need airway assessment prior to surgery. Fortunately, not a lot of our patients are elderly or frail but there are a few, and these obviously require special consideration regarding anesthesia and perioperative management.

The drug medication history is one of the most important areas to consider during preassessment. Quite a significant number of our patients are on complex antiplatelet medication prior to surgery. It is imperative that these are reviewed and if at all possible stopped or reduced in dosage. Aspirin, clopidogrel, and nonsteroidal anti-inflammatory drugs (NSAIDs) can all have significant perioperative effects and can preclude the use of epidural and spinal blocks. Antihypertensive drugs such as beta-blockers and ACE-inhibitors can also have significant interaction with neuraxial blockage potentiating the hypotension and also affecting renal function.

Other areas of concern include the relatively rare but ever increasing serious allergies that individuals may present with. The obvious ones of note relate to antibiotics and anesthetic drugs, but we are seeing an increasing number of individuals who are latex sensitive or who have metal ion allergies. These sensitivities and allergies are all investigated thoroughly, are taken very seriously, and a management plan is worked out for each individual.

During preoperative assessment, routine blood profiling is undertaken, including full blood count, hemoglobin level, platelet count, prothrombin time, and international normalized ratio (INR). Blood is taken for grouping, but we no longer cross-match our patients unless their hemoglobin is lower than 11.5 g/dL. It has been several years since we have transfused blood in the operating room to a patient undergoing primary joint arthroplasty, and as mentioned previously our inpatient transfusion rate for BHR is currently only 1.4%, which we believe relates to improved surgical technique, perioperative hypotension, and a higher threshold to transfuse. Other blood chemistry requested includes urea, creatinine, electrolytes, and blood glucose. An ECG and CXR are performed as routine as is urinalysis.

Choice of Anesthetic

As explained earlier, hip arthroplasty can be performed under general, spinal, or epidural anesthesia, and we tend to use a combination of these techniques. We have altered our anesthetic protocol on many occasions in response to reviewing others' work, the literature, and patient request. It has been argued for years that the choice of anesthetic makes little difference to patient outcome as regards mortality in elective surgery [1–3]. There is however sufficient evidence that the technique can affect perioperative management, blood loss, and postoperative pain relief and mobilization, and a recent meta-analysis showed that compared with general anesthesia (GA), neuraxial block reduces many serious complications in patients undergoing a variety of surgeries [4–6]. Choice of technique can also dramatically affect the patient's postoperative course. Evidence exists to suggest that early mobilization after some types of anesthesia is better than with others. Obviously, a technique that confines someone to bed for several days, such as a prolonged neuraxial block, may delay mobilization and early discharge from hospital but conversely one that causes postoperative nausea and vomiting and delayed return of psychomotor function, as may be seen with opiate anesthesia, will also delay patient progress [7]. In a Cochrane Database Systematic Review comparing the efficacy of epidural analgesia with other postoperative modalities for pain relief after hip or knee replacement, Choi et al. concluded that epidural analgesia may be useful for postoperative pain relief after major joint replacements, however, the benefit may be limited to the early (4 to 6 hours) postoperative period and that it may be beneficial to convert to some other form of analgesia after this time [8].

These reviews suggest that a variety of appropriate anesthetic techniques can be used for hip arthroplasty and that it is best to distil the benefits and advantages of all techniques, which is what we have done. To this end, we have settled on using a low thoracic hypotensive epidural anesthetic technique (HEA), which we believe provides the benefits of good analgesia, reduced blood loss and transfusion, low incidence of postoperative nausea and vomiting (PONV), rapid return of psychomotor function, early mobilization, reduced incidence of postoperative venous thrombosis and pulmonary embolism, maintained pulmonary function, and a reduced stress response to surgical trauma. Spinal and epidural anesthesia are not without their complications, however, and there is a need for continued monitoring and attention to the block level. Minor complications are frequently seen, including inadequate pain relief, failure of block or unilateral blockade, and troublesome side-effects such as urinary retention and incontinence. We have had our fair share of minor and moderate complications during this time. These include the occasional dural tap headache after inadvertent or covert dural puncture, at the time of performing the epidural, but these can be readily treated by epidural blood patch if picked up early postoperatively. It has to be accepted, however, that although this is considered a minor complication, it can cause quite marked patient distress. Severe complications are fortunately rare but have been well documented in the literature. These include temporary or even permanent neurologic sequelae, chronic back pain, and probably more importantly the masking of acute problems such as blood loss, nerve damage after surgery, or even postoperative joint dislocation.

In comparison, GA offers some very important advantages over neuraxial blockade. Hemodynamic status is probably more stable under a "gentle" and carefully administered GA and can avoid marked blood pressure swings seen in patients with cardiac comorbidity such as aortic stenosis with the rapid establishment of a spinal or epidural block. GA also avoids having to position the conscious patient in an uncomfortable lateral position, which most find difficult for the duration of surgery under sole neuraxial blockade. Others who cannot tolerate lying flat are also best sedated or given a GA.

It is with these considerations in mind that over the past 14 years, we have developed a continually evolving anesthetic technique that we believe works best for most of our patients and combines the benefits of both neuraxial blockade with the calmness of light general anesthesia. Most of our patients tolerate this technique well and mobilize early.

The Technique Currently Used in Birmingham

Unless specifically indicated or requested by overly anxious patients, the only premedication is that of gentle and considerate counseling and reassurance along with a "night-cap" of their choice or an early retirement to bed. We rarely give preemptive analgesia, but if there is some preexistent discomfort or pain, which is not uncommon, then an oral analgesic (paracetamol, NSAID, or codeine) of the patient's choice is administered.

Patients are brought to the anesthetic room (a much hallowed anesthetic domain in U.K. practice) where they are fully monitored with pulse oximetry, noninvasive blood pressure, and five-lead ECG with three-lead ST segment analysis. After normal preoperative checks and final discussions with the surgical team, they are given preoxygenation via a face mask, an intravenous line is established in the upper arm for lateral surgery (the side of the surgery), and a light general anesthetic is induced with propofol either by infusion or as a bolus. We now always protect the airway with endotracheal intubation after paralysis with a relaxant and intermittent positive ventilation is commenced. We have in the past allowed spontaneous ventilation with face mask oxygen or with a laryngeal mask airway, but there is evidence that the lateral position, especially the left lateral, is more associated with passive gastric reflux, and we feel that securing the airway is important to prevent pulmonary aspiration.

Once anesthesia has been induced, a second intravenous cannula (14 gauge) is inserted followed by an internal jugular central venous line and a radial artery invasive blood pressure line. A low thoracic epidural (T10–12) catheter is then inserted under aseptic conditions and a neuraxial block is established with a large-volume, low-concentration local anesthetic solution. We currently use between 15 and 30 mL of a 50:50 mix of 2% lidocaine and 0.5% Levo-bupivacaine depending on age, body mass index, and height of patient. This dose is added incrementally, to achieve the desired sympathetic block and level of hypotension.

Monitoring of invasive blood pressure and three ST segment analysis is important during the establishment of the neuraxial block, and as per the regimen outlined by Sharrock

et al. an infusion of vasoconstrictor (usually epinephrine) is commenced early down the central venous line to prevent precipitous blood pressure swings [9]. This technique combines an extensive epidural blockade that results in a controlled hypotension, but with preservation of central venous pressure, heart rate, stroke volume, and cardiac output. The technique does not appear to adversely compromise cardiac, renal, or cerebral function. Sharrock and others however have gone on to document several case reports of bradycardia and even asystole using this technique, and care must be taken with high-risk patients [10–12]. In our practice, we have found this technique to be extremely effective at reducing the blood pressure and extremely controllable. We have not had any complications attributable to this hypotensive technique. The benefits as previously alluded to include a relatively bloodless field for surgery and reduced intraoperative blood loss.

After a preliminary skin preparation and sterile draping, the patient is transferred from the anesthetic room into the operating room. Here, a final skin preparation and secondary draping occurs, and we commence the final reduction in mean arterial pressure prior to the start of surgery. We try to maintain the mean blood pressure around 45 to 55 mm Hg with a systolic of approximately 55 to 65 mm Hg. during the initial dissection phase. The central venous pressure is kept low (0 to 4 mm Hg) during this time as a rise can contribute to venous oozing. The heart rate is maintained around 55 to 65 beats per minute if necessary by administering small increments of intravenous beta-blockade such as labetalol or sotalol. The blood pressure is eventually elevated by increasing the epinephrine infusion once the acetabular component has been located and attention is turned to the femoral head. Relative hypotension, a mean of 55 to 60 mm Hg, is maintained however until the prosthesis is reduced into the cup and closure of the wound is commenced (Fig. 15.1).

In an attempt to allay our own concerns over hemodynamic and cardiac function during the use of hypotensive anesthetic

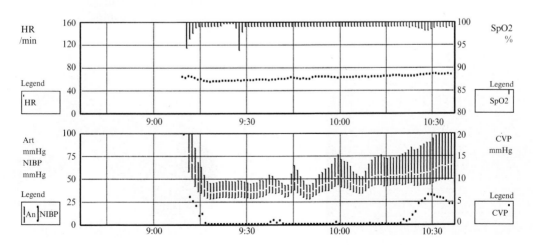

Fig. 15.1. Anesthetic record showing induced hypotension and low central venous pressure during the main operative period

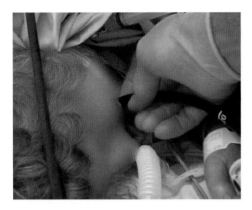

FIG. 15.2. Transesophageal echocardiography (TOE) being inserted.

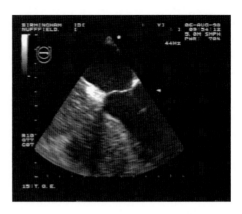

FIG. 15.4. Image of transesophageal echo with intravascular debris

techniques, we have performed a study on 20 BHRs and 20 THRs using transesophageal echocardiography along with invasive arterial pressure monitoring (Figs. 15.2–15.4).

In both patient groups that we monitored, cardiac function and ejection fraction were maintained during hypotensive anesthesia. However, the most interesting events observed concern the return of intravascular debris (clots and microbubbles) to the heart during intramedullary reaming for THRs and pressuring of the femoral component with insertion of the prosthesis whether it is the complete femoral component with THRs or just the centralizing pin of the BHR (Fig. 15.4). We, like others, have subsequently shown that venting of the femur with a trochanteric cannula reduces this effect in the THRs and renders it insignificant when we perform this with our BHRs. We now vent the femur as a routine in all our cases.

Other factors that appear to contribute to hemodynamic instability and problems such as venous oozing during the operative dissection phase include poor positioning of the patient, increased abdominal pressure, and vena-caval compression from the support props and raised positive pressure ventilation (Fig 15.5).

Other attention to detail during the operation includes the monitoring of body temperature by using an esophageal temperature probe and the provision of added warmth in the form of a forced convection blanket and warmed intravenous fluids. The combination of a vasodilated patient secondary to a high thoracic sympathetic block from the epidural, the use of several liters of pulse lavage to wash the joint, and a forced air Charnley tent can rapidly drop patient temperature. Every effort is made to return the patient's temperature to within the normal range before waking, as shivering increases oxygen consumption postoperatively and heightens any discomfort felt by the patient. Aggressive warming may also have benefits in reducing postoperative blood loss [13].

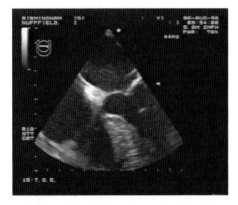

FIG. 15.3. Normal transesophageal echo

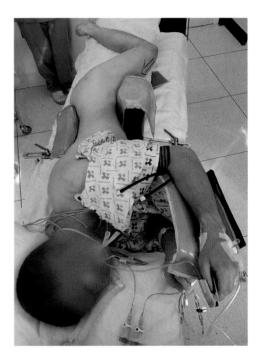

FIG.15.5. Positioning of patient taking care with props

Pain Control

The maintenance of good postoperative pain control has always been a difficult area to address as there is always a conflict of the provision of adequate pain relief but with the need for early mobilization. We have tried many combinations of intramuscular opiates, intravenous bolus of opiates, and PCA techniques along with supplemental, regular oral analgesics including NSAIDs, opiates, and simple drugs such as paracetamol and aspirin. Postoperative nausea and vomiting are frequent sequelae to high-dose opiate use with early mobilization, and the delay in psychomotor function associated with intraoperative opiates has already been mentioned. Regional neuraxial blocks are an obvious advantage if their use is continued into the postoperative period, but prolonged usage may delay mobilization, require attentive monitoring, and may not be liked by the patient. Prolonged neuraxial blockade also has attributable complications such as poor mobility in bed, loss of skin sensation, and pressure sores [14]. Conversely, early cessation of neuraxial blockade allows mobilization and reduces the requirement for urinary catheterization [15]. We have also experimented with femoral 3:1 block or psoas lumbar plexus blocks as a sole technique or even to potentiate central neuraxial blocks that have been used intraoperatively but discontinued in the postoperative period. All these techniques have their failure rates and complications, need a certain level of technical expertise, and take time to establish [16,17]. We have also had several of our own complications from this technique including one case of a total spinal block with hypotension and respiratory arrest requiring ventilation for 3 hours after inadvertent nerve root dural cuff puncture! Other complications relating to the unilateral neural block provided by such techniques as psoas sheath block include the inevitable confusion regarding the cause of postoperative foot drop, and we have stopped doing these blocks as a routine so that nerve assessment can be made early in the postoperative period. We even allow our central neuraxial blocks to wear off enough to assess early limb function and neural integrity in the recovery ward before recommencing them for postoperative pain relief.

Our current postoperative pain control regimen is to use the epidural established during the operation for a period of 4 to 8 hours into the postoperative period. This is achieved by connecting the epidural catheter to a PCEA and allowing the patient to establish their own level of block. In an attempt to reduce the need for the PCEA, local anesthesia is also infiltrated at the site of the arthroplasty at the time of surgery as outlined in Chapter 16, although we have no experience with intraarticular injection of local anesthesia postoperatively through a catheter. Local anesthesia infiltrated into the wound during surgery has proved to be effective and allows early discontinuation of the epidural but with good maintained pain relief. We supplement these local techniques with simple oral

analgesics and mobilize the patient on the first postoperative day at around 18 to 24 hours, and we try to keep parenteral or oral opiate use to a minimum. If a patient is unable to pass urine in the early postoperative period, he or she is allowed to stand with nurse assistance.

Thromboprophylaxis

There is no doubt that venous thromboembolism (VTE) is a life-threatening event with serious perioperative morbidity and mortality, and those undergoing elective orthopedic surgery are known to be a population at increased risk. The problem of thromboprophylaxis is one that is continually being addressed, but the search for the ideal combination of agents continues. There is always the dilemma of balancing increased blood loss, bruising, and transfusion rates secondary to prophylaxis against the need to reduce a well-recognized complication of surgery. Recent data from the U.K. Government Health Select Committee provide up to date accurate figures of the estimated extent of the problem. Each year in England, more than 25,000 people die from VTE in hospital from all causes [18]. This is more than the combined total of deaths from breast cancer, AIDS, and traffic accidents! The problem with this data is that it is retrospective and includes all patients regardless of premorbidity, underlying disease status, and current active treatment. The U.K. National Institute of Health and Clinical Excellence (NICE) has recently produced guidelines that recommend the use of low-molecular-weight heparin (LMWH) or fondaparinux (a selective factor Xa inhibitor) for thromboprophylaxis after elective orthopedic surgery, but they are based on historic data regarding the actual VTE risk [19]. There is evidence that although VTE is still a problem in the orthopedic population, there have been numerous changes in patient management over recent years that reduce this risk. These include changes in surgical technique, anesthetic practice, early mobilization, reduced blood transfusion, and the wide use of mechanical measures such as compression stockings and early in-bed exercises. It may be that the current incidence of VTE in elective orthopedic surgery undergoing active treatment and mobilization, with or without aggressive chemical prophylaxis, is exaggerated.

Understanding the etiology of this condition is part way to evolving methods of countering the problem. We know that the pathogenesis is multifactorial and includes the triad of hypercoagulability, venous stasis, and endothelial damage. Any interventional modality that tries to address these factors must go some way to reducing the risk. Historically, we have tried to approach these by direct pharmacologic treatment of the coagulation cascade process in an attempt to prevent thromboembolic progression. This has meant the use of intravenous heparin and or oral warfarin during inpatient treatment in doses that significantly alter the patients bleeding time and may be associated with unacceptable complications, including mortality. Over the past few years, we have tried to deviate from the time-honored therapeutic regimens and try a different approach. Our thromboprophylactic management differs considerably from both that of the recommendations of the American College of Chest Physicians and those of NICE in the United Kingdom. These recommendations have already been contested by others as well as ourselves [19,20].

We are fully aware that release of tissue thromboplastin occurs early in the dissection phase of any major surgery. Our own studies looking at tissue thromboplastin and thromboelastography (TEG) indicate that this effect occurs within 10 minutes of major muscle dissection, and the clotting cascade becomes acutely activated. The TEG is a viscoelastic measure of clot formation with definable parameters that can be used to assess the coagulation cascade and record a hyper- or hypothrombotic state (Fig. 15.6). The parameters of particular note are the reaction time R and the alpha angle α. As the reaction time shortens and the alpha angle increases, a more prothrombotic activated state is seen (Figs. 15.7 and 15.8). These traces are from one patient with baseline trace and repeated approximately 15 minutes after commencing surgery.

Any therapeutic modality aimed at the prevention of this effect obviously needs to be commenced prior to the insult, and pretreatment with anticoagulant therapy and early techniques to reduce the effect are paramount. There is evidence that maintained peripheral blood flow, reduced stasis, and the use of epidurals may be helpful in reducing the stress response

to trauma and ultimately the overall risk. More studies are required to investigate the effect of different anesthetic techniques and therapeutic modalities on thrombogenesis.

In Birmingham UK, we have embarked on an active non–anticoagulant regimen of thromboprophylaxis (nACT), which combines hypotensive epidural anesthesia (HEA), early mobilization, elastic graded compression stockings, and an oral antiplatelet agent (usually aspirin unless contraindicated), and we have reported safe and effective thromboprophylaxis in a consecutive group of patients undergoing unilateral primary hip arthroplasty [21]. The addition of adjuvant intermittent pneumatic calf compression has significantly reduced the asymptomatic DVT rate even further [22].

These recent results are very encouraging, and we have just submitted a retrospective analysis of our last 463 consecutive primary hip arthroplasty patients managed without conventional anticoagulants. In approximately half of these patients, a mechanical leg compression device was also used. All were reviewed as in-patients and for up to 6 to 10 weeks postoperatively. In addition, all patients completed a questionnaire at a minimum of 3 months postoperatively, to ensure that no thromboembolic events had occurred after their first outpatient consultation. There were no cases of symptomatic DVT. The incidence of asymptomatic Doppler ultrasonic screened DVT was 10.2% in the group without pneumatic calf compression and 4.3% in those with. There were no cases of symptomatic PE. This combination we believe offers a low

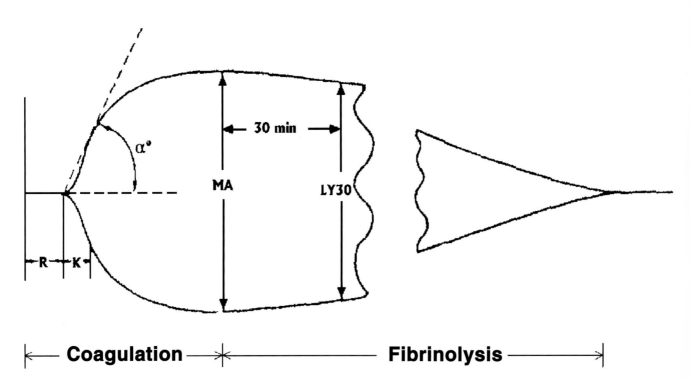

FIG. 15.6. Stylized normal TEG trace. R, reaction time or rate of fibrin formation; K, clot formation time, measured from end of R to when the trace reaches 20 mm from baseline. Alpha angle is the angle formed by the slope of the TEG trace from the end R point to the K value and indicates rate of clot formation. MA, maximum amplitude, reflects absolute fibrin clot strength

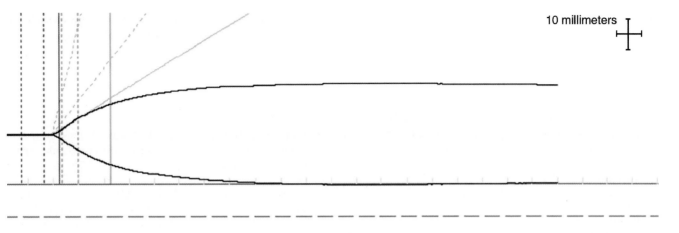

10 millimeters

FIG. 15.7. Baseline thromboelastograph prior to surgery with normal thromboplastin activation as indicated by normal start point, reaction time, and alpha angle (solid blue tangential line)

incidence of VTE without the complications and higher risks associated with anticoagulant use and should be considered as an alternative treatment method for those patients undergoing primary joint arthroplasty. An interesting observation for these patient groups was the incidence of homologous blood transfusion. Only 1.4% of our unilateral BHR patients required a blood transfusion for symptomatic anemia and only 8.3% for those undergoing THR. There is no doubt that this combination of hypotension and non-usage of conventional anticoagulation reduces perioperative and postoperative bleeding and is worthy of consideration. We have resorted over the past few years to the use of rescue tranexamic acid or aprotinin perioperatively in the presence of what is apparent marked operative bleeding, but there is little evidence that this reduces our overall blood loss unlike in liver and cardiac surgery. Numerous publications have extolled the virtues of protease inhibitors to reduce blood loss, but most have indicated that pretreatment rather than administration at the time of blood loss is the treatment of choice [23,24]. The risks of increased thrombogenesis, clot stabilization, increased possibilities of VTE and allergic reactions to therapeutic modalities raise questions marks over their use in operations where the incidence of thrombogenesis and clot progression is so high. Their routine use, as recommended in some centers, is debatable.

Like all our management protocols, the use of anesthetic techniques, pain control, and prophylaxis are constantly evolving. The questions relating to routine anticoagulation, blood loss reduction, and transfusion rates are always in our minds. There is no doubt that we shall modify our management strategies as time and knowledge evolve, but up to now the journey has been interesting and constantly challenging.

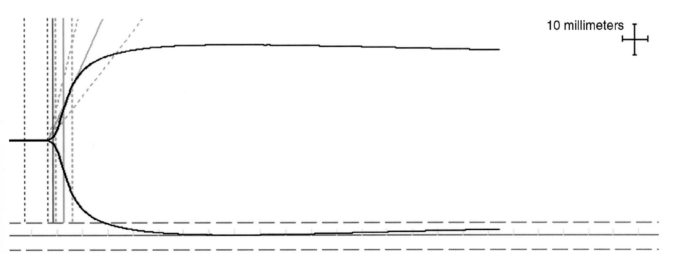

10 millimeters

FIG. 15.8. Activated thromboelastograph showing early start-point, shortened reaction time, and a more acute alpha angle

References

1. Rodgers A, et al. Reduction in postoperative mortality and morbidity with epidural or spinal anaesthesia: results from overview of randomised trials. BMJ 2000;321:1–12.

2. Rigg JR, et al. Epidural anaesthesia and analgesia and outcome of major surgery: a randomised trial. Lancet 2002;359:1276–82.

3. Park WY, et al. Effect of epidural anaesthesia and analgesia on peri-operative outcome: a randomised, controlled veteran affairs cooperative study. Ann Surg 2001;234:560–9.

4. Thompson GE, Miller RD, Stevens WC, Murray WR. Hypotensive anaesthesia for total hip arthroplasty: a study of blood loss and organ function (brain, liver and kidney. Anesthesiology 1978;48(2):91–6.

5. Rashiq S, Finegan BA. The effect of spinal anesthesia on blood transfusion rate in total joint arthroplasty. Can J Surg 2006;49(6):391–6.

6. Mauermann WJ, Shilling AM, Zuo Z. A comparison of neuraxial block versus general anaesthesia for elective total hip replacement: a meta-analysis. Anesth Analg 2006;103(4):1018–25.

7. Sharrock NE, Fischer G, Gross S, Flynn E, Go G, Sculco TP, Salvati EA. The early recovery of cognitive function after total hip replacement under hypotensive epidural anaesthesia. Reg Anesth Pain Med 2005;30(2):123–7.

8. Choi PT, et al. Epidural analgesia for pain following hip or knee replacement. Cochrane Database Systematic Review 2003;3: CD003071.

9. Sharrock NE, Salvati EA. Hypotensive epidural anesthesia for total hip arthroplasty: a review. Acta Orthop Scand 1996;67(1):91–107.

10. Liguori GA, Sharrock NE. Asystole and severe bradycardia during epidural anaesthesia in orthopaedic patients. Anesthesiology 1997;86(1):250–7.

11. Sharrock NE. Asystole under hypotensive epidural anesthesia. Anesth Analg 1998;87(4):982.

12. Heidegger T, Kreienbuhl G. Unsuccessful resuscitation under hypotensive epidural anesthesia during elective hip arthroplasty. Anesth Analg 1998;86:847–9.

13. Winkler M, et al. Aggressive warming reduces blood loss during hip arthroplasty. Anesth Analg 2000;91:978–84.

14. Shah JL. Lesson of the week: Postoperative pressure sores after epidural anaesthesia. BMJ 2000;321:941–2.

15. Macdowell AD, Robinson AHN, Hill DJ, Villar RN. Is epidural anaesthesia acceptable at total hip arthroplasty. A study of the rates of urinary catheterization. J Bone Joint Surg (Br) 2004;86:1115–1117.

16. Somayaji H, Hassan A, Reddy K, Heatley F. Bilateral gluteal compartment syndrome after total hip arthroplasty under epidural anaesthesia. J Bone and Joint Surg (Br) 2005;20:1081–83.

17. Lee LA, Posner KL, Domino KB, Caplan RA, Cheney FW. Injuries associated with regional anesthesia in the 1980s and 1990s: a closed claims analysis. Anesthesiology. 2004;101(1):143–52.

18. House of Commons Health Committee. HC 99 2005. The Stationary Office, London.

19. NICE Clinical Guideline 46. Venous thromboembolism. U.K. National Institute for Health and Clinical Excellence. 2007.

20. Callaghan JJ, et al. Editorial. Prophylaxis for thromboembolic disease: Recommendations from The American College of Chest Physcians – Are they appropriate for Orthopaedic Surgery? J Arthroplasty 2005;200:273–4.

21. Daniel J, Pradhan A, Pradhan C, Ziaee H, McMinn DJW. Thromboprophylaxis without routine anticoagulation in primary arthroplasty: Is it safe. Poster presented at: International Society for Technology in Arthroplasty, 2007, New York, NY, USA.

22. Daniel J, Pradhan A, Pradhan C, Ziaee H, Moss M. Freeman J, McMinn DJW. Multi-modal thromboprophylaxis following primary hip arthroplasty: The role of adjuvant intermittent pneumatic calf compression. J Bone Joint Surg (Br) 2008; 90-B:562–9.

23. Ekback G, et al. Tranexamic acid reduces blood loss in total hip replacement surgery. Anesth Analg 2000;91:1124–31.

24. Lemay E, Guay J, Cote C, Roy A. Tranexamic acid reduces the need for allogenic red blood cell transfusions in patients undergoing total hip replacement. Can J Anesthesia 2004; 51:31–7.

16
Anesthesia with Special Emphasis on Pain Control

Dennis R. Kerr and Lawrence Kohan

Pain management has an important influence on short-term outcomes after hip surgery particularly in relation to thrombo-embolism, hospital length of stay, nosocomial infection rate, and cost. Conventional pain management techniques including epidurals, nerve blocks, and patient-controlled analgesia using opioids make it difficult to mobilize patients quickly and characteristically require hospitalization for 3 to 10 days to achieve effective analgesia. However, this approach has often been the root cause of certain undesirable outcomes. Specifically, immobilization of the patient in bed often invites deep vein thrombosis (DVT), and prolonged hospital stays invite nosocomial infection.

To solve these problems, we have developed a key technique for the control of acute postoperative pain called local infiltration analgesia (LIA), which is based on systematic infiltration of a mixture of local anesthetic (ropivacaine) and a directly acting anti-inflammatory drug (ketorolac) around all structures subject to surgical trauma [1]. The initial infiltration is followed by top-ups as required and finally extensive reinjection by hand through a fine catheter after approximately 20 hours. The technique was developed specifically to avoid sedation and facilitate rapid physiologic recovery after lower-limb arthroplasty so as to enable early mobilization and discharge. In contrast with conventional acute pain management, opioid drugs are used only sparingly or not at all. The technique is particularly appropriate for patients having the Birmingham Hip Resurfacing (BHR) procedure because they are typically in good health and younger (mean age 53.8 years in our series) than those presenting for total hip replacement (mean age 69.8 years in our series), and there is generally no reason to confine them to bed. Also, the BHR prosthesis is stable, difficult to dislocate, and suitable for immediate mobilization.

Injectant

The injectant mixture (RKA mixture) consists of 150 mL (300 mg) ropivacaine HCl 0.2% (Naropin; Astra Zeneca Pty Ltd, North Ryde, NSW), mixed with 30 mg ketorolac tromethamine (Toradol; Roche Products Pty Ltd, North Ryde, NSW) and 5 to 10 µg/mL adrenaline (1 mg in a 100- or 200-mL bag). If the wound is large and more than 150 mL of injectant is required to adequately infiltrate the surgical field, the mixture is diluted with normal saline for volumes in excess of 150 mL to limit the total dose to a maximum of 300 mg. The total dose of ropivacaine is reduced to 250 mg if the patient is unusually small (<55 kg), very elderly (>85 years), infirm (American Society of Anesthesiologists [ASA] class 3 and 4), or has a history of unusual sensitivity to analgesics or anesthetic agents. In patients with contraindications to the use of nonsteroidal anti-inflammatory drugs (NSAIDs), especially renal failure, ketorolac is eliminated from the mixture and other oral or parenteral analgesics are used. All infiltration is done using 50-mL syringes and 10-cm-long, 19-gauge spinal needles. Injections are made using a "moving needle" technique, to avoid depositing large volumes of drug intravascularly, and they are spread over about 1 hour, injecting one layer at a time, to keep the blood levels of local anesthetic to a minimum.

Catheter

A 16-gauge Tuohy needle, 18-gauge epidural catheter ("pain catheter") (Portex; Smiths Group Plc, Smiths Medical International Ltd, Hythe, Kent, UK), and a 0.22-µm high-performance antibacterial flat epidural filter (SIMS-Portex Co.,

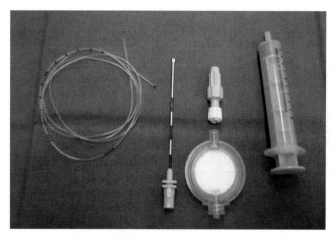

Fig. 16.1. Catheter setup.

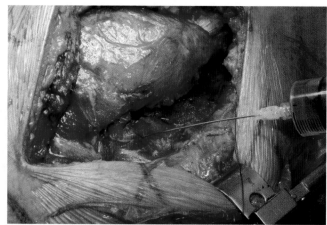

Fig. 16.3. Injection of the posterior capsule, and the short external rotator muscles.

Hythe, Kent, UK) are used (Fig. 16.1). Care is taken to ensure that the catheter is not caught in the joint mechanism and that the catheter lies in a position such that the RKA mixture can be delivered to all parts of the joint, tissue planes, and under the wound by injecting as the catheter is withdrawn during reinjection (see below).

Injection Technique

Depending on the size of the surgical incision, a total of 150 to 200 mL of injectant is injected in three stages in equal 50- to 70-mL doses. The first injection is made after completion of the acetabular surgery (Fig. 16.2), the second after femoral component insertion (Fig. 16.3), and the final immediately before the skin is sutured (Fig. 16.4). The first injec-

tion is made into the tissues around the rim of the acetabulum, focusing on both the joint capsule if it remains and around the exposed gluteal and adductor muscles. The injection is made using a systematic sequence around the acetabular rim to ensure uniform delivery to these tissues. The second injection is made into the external rotators, gluteus tendon, and iliotibial band. Multiple injections are made in a systematic sequence every 25 mm or so along the length of the exposure. Care is taken to infiltrate in a fanwise fashion around the apices of the wound so that tissues traumatized in these locations are covered. The third injection is made into the subcutaneous tissues under the wound. Multiple injections are made in a systematic sequence every 25 mm around the wound. The needle is inserted each time perpendicular to the wound edge to a depth of about 25 mm and injection made as the needle is withdrawn.

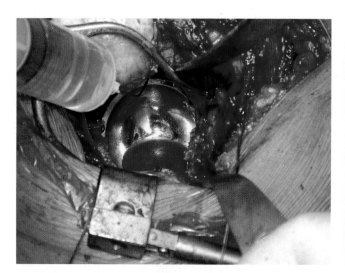

Fig. 16.2. Circumferential injection of the local anesthetic mixture around the acetabular component, once the acetabular component is fixed.

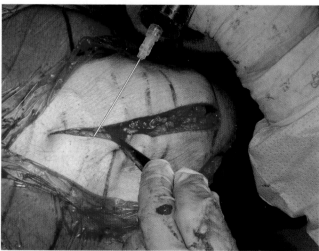

Fig. 16.4. Injection of the subcutaneous tissues.

Catheter Placement

Immediately before wound closure, a Tuohy needle is inserted about 10 cm below the inferior apex of the incision through the fascial layers and iliotibial band (Fig. 16.5). The tip of the catheter is then inserted through the hub of the needle from the outside into the surgical field, advanced to the superior apex of the wound, and placed with forceps above the piriformis tendon such that its tip lies anterosuperior to the joint (within the capsule for BHR) (Fig. 16.6). The slack is taken up so that the catheter lies over the long axis of the wound in the plane over the external rotator muscles. The needle is then removed so that the catheter exits through the skin about 10 cm below the distal end of the incision, and the catheter is cut to a convenient length such that only about 20 cm protrudes from the skin (Fig. 16.7). The hub and bacterial filter are then connected and 1 to 2 mL is injected through the catheter to ensure patency. After wound closure, a further 10 to 15 mL is injected through the catheter to flood the joint with RKA mixture.

Ancillary Measures

Measures to Restrict Drugs to Site of Injection

To minimize drug absorption and systemic toxicity, a vasoconstrictor (adrenaline 10 μg/mL), compression, cooling, and splinting of the injection site are used [1]. Because hip wounds are difficult to compress with a bandage, a surgical sponge roll is placed along the wound (Fig. 16.8) and compressed onto the wound with an elastic binder around the lower part of the pelvis (Dale Abdominal Binder: [Dale Medical Products, 7 Cross Street, Plainville, MA USA] 4 panel, 30-cm, white, code 811; Cosmac Surgical Pty. Ltd). (Fig. 16.9). In addition, ice packs are applied on the incision for the first 4 hours.

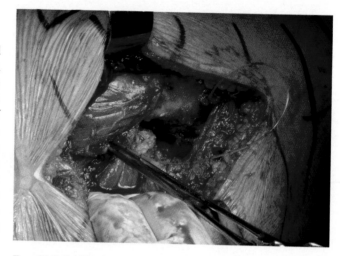

FIG. 16.6. Positioning of the catheter, above the the piriformis tendon, into the joint.

Wound Drains

Wound drains are not routinely used, but on rare occasions when a drain is used, it may be an important source of pain and it is important to anesthetize the area. Injection is made along the line of the drain and pain catheter by inserting the needle through the wound from inside to outside under direct vision.

Postoperative Management

Recovery Room

If the patient has pain in the recovery room, options for treatment include catheter top-up and direct injection of painful spots as well as conventional analgesics. Before leaving

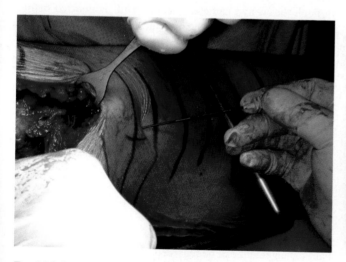

FIG. 16.5. Insertion of catheter, approximately 10 cm distal to the end of the surgical incision.

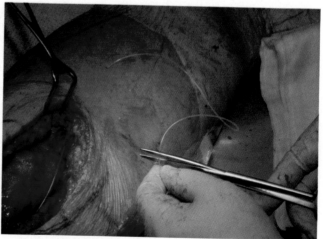

FIG. 16.7. Excess slack in the catheter is taken up, and patency is tested.

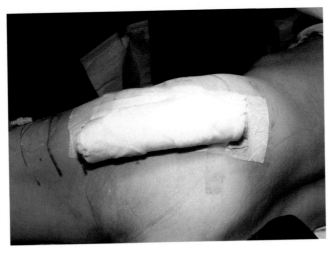

FIG. 16.8. Pressure dressing applied to the surgical incision.

the recovery room, a loading dose of ibuprofen (400 mg) or celecoxib (200 mg) is given.

Opioids

All patients are routinely prescribed rescue doses of up to 10 mg of morphine to be administered intravenously according to our recovery room pain protocol as the need arises (e.g., pain arising from outside the surgical site such as back pain or pain in other arthritic joints) and a single rescue dose of intramuscular morphine 10 mg for use in the ward. The nursing staff are also encouraged to exercise this option overnight if patients are uncomfortable and finding it difficult to sleep. Further doses of morphine are available after consultation with the anesthetist. However, parenteral opioids are avoided during the day where possible because they delay mobilization and may result in nausea and vomiting.

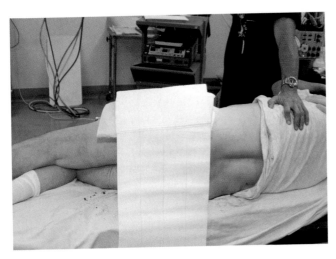

FIG. 16.9. Abdominal blinder is applied, and tensioned once the patient is rolled off the operating table.

Oral and Transdermal Medication

Unless contraindicated, ibuprofen 400 mg is given by mouth 4 hourly, for 24 hours, then patients self-medicate as required with a view to stopping the drug over a 2- to 3-day period. Oral analgesics, usually paracetamol 1 g alone or together with tramadol 50 to 100 mg or Codeine Phosphate 30-60mg, are provided for use not more than 4 hourly as required. After 36 hours, residual pain is managed with conventional oral analgesics and/or buprenorphine skin patches. Patients are instructed to cease the tramadol or codeine and take only paracetamol as soon as the pain had decreased to an acceptable level. Aspirin 300 mg is given daily for 6 weeks for thromboprophylaxis. However, when patients cannot or will not comply with the aggressive mobilization regimen, or have a history of hereditary or acquired predisposition to thrombosis, or previous thromboembolic events, we use conventional thromboprophylaxis with enoxaparin and warfarin on an outpatient basis. An H_2 blocker such as ranitidine or a proton pump inhibitor such as esomeprazole is also given for the first 24 hours to cover the high dose of NSAID, and a psyllium husk preparation such as Metamucil is given to prevent constipation.

Top-up

Occasionally, if we expect the block to recede overnight or to relieve discomfort at any time, we give a small top-up dose of about 10 to 15 mL of the RKA mixture through the pain catheter to flood the joint with local anesthetic. Ketorolac is omitted if 6 hours have not elapsed from the time of the last dose.

Reinjection

Extending the duration of pain control by reinjecting the surgical site is a central feature of this pain management technique. Fifteen to 20 hours postoperatively, the surgical field is reinjected with approximately 50 mL of the RKA mixture by hand through the wound catheter. About 15 mL is injected before the catheter is moved and the rest spread evenly throughout the wound as the catheter is withdrawn and removed. If a wound drain was used, it is removed before reinjection through the pain catheter so as to prevent drug loss through the drain. Our intention is to again flood the joint capsule and all the tissue planes through which the catheter passes with the RKA mixture. This approach differs conceptually from slow infusion techniques ("painbusters") in that it is designed to extensively flood the tissues throughout the surgical field once only as the initial block recedes.

Comments

Pain management can be regarded as falling into four distinct phases, namely preoperative (education, building confidence, and motivation), operative (suitable anesthesia), acute postoperative, and residual periods. It is important to appreciate that local infiltration analgesia is merely one piece of this jigsaw puzzle of important contributing elements. Specifically, it is the element designed to manage the acute postoperative pain phase lasting about 36 hours. Its importance derives from the fact that it is a key *enabling* technique promoting rapid return to normal activities of daily living and facilitating discharge from hospital. However, one can *only* expect surgical outcomes to be improved by this technique *if its benefits are exploited by such further measures as reduced invasive interventions (e.g., PCA, urinary catheters), early mobilization, and early discharge*, all of which require appropriate attitudes and organization. Improved outcomes also rely on adequate management of the residual pain phase, which often lasts for a further 1 to 2 weeks. Although there are various alternatives, we use Buprenorphine '5' (5 micrograms per hour) skin patch plus supplementation with occasional oral analgesics (predominately paracetamol) to manage this phase.

The use of ketorolac in the RKA mixture is seen by some as controversial because of possible renal and gut toxicity [3,4] and especially as there is a suggestion from animal studies (not replicated in humans) that NSAIDs may inhibit bony ingrowth and adversely influence endoprosthetic fixation. Also, local infiltration of NSAIDs has not been widely used and the literature is equivocal as to their efficacy when used in this way [5–7]. Nonetheless, sensitization of pain nerves by locally active mediators derived from damaged tissue is believed to be a major mechanism amplifying and sustaining pain intensity. Synthesis of the prostanoid components of this biological soup can be blocked by NSAIDs, and the infiltration technique that we have described appears to be effective in delivering locally high concentrations of drugs to the appropriate site. If the local anesthetic in the RKA mixture successfully blocks pain nerve conduction, then the NSAID molecules must also be in the immediate vicinity of the nerve endings and in a perfect position to inhibit prostaglandin synthesis and subsequent nerve sensitization. Clinical experience with the technique (spanning 10 years and more than 850 Birmingham hip procedures) has not been associated with clinical or laboratory evidence of renal toxicity or inadequate endoprosthetic fixation. This may be explained perhaps by very slow systemic uptake of the NSAID as a result of vasoconstriction, cooling, and firm bandaging. To be useful for local infiltration, a drug must act directly at the site of injection. Ketorolac was chosen because it was the only directly acting injectable nonselective NSAID available to us. It is noteworthy that the COX-2

inhibitor prodrug paracoxib is unsuitable for local infiltration because it is pharmacologically inactive until it is absorbed and activated in the liver.

For the intraoperative phase of pain control, we have used a short-acting spinal anesthetic technique (3.0 mL bupivacaine 0.25%). This ensures that no pain signals reach the CNS at any time before the infiltration block has been initiated, had time to spread and become fully established. Emergence from spinal blockade is timed to occur at approximately 2 hours postoperatively, so as to allow early mobilization. This approach provides a smooth transition from central blockade to infiltration blockade. Secondary benefits of using spinal blockade include facilitation of moderate controlled hypotension and reduction of thromboembolic complications [8,9].

References

1. Kerr DR, Kohan L. Local infiltration analgesia: a technique for control of acute postoperative pain following knee and hip surgery. A case study of 325 patients. Acta Ortho 2008;79.
2. Sutherland SK, Leonard RL. Snakebite deaths in Australia 1992–1994 and a management update. Med J Aust 1995;163:616–618.
3. Jaquenod M, Ronnhedh C, Cousins MJ, Eckstein RP, Jordan V, Mather LE, et al. Factors influencing ketorolac-associated perioperative renal dysfunction. Anesth Analg 1998;86:1090–1097.
4. Smith K, Halliwell RMT, Lawrence S, Klineberg PL, O'Connell P. Acute renal failure associated with intramuscular ketorolac. Anaesth Intens Care 1993;21:700–703.
5. Ben-David B, Katz E, Gaitini L, Goldik Z. Comparison of IM and local infiltration of ketorolac with and without local anaesthetic. Br J Anaesth 1995;75:409–412.
6. Garcia-Enguita MA, Ortega-Lahuerta JP, Arauzo-Perez P, Laglera-Trebol S, Giron-Mombiela JA, Lopez-Sicilia S, et al. The utility of digital infiltration of mepivacaine and ketorolac in postoperative analgesia of the unilateral hallux valgus. Rev Esp Anestesiol Reanim 1997;44:345–348.
7. Romsing J, Moiniche S, Ostergaard D, Dahl JB. Local infiltration with NSAIDs for postoperative analgesia: evidence for a peripheral analgesic action. Acta Anaesthesiol Scand 2000;44:672–683.
8. O'Reilly RF, Burgess IA, Zicat B. The prevalence of venous thromboembolism after hip and knee replacement surgery. Med J Aust 2005;182:154–159.
9. Heit JA, O'Fallon WM, Petterson TM, Lohse CM, Silverstein MD, Mohr DN, et al. Relative impact of risk factors for deep vein thrombosis and pulmonary embolism. Arch Intern Med 2002;162:1245–1248.

17

Templating for the Birmingham Hip Resurfacing from Conventional X-Rays

Derek J.W. McMinn

I am going to make this section brief as in some respects templating from conventional x-rays has been overtaken by events. I still work from conventional x-rays, but most hospitals throughout the world have abandoned these and gone to digital x-rays. I have had the misfortune of operating in a number of hospitals in various countries working from digital x-rays. I have had the x-rays printed out at an alleged 115% magnification only to find during the surgery that the magnification factor from these films is completely astray. If digital x-rays are going to be used for templating, then the magnification factor must be controlled.

Some aspects of templating from both digital and conventional x-rays are common, and I am going to address these issues. The first problem is that there seems to have been a complete misunderstanding in relation to valgus positioning of the femoral component. The source of this misunderstanding seems to have come from my 3 AM telephone friend Dr. Harlan Amstutz. When one looks at Harlan's published x-ray films over the past 30 years, it seems he routinely placed the femoral component in varus. For some reason, Harlan has now decided that placing the femoral component with its long axis 140 degrees to the shaft of the femur is a better idea than that of his previous 30 years of practice. Picking a certain angle at which to insert the femoral component, particularly when one is supposedly "measuring" that angle by an externally applied goniometer, is not recommended. I would urge the users of the Birmingham Hip Resurfacing (BHR) system to apply much simpler and practical alternatives for femoral component positioning. In Chapter 22, I describe the preparation and implantation of the BHR component. The thought process that underpins that practical embodiment will now be described. Each individual patient's x-ray needs to be templated. A patient with coxa vara whose femoral component is implanted at a 140-degree angle to the shaft of the femur will almost certainly get notching of the superior femoral neck. A patient with coxa valga will require a femoral component insertion angle of greater than 140 degrees. The x-ray of the patient I am going to demonstrate this templating on is shown in Fig. 17.1.

A suitable-sized template is offered up to the x-ray. The size of this template must be sufficient to span the width of the femoral neck. Even with conventional x-rays, it is clear that in big men with lots of buttock muscle, the bone is lifted away from the x-ray plate (increased object-film distance) and the x-ray gives an artificially enlarged dimension. The template should be placed with the femoral component medial side at the medial head-neck junction (Fig. 17.2).

It can be seen that if the femoral head was prepared in this position, then it would leave cancellous bone exposed in the lateral femoral head. This is highly undesirable. The cancellous bone is poor at coping with shear stress and a fracture of the femoral neck starting in this exposed cancellous bone region can follow. Surgeons seem to understand now that a valgus position of the femoral component is good. However, as can be seen in Fig. 17.3, too much valgus is bad.

When an extreme valgus position is chosen, if the femoral head was prepared in this position, then gross notching of the lateral femoral neck would occur. Clearly, a position between these two extremes is desirable (Fig. 17.4).

In this ideal position, the superior part of the femoral component lies covering the superior cortical femoral neck. It is known from finite element analysis that strain concentration occurs at the periphery of the femoral component, and if strain is going to be concentrated, it is better to do this in cortical rather than cancellous bone. Figure 17.4 represents the ideal position for the femoral component. There is no need to measure its angle to anything, the angle it makes with any other structure is of supreme irrelevance. The femoral head can be prepared in this position without damaging the femoral neck, and the femoral component covers all the cancellous bone, particularly in the critical superolateral region. The goal of the surgeon is now to translate that position into his surgery. With the BHR, this has been traditionally done by measuring down from a fixed point, namely the tip of the greater trochanter. Two errors are possible with this measurement. Figure 17.5 shows that the tip of the greater trochanter is a posterior structure, and it is even more posterior in a patient with an arthritic hip and an external rotation deformity. If the external

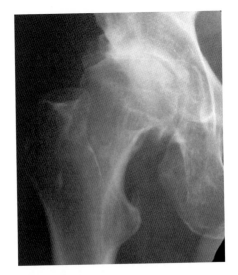

FIG. 17.1.

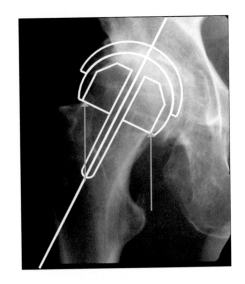

FIG. 17.4.

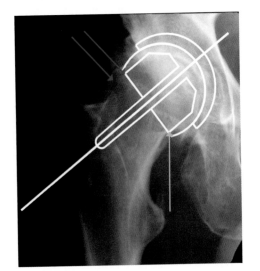

FIG. 17.2.

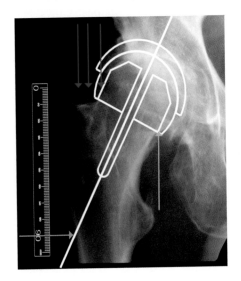

FIG. 17.5.

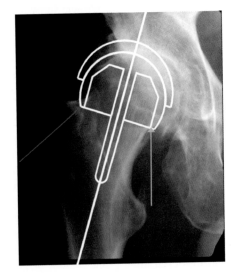

FIG. 17.3.

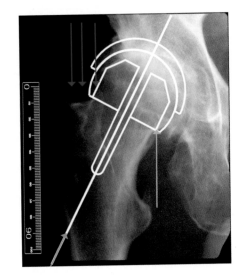

FIG. 17.6.

rotation deformity is severe, the surgeon has two templating choices. He can template the unaffected side if he believes that the upper femoral anatomy is symmetric. If he has reason to believe that the upper femoral anatomy is not symmetric, then a further anteroposterior radiograph of the affected hip should be taken with the x-ray beam externally rotated to match the deformed femur. The tip of the greater trochanter is most reliably delineated by inserting a hypodermic needle in the posterior aspect of the tip of the greater trochanter to outline it (see Chapter 24).

From the tip of the greater trochanter marked by the hypodermic needle, the surgeon measures down to the entry point for the guide pin in the lateral femoral cortex (Fig. 17.5).

This is another area where error can occur. Because the pin is being inserted through the vastus lateralis muscle, which in young men is of substantial thickness, then the guide pin at surgery must be angled from the entry point toward the center of the patient's femoral head (Fig. 17.6).

Following these simple rules will place the femoral component in the correct varus-valgus alignment, provided the x-ray magnification is correct. This method of templating and pin insertion has been in use since February 1991 and it works.

I have not used a pin in the lateral femoral cortex for some 5 years now as my incision length does not allow me access to the lateral part of the femur. Instead, I use a short-arm jig, which is described in Chapters 22 and 24. With the use of this jig, we take our fixed point from the tip of the lesser trochanter, and this achieves exactly the same position as the long-arm jig with a pin in the lateral femoral cortex (Fig. 17.7).

When templating for the short-arm jig, a measurement is taken from the long axis of the femoral component to the tip of the lesser trochanter, and this is transferred into the operation to give the desired varus-valgus alignment. The acetabular component positioning is no different for a hip resurfacing than for

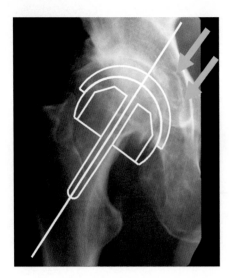

FIG. 17.8.

any other cementless total hip replacement shell. It is desirable to have the inclination angle around 40 degrees, and it is desirable not to have the component resting on floor osteophyte.

Figure 17.8 shows two arrows indicating the true floor of the acetabulum. All the floor osteophyte in this man needs to be reamed to allow satisfactory positioning of the acetabular component (Fig. 17.9).

All of the above is only achievable if the magnification factor is known. Without this, the size of components templated will be wrong, and the measurements from the bony prominences will also be incorrect. Because of the widespread use of digital x-rays in the modern era, I have asked Dr. Henrik Malchau and his colleagues to present their system of templating these digital x-rays. I do like the look of their system, and, critically, it controls for magnification factor.

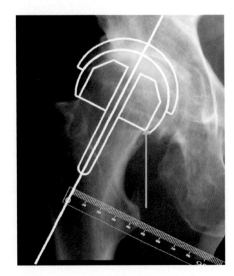

FIG. 17.7.

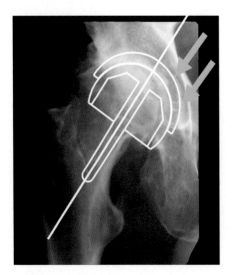

FIG. 17.9.

18
Computer Templating of Hip Resurfacing Arthroplasty

James Slover, Erik Wetter, and Henrik Malchau

Introduction

The goals of conventional hip replacement surgery typically include restoration of leg length and femoral offset, and preoperative templating has been an essential component of achieving these goals with surgery. Hip resurfacing has more limited ability to alter these variables than does conventional hip replacement [1,2]. Despite this, preoperative templating may be even more critical when planning for a hip resurfacing procedure for several reasons. First, not all patients with osteoarthritis of the hip are appropriate for resurfacing, and templating can assist in determining if a patient's anatomy is suitable for hip resurfacing [3]. Like any hip replacement procedure, the positioning of the femoral and acetabular components is critical to the long-term success of a hip resurfacing procedure [4]. The acetabular component must be positioned with appropriate anteversion and verticality for postoperative hip stability and avoidance of impingement. Excessive vertical positioning of the acetabular component can lead to increased contact stresses and rapid wear of the metal on metal bearing. The femoral component must also be positioned properly to ensure success. Neutral or slight valgus orientation is optimal. Varus positioning or notching of the cortex of the femoral neck, particularly on the tension side, can lead to femoral neck fracture [5,6]. Furthermore, the acetabular and femoral components can only match each other within select ranges. Because of the limitations the retained femoral head presents, the acetabular component must be implanted first. However, it is important to understand the femoral component sizes that can be matched to a particular acetabular component. Typically, each acetabular component can be matched with only two femoral sizes. If the femur cannot accommodate these sizes, then the acetabular component size must be altered or the plan for hip resurfacing must be abandoned in favor of a total hip replacement construct. It is more difficult to change these parameters than in conventional total hip replacement, where a wider variety of stem and neck length options are possible. In addition, it is far easier and more efficient to plan for any alteration in the operative plan before undertaking an operative procedure. Finally, it is crucial to plan for the possibility of intraoperative conversion from hip resurfacing to total hip replacement. This may become necessary for several reasons. For example, if excessive femoral head cysts become evident, such that the stability of the femoral component comes into question, or if a technical error such as creation of a significant notch or fracture in the femoral neck occurs, then conversion to a total hip construct is necessary. This possibility should be planned for and discussed with the patient beforehand. The purpose of this chapter is to discuss the use of computer templating for preoperative planning of hip resurfacing arthroplasty.

Methods

Templating is performed using an anteroposterior (AP) pelvis film. The first step in using computer templating to plan a hip resurfacing is to determine the precise magnification of the computer images. This can be accomplished in a number of ways. For example, the mdesk system by RSA Biomedical (Umeå, Sweden) [7] uses a radiopaque metal ball of known diameter, which is placed beside the patient at the time of his or her x-ray. The known true dimension of the ball is then used to precisely calibrate the image magnification. Use the mouse to click once on the calibration object, and the software will automatically adjust the image scale. Once the image has been appropriately calibrated, templating can begin. Leg length differences are established using known vertical references from the AP pelvis film (Fig. 18.1). A horizontal line across the inferior border of the pelvic teardrops or across the pelvis tangent to the inferior border of the pubic rami is drawn for vertical reference. Any leg length discrepancy is then determined by reference points on the lesser trochanter on each side. The distance between the reference point on the lesser trochanter and the reference line is then used to establish the leg length discrepancy, although hip resurfacing only allows for minimal correction of any discrepancy. A conventional total hip replacement should be considered for patients with a large leg length discrepancy.

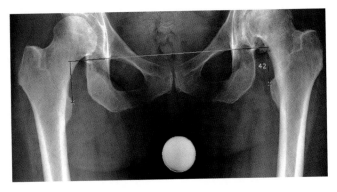

Fig. 18.1. Scale image and determine leg length discrepancy

The next step is to determine the placement of the femoral component. The software places a sample femoral head over the underlying image, which is calibrated to the same scale as the image (Fig. 18.2). The image of the head contains an extended line across the vertical and horizontal axis of the implant to assist with appropriate orientation. The first step in templating the femoral component is to select the appropriate size. This is typically done by using the cursor to move the femoral component such that the base of the cap is at the femoral head neck junction. A size that provides appropriate resurfacing and coverage without notching the femoral neck is selected. The vertical orientation line extends through the stem of the implant and reflects the angle of the stem within the femoral neck. The femoral component can be rotated into the appropriate orientation using these lines as a guide. A neutral or slight valgus position is ideal.

One of the most important measurements is the distance from the tip of the greater trochanter to the point where the vertical orientation line of the femoral component, which extends distally from the tip of the femoral stem, exits the lateral cortex of the femur. This point represents the point where the guide pin

should be placed in order to orient the femoral component consistent with the computer template. The pin position is marked while the stem extension line is still shown as well as a marker on the greater trochanter for reference during surgery.

Once templating of the femoral component is complete, attention is again turned to the pelvis. The next step is to determine the placement of the cup component. The cup is moved to the appropriate location along the medial wall of the pelvis where it will sit after appropriate reaming of medial osteophytes. The angle formed where these lines cross the horizontal reference line previously placed determines the vertical angle of inclination of the implant, and the cup is rotated with the cursor until this angle is 40 to 45 degrees (Fig. 18.3). The cursor can also be used to easily size the cup up or down until an appropriate size with adequate coverage and lack of impingement is achieved.

Once the cup component position is selected, the remaining measurements which help with appropriate placement are automatically calculated by the software. If desired, the femur can be cut out and moved into correct position where the leg length discrepancy is corrected; see complete planning image (Fig. 18.4). After the templating is complete, the image with the templated components and their sizes, along with the magnitude of the distance from the tip of the greater trochanter to the entry point for the lateral guide pin, is saved and printed so that it can be appropriately shared and brought to the operating room for reference.

There are a few essential measurements as a result of the preoperative planning, and they are listed in Fig. 18.5.

After the hip resurfacing template is complete, it is recommended to template for the contingency that a conventional total hip is necessary. The goal of templating a conventional total hip replacement is to choose an implant of adequate size in order to ensure the ability to gain fixation and to restore

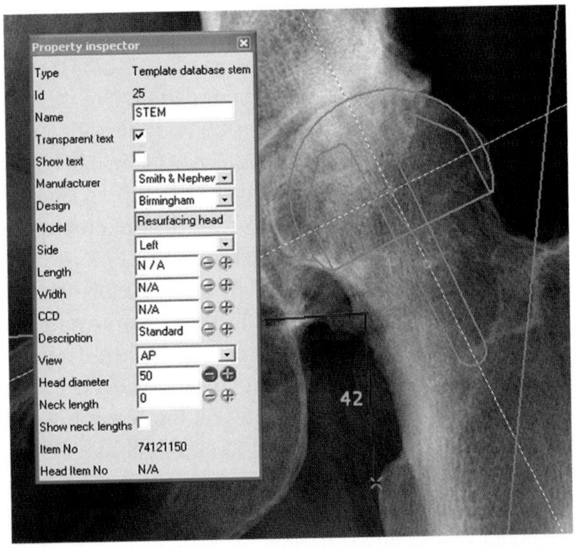

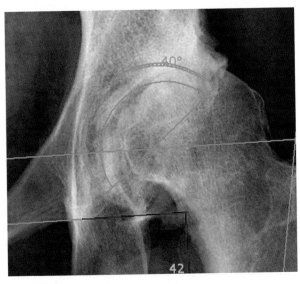

Fig. 18.3. Place the cup component, select size, and adjust inclination. Note guideline indicating optimal vertical position for leg length discrepancy correction.

Fig. 18.2. Femoral component placement and selection of size.

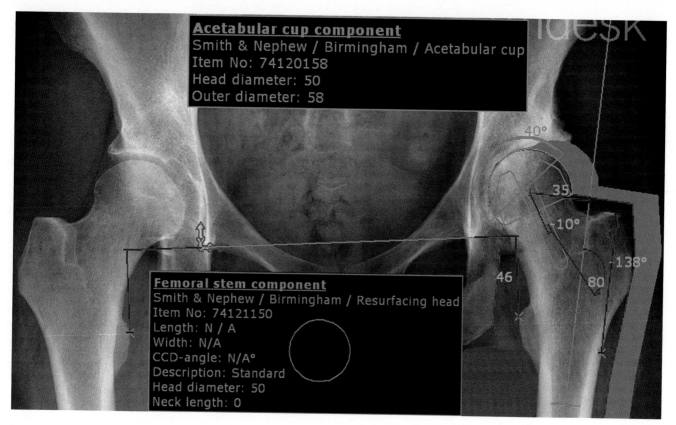

FIG. 18.4. A complete planning. Note that the femur is cut out and repositioned and aligned with the cup; the simulation shows a reduced leg length discrepancy.

leg length and offset. To template a conventional total hip, the acetabular component is templated as discussed above. The center of the cup, indicated by the point where the horizontal and vertical orientation lines cross, is marked. This point represents the center of the acetabulum and femoral head of the hip arthroplasty implant. An appropriate femoral component is chosen and sized to fit the femoral canal. The possible positions for the center of the femoral head obtained with the various neck length options are shown. The neck length, which restores any leg length discrepancy measured as previously described, and which re-creates the appropriate offset, determined by measuring the distance from the center of the femoral head to the tip of the greater trochanter on the opposite side, is selected. This plan is also saved and printed for distribution to appropriate personnel and brought to the operating room for reference.

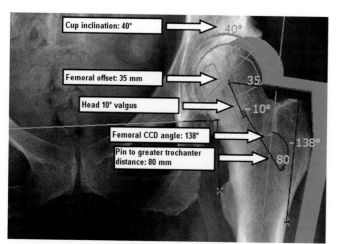

FIG. 18.5. Explanations of planning made with mdesk.

Discussion

Although it is certainly possible to template for a hip resurfacing procedure using conventional templates and printed x-rays, it also currently possible to use computer templating programs to perform this important part of the preoperative planning. Computer templating programs have several advantages in planning a hip resurfacing arthroplasty. Most importantly, they provide a method for formally determining the x-ray magnification of the images. This is particularly important in planning a hip resurfacing procedure. As previously discussed, the available femoral sizes for each acetabular size is more limited than in conventional total hip replacement. If the available sizes will not allow for an adequate reconstruction, then adjustments to the acetabular component or an alteration in the type of femoral component can be anticipated. In addition, preoperative computer templating allows for more precise determination of landmarks and measurements to be used for guide pin and implant placement, which will be used intraoperatively to help ensure appropriate implant position, which is key to the short-term and long-term success of this procedure. They also allow for easy generation of multiple plans, including a plan for an intraoperative change to a total hip construct if it becomes necessary. As medical centers increasingly move to digital imaging systems, computer templating makes practical sense as well reducing the need for printing of films already available on computer. Opportunities for enhanced education and sharing of preoperative plans is also possible as computer-generated plans are more easily shared with appropriate personnel. Surgeons performing hip resurfacing should strongly consider adoption of computer templating for this essential step in the preparation of this technical procedure as precise preoperative planning for multiple contingencies is essential to the success of this procedure.

References

1. Loughead, J. M.; Chesney, D.; Holland, J. P.; and McCaskie, A. W.: Comparison of offset in Birmingham hip resurfacing and hybrid total hip arthroplasty. J Bone Joint Surg Br, 87:163–6, 2005.

2. Silva, M.; Lee, K. H.; Heisel, C.; Dela Rosa, M. A.; and Schmalzried, T. P.: The biomechanical results of total hip resurfacing arthroplasty. J Bone Joint Surg Am, 86:40–46, 2004.

3. Eastaugh-Waring, S. J.; Seenath, S.; Learmonth, D. S.; and Learmonth, I. D.: The practical limitations of resurfacing hip arthroplasty. J Arthroplasty, 21:18–22, 2006.

4. Schmalzried, T. P.; Fowble, V. A.; Ure, K. J.; and Amstutz, H. C.: Metal on metal surface replacement of the hip. Technique, fixation, and early results. Clin Orthop Relat Res, 329(Suppl):S106–114, 1996.

5. Mont, M. A.; Ragland, P. S.; Etienne, G.; Seyler, T. M.; and Schmalzried, T. P.: Hip resurfacing arthroplasty. J Am Acad Orthop Surg, 14:454–63, 2006.

6. Shimmin, A. J., and Back, D.: Femoral neck fractures following Birmingham hip resurfacing: a national review of 50 cases. J Bone Joint Surg Br, 87:463–4, 2005.

7. mdesk software suite. RSA Biomedical, Umeå, Sweden. Available at http://www.mdesk.com. Accessed August 15, 2007.

19
Patient Positioning and Exposure

Derek J.W. McMinn

Surgical exposure of the hip is a little more difficult for hip resurfacing than for standard total hip replacement (THR), as the femoral head and neck are obviously not resected in resurfacing. The other difficulty is that one is often operating on young, muscular men with stiff hips, and this adds much more difficulty than newcomers to the resurfacing operation expect. Obese patients also add a degree of difficulty with the surgical exposure but are not as much of a problem as muscular men. Previous surgery adds problems, particularly when metalwork is still *in situ* from childhood developmental dysplasia of the hip (DDH) surgery or when there is retained metalwork from previous pelvic fractures. The scarring from previous surgery often stiffens the hip making exposure more difficult. Previous scars must be considered in order to avoid tram lines and skin necrosis. All this has to be taken into account in positioning and surgical approach.

I am going to deal with the patient positioning and posterior surgical approach, and this is covered in more depth in the accompanying DVD. Also in the DVD, Mr. Andrew Thomas, FRCS, shows the patient positioning and surgical technique required for performing the Birmingham Hip Resurfacing (BHR) through an anterolateral approach. Andrew was my senior registrar in 1991, and at that time I was carrying out the hip resurfacing operation through an anterolateral approach, a procedure that Andrew has continued to use and perfected. His tips will be very useful to those surgeons who normally perform their THRs through an anterolateral approach. I gave up this approach as I blamed it for causing a permanent limp in too many patients, I presumed from damage to the superior gluteal nerve. It was a struggle to perform hip resurfacing in large muscular men using an anterolateral approach. It was these patients who tended to limp. I found the posterior approach much easier for resurfacing as I used this for my THRs. I only used the anterolateral approach to avoid damage to the ascending branch of the medial circumflex femoral vessels when performing hip resurfacing. I preserved these vessels but ruined several patients' function by nerve or muscle damage. I reasoned that if a patient developed avascular necrosis and collapse of the head after a posterior approach resurfacing,

I could easily rectify the situation with a stem and modular head and still give the patient good function. Happily, this has rarely been required in the past 15 years.

By the time Ronan Treacy joined my team as senior registrar, the posterior approach for hip resurfacing was the norm. He has continued to carry out his resurfacings through this approach. There is nothing that gets surgeons worked up so much as a discussion on which surgical approach is best. I participated in a debate a few years ago making the case for the posterior approach. Kevin Hardinge annoyed me by asserting that the posterior approach was only useful in draining a septic arthritis and said that I was exposing the hip from the "tradesman's entrance." I retorted that his direct-lateral approach was the "burglar's entrance" where the emphasis is on plunder and scant regard is paid to collateral damage!

I was amused to read the draft of a paper from the Research Centre at the Royal Orthopaedic Hospital recently where they had compared 10 years of work from Andrew Thomas and Ronan Treacy, looking at outcomes of the BHR in unilateral osteoarthritis patients. For those anterolateral addicts who believe that the posterior approach ruins the femoral head blood supply, the 10-year survivorship figure was the same with both approaches. For those posterior approach addicts who believe that the anterolateral approach ruins the abductor muscles, the hip scores were the same with both approaches.

Both these men are exceptionally talented surgeons, and the fact is that a great outcome can be achieved with either approach provided the operation is done well.

The direct anterior approach is much talked about at present. The attractions of not cutting muscle and not damaging nerves or vessels are obvious. Despite excellent one on one training from Prof. Thierry Judet, one of the most experienced surgeons in the world with this approach, I find this approach for hip resurfacing very stressful and almost impossible without significant collateral damage. I hear reports from various corners of the world that certain surgeons have perfected this approach for hip resurfacing, so it may emerge as a viable alternative in the future. No further discussion of this approach will be presented in this book. Trochanteric osteotomy is also much talked about. It is not new, as Sir John Charnley performed his Teflon on Teflon resurfacings through this approach in the 1950s and it at least has the advantage of giving an extensile exposure. I have performed a few BHRs through this approach in very special circumstances (Figs. 19.1 and 19.2).

The issue with this exposure relates to the patient population being treated with hip resurfacing. These young patients want a rapid return to work and, soon after, return to sport.

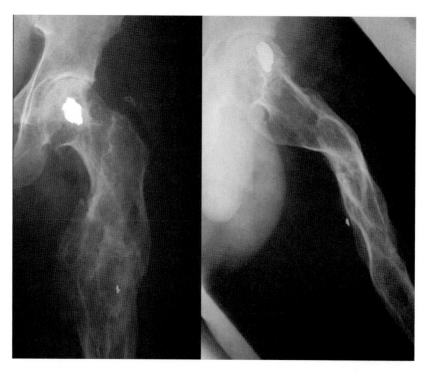

FIG. 19.1. Anteroposterior and lateral x-rays of a patient with missile injury to his hip 5 years before. Shrapnel in anterior femoral head.

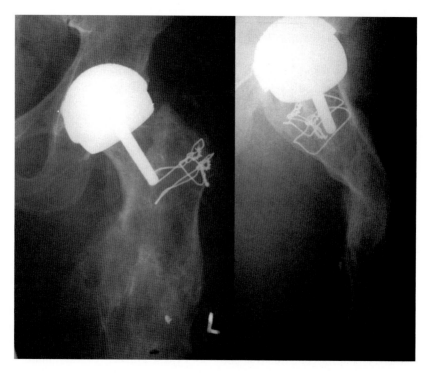

FIG. 19.2. Because of extreme stiffness, trochanteric osteotomy approach was used. Good function and trochanteric union 4 years postoperatively.

As a surgeon who was trained on the Charnley THR through a trochanteric osteotomy, I cannot imagine that this approach will gain wide acceptance. I fear that the trochanteric nonunion rates in this active population will be unacceptable. Trochanteric osteotomy will not be considered further.

The first task is to position the patient correctly. The surgeon should do this himself or herself in view of its importance. The patient needs to be well supported in the lateral position and the details are important. There is a large variety of supports available. I use an old-fashioned support system for the vast majority of my patients (Fig. 19.3).

An Innomed (Innomed Orthopaedic Instruments, Savannah, GA, USA) pelvic positioner is used for grossly obese patients in order to prevent abdominal compression (Fig. 19.4).

On the unoperated leg, we use a T.E.D (The Kendall Company, Mansfield, MA, USA) stocking and intermittent pneumatic calf compression (Fig. 19.5).

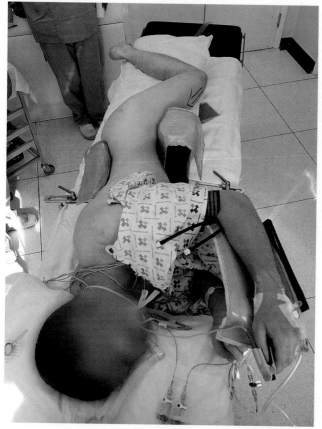

Fig. 19.3. Pelvis is fixed anteriorly and posteriorly and upper body is stabilized with upper arm in gutter support.

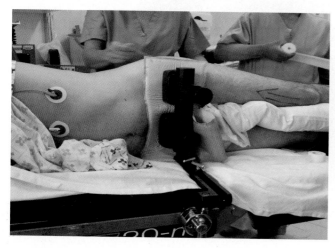

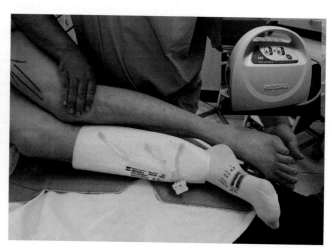

Fig. 19.4.

Fig. 19.5.

The anterior pelvic support should apply compression on the anterior superior iliac spines. To give the best support, this should take purchase on the uppermost anterior superior iliac spine (ASIS) (Fig. 19.6).

In recent years, with the use of navigation, we have had to compromise sometimes and not support the uppermost anterior superior iliac spine. Instead we attempt to gain purchase on the region of the symphysis pubis, but this is a compromise and does not give as good support to the pelvis (Fig. 19.7).

When the uppermost ASIS is not supported, the pelvis can tilt forward during acetabular exposure altering the intra-operative acetabular alignment that the surgeon sees. Whatever support is used for the anterior pelvis, under no circumstances should the support be allowed to migrate up onto the abdomen as this will increase intraabdominal pressure and increase bleeding at surgery. The anterior pelvic support should be arranged so that flexion of the uppermost hip past 90 degrees can still be comfortably accomplished.

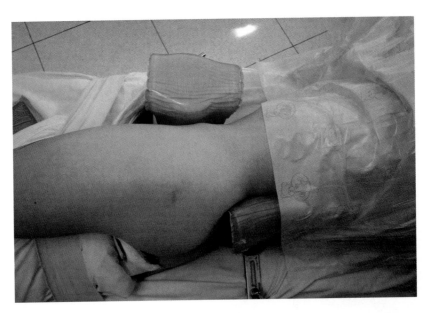

FIG. 19.6.

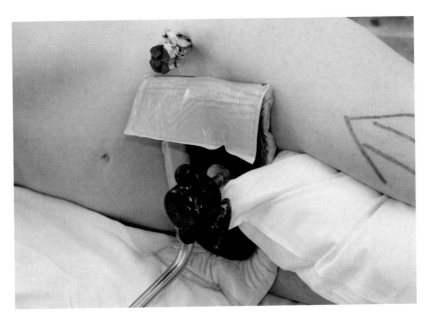

FIG. 19.7.

There are two alternatives with regard to posterior pelvic support. Either one chooses a short paddle that does not extend upwards any further than the sacrum or one uses a more traditional posterior support more superiorly to gain support not only on the posterior pelvis but also on the lumbar spine (Fig. 19.8).

It is important that the posterior pelvic support and the draping that follows does not encroach into an area where the surgeon might want to extend a more traditional poste-

rior approach incision. One also must be careful, particularly in young, flexible women with DDH, that the lumbar spine does not become hyperlordosed as this will flex the pelvis and alter the intraoperative view of the acetabulum that the surgeon sees. Anterior and posterior chest supports can also be used, but our anesthesiologists do not favor compression on the chest. Instead, we find that the whole of the upper body is stabilized satisfactorily by a gutter support for the forearm (Fig. 19.9).

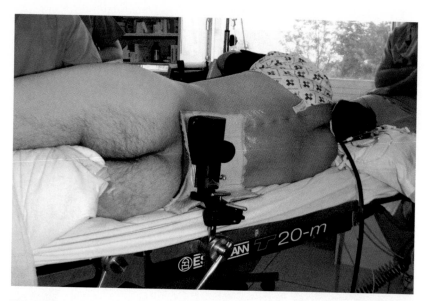

FIG. 19.8.

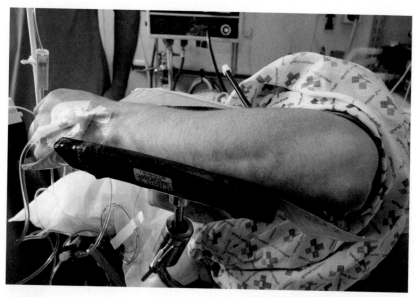

FIG. 19.9.

The patient's head and neck must be supported. This is particularly important in patients with ankylosing spondylitis and rheumatoid arthritis. Padding needs to be applied to protect the ulnar nerve, the genitalia, and the peroneal nerve in the lower leg (Fig. 19.10).

We only flex the lower hip to about 20 degrees, and we use a thin pillow strapped between the legs. It is important to keep the lower knee exposed so that an intraoperative estimation of leg length can be obtained. More importantly, it is very useful to be able to drop the operated leg knee in front of the lower knee during femoral preparation to get better femoral head and neck exposure (Fig. 19.11).

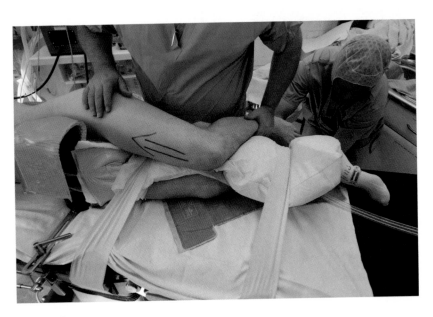

Fig. 19.10.

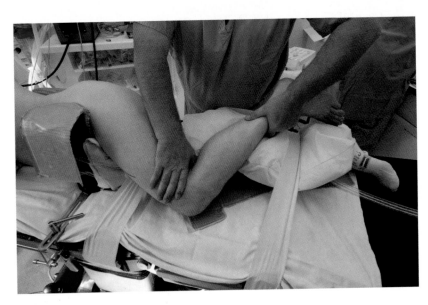

Fig. 19.11.

In the United Kingdom, we have anesthesia rooms where we carry out a first skin preparation and a first draping (Fig. 19.12).

The patient is then wheeled into the operating room where a second skin preparation and a second draping are then performed (Fig. 19.13).

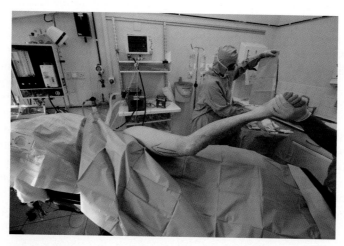

FIG. 19.12.

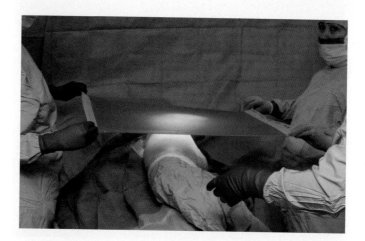

A

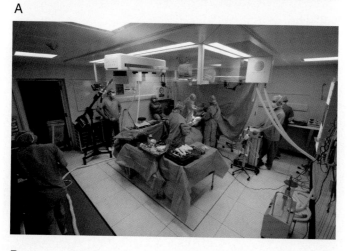

B

FIG. 19.13. (A, B)

We take all precautions to try and reduce our infection rate. At the induction of anesthesia, we give intravenous antibiotic, and for cement fixation of the BHR femoral component I use antibiotic Simplex cement (Stryker Corporation, Kalamazoo, MI). We operate in a Charnley-Howarth (Howarth Airtech - Bolton, UK) vertical downflow clean air enclosure. I use a Charnley body exhaust suit, and my team use mandarin exhausts. The skin is covered with adhesive drape, and we use pulsed lavage throughout the operation. I use meticulous diathermy hemostasis and I still use two suction drains for the first 10 hours after surgery. As can be seen from Chapter 28, our infection rate is low but unfortunately not zero.

In the surgical technique chapters that follow, I make an attempt to use photographs from the same patient's surgical procedure in order not to disorientate the reader. However, surgeons know that getting good-quality photographs of every step from the beginning to the end of an operation is almost impossible. Where necessary therefore to show particular steps in a procedure, I have used photographs from other patients' surgical procedures.

For hip arthroplasty, I use a small posterior approach nowadays. In the past I have used an extensile posterolateral approach but no longer find this necessary to do a hip resurfacing operation. However, for surgeons new to this resurfacing procedure, it is a good idea to initially start with a longer incision and then reduce the incision length as one's experience grows. The tip of the greater trochanter and the posterior aspect of the greater trochanter are marked (Fig. 19.14).

A position 5 cm down from the tip of the trochanter is marked along the posterior border of the trochanter, and a 10-cm incision is marked from this point posterosuperiorly angled about 20 or 25 degrees to the long axis of the femoral shaft. This is adequate for performing a total hip replacement, but with hip resurfacing it is advisable to continue the incision distally 2 or 3 cm, depending on the size of the patient, so that the lesser trochanter can be visualized. It is important when using a reduced-length incision for a posterior approach in hip resurfacing that it is much more posterior than a traditional posterolateral incision (Fig. 19.15).

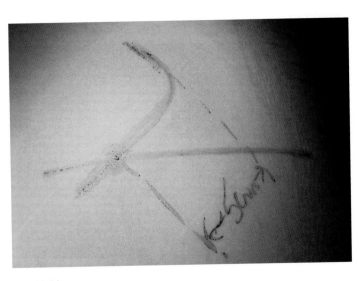

Fig. 19.14.

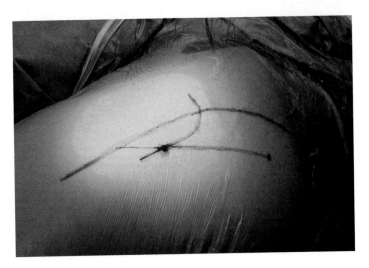

Fig. 19.15.

This ensures that good access to the acetabulum can easily be achieved and it also means that the dislocated femoral head is delivered into the center of the wound.

The incision is deepened through the fat, and electrocautery of bleeding vessels performed (Fig. 19.16). I find it well worthwhile coagulating vessels in the muscle and fat layer as superficial hematoma formation is a problem. Patients are disturbed by persistent drainage from their wound, and of course a draining wound represents a risk of organisms entering the surgical site.

The fibers of gluteus maximus are divided along the line of their fibers, and the fascia lata 2 to 3 cm distal to this is divided.

A small self-retaining retractor is placed to open the gluteus maximus incision (Fig. 19.17). Using blunt dissection with a finger, the fibers of gluteus maximus are gently separated in the proximal extent of the wound. It is important not to carry the gluteus maximus proximal separation too far as this may injure the inferior gluteal nerve supply to gluteus maximus. This can cause weakness and can leave an ugly cosmetic problem with a dip in the buttock from muscle atrophy. Dissection is also carried posteriorly, lifting the undersurface of gluteus maximus away from the greater trochanteric bursa. Any vessels in the connecting fibers between gluteus maximus and the greater trochanteric bursa are coagulated.

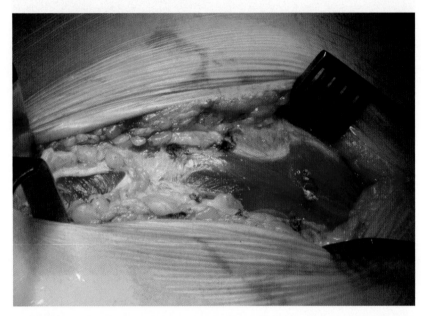

Fig. 19.16.

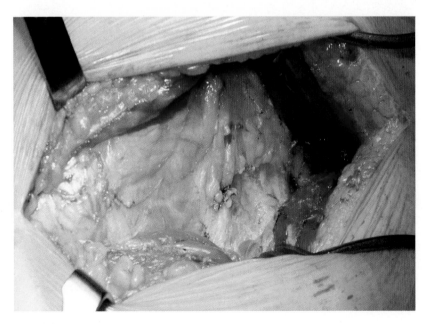

Fig. 19.17.

The posterior dissection between the undersurface of gluteus maximus and the greater trochanteric bursa should be continued far enough posteriorly so that the sciatic nerve can easily be palpated.

A Charnley retractor is substituted for the small self-retaining retractor, taking care not to catch the sciatic nerve with the posterior limb of the retractor (Fig. 19.18).

For the purposes of illustration, the greater trochanteric bursa has been divided so that the sciatic nerve can be visualized clearly in the posterior aspect of the wound (arrow, Fig. 19.19).

I do not expose the sciatic nerve in routine cases, but I do expose it in all cases of complex anatomy and in revision surgery.

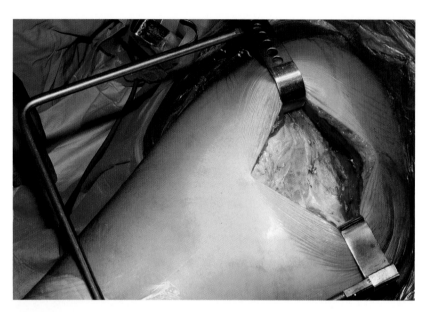

FIG. 19.18.

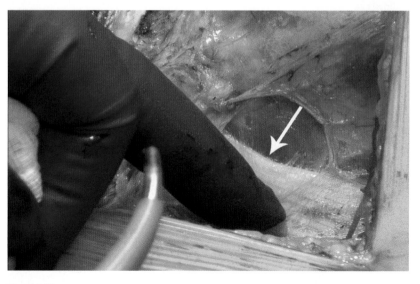

FIG. 19.19.

In patients with DDH, it is particularly important to expose the sciatic nerve. In addition, the tension in the sciatic nerve is assessed with finger pressure and compared with the tension in the nerve after hip reconstruction and leg lengthening.

The assistant uses two Langenbeck-type retractors and the tendinous insertion of gluteus maximus (gluteal sling) can easily be visualized. In former years, I used to divide all of the tendinous insertion of gluteus maximus (TGM) but now I divide only the sharp upper border of gluteus maximus with division of 1.0 to 1.5 cm of the upper part of the tendon (Fig. 19.20). The upper part of the tendon is divided with electrocautery (Fig. 19.21). An attempt is made not to dam-

age the underlying first perforating vessels. It is sometimes difficult to control the bleeding if these vessels are divided, and as they do provide an intraosseous blood supply to the proximal femur, they may be of importance in blood supply to the resurfaced hip.

It is possible to carry out the resurfacing operation without dividing the tendon of gluteus maximus, but Dr. Chit Ranawat has shown that division of this structure is important when performing a hip arthroplasty through a posterior approach. If the tendon is not divided, then pinching of the sciatic nerve can occur with leg rotation causing a sciatic nerve palsy. As can be seen in the figures, the tendon of gluteus maximus can

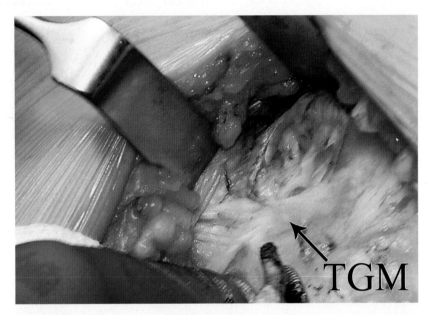

Fig. 19.20.

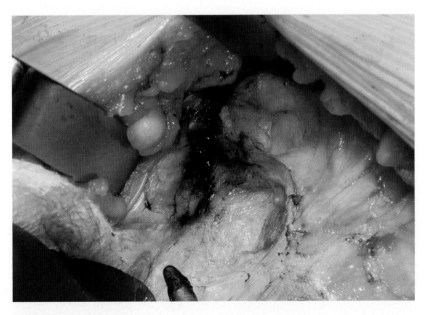

Fig. 19.21.

easily be visualized in the inferior aspect of the wound. At the beginning of my small-incision experience, I was using a shortened version of a standard posterolateral approach, and it is not possible to get to the tendon of gluteus maximus through such an incision. It is worth noting that in Fig. 19.15, the short posterior approach incision lies inferior and posterior to the standard incision. This more posteriorly sited incision does take a little getting used to on the part of the surgeon, but having used this approach for several years, I would now never return to the traditional incision.

The greater trochanteric bursa is divided along the posterior aspect of the greater trochanter using electrocautery (arrows, Fig. 19.22).

This incision in the greater trochanteric bursa is continued along the posterior edge of the gluteus medius muscle (GMED). In this aspect of the incision, there are always vessels that require electrocautery (Fig. 19.23). This is where the operation starts to go wrong for the learner surgeon. It is very important to carefully identify the piriformis tendon. A common mistake is that the obturator internus is mistaken for the piriformis tendon. The learner surgeon proceeds with the posterior approach but leaving the piriformis attachment intact. This greatly limits the amount of rotation possible. Unless massive force is used and the muscle belly of piriformis ruptured, the operation will be very difficult from here on in. Two variants of anatomy deserve mention.

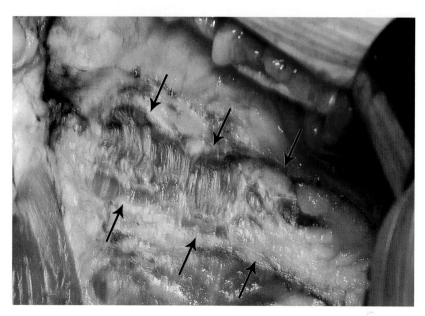

Fig. 19.22.

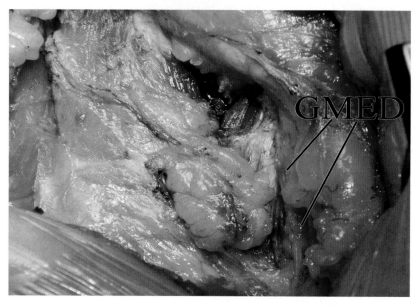

Fig. 19.23.

The piriformis tendon insertion can blend with the insertion of obturator internus, this is no problem for the hip surgeon. The piriformis tendon can blend with the posterior fibers of gluteus medius. This can be a major problem for the hip surgeon, for if it is not recognized then the piriformis tendon will be left intact. It is important to divide the connection between piriformis and gluteus medius fibers.

A large Langenbeck-type retractor is used by the second assistant to retract forwards the posterior edge of the gluteus medius muscle (Fig. 19.24).

Retraction of the posterior edge of the gluteus medius forwards reveals the gluteus minimus muscle (GM) and the piriformis tendon (P). The learner surgeon must resist the temptation to insert a large lever retractor at this stage.

The interval between piriformis and the posterior edge of gluteus minimus is opened using electrocautery, and a combination of electrocautery and heavy Muller scissors are used to cut the connecting fibers between the undersurface of gluteus minimus and the superior acetabulum and superior capsule (Fig. 19.25).

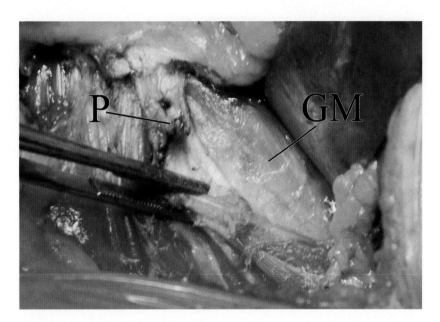

FIG. 19.24.

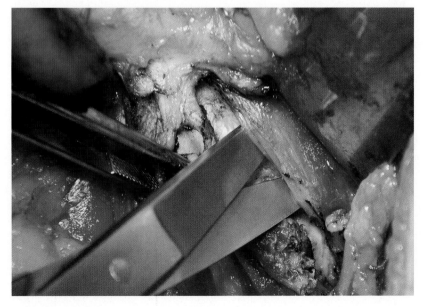

FIG. 19.25.

Division of connecting fibers mobilizes the gluteus minimus muscle and allows it to safely be retracted forwards without tearing its fibers (Fig. 19.26).

If a large lever-type retractor is used to retract the abductor muscles without division of these connecting fibers, then tearing of the gluteus minimus muscle, in particular, occurs and we have seen that tearing of the gluteus minimus muscle leads to heterotopic ossification. Pelvic fracture surgeons understand this issue very well and they recognize that trauma to gluteus minimus is a major risk factor for heterotopic ossifica-tion. Some fracture surgeons go so far as to excise portions of the gluteus minimus in an attempt to reduce ossification. This is not required for hip arthroplasty but great care should be taken not to traumatize the abductor muscles.

A pin (PN) is hammered into the posterosuperior acetabulum retracting forwards the fibers of gluteus medius and gluteus minimus. It is, of course, important that this pin is inserted superior enough so that the femoral head is not impaled (Fig. 19.27). This is checked by the first assistant rotating the femur, and the pin retractor should not rotate!

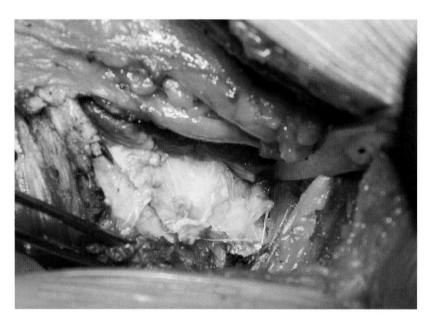

Fig. 19.26.

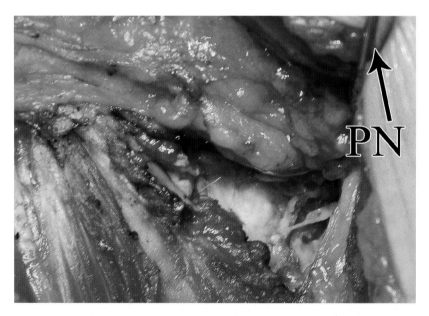

Fig. 19.27.

The piriformis tendon (P) and attached capsule are sharply divided very close to the posterosuperior edge of the greater trochanter. The capsular incision is carried along the superior border of piriformis to the edge of the acetabulum (Fig. 19.28). It is important to divide the piriformis tendon as close as possible to the greater trochanter as failure to do so can lose valuable length in this tendon and make closure of this structure unnecessarily tight leading to either an external rotation deformity or rupture of the suture line.

The femoral head (FH) and posterosuperior edge of acetabulum (A) can now be visualized (Fig. 19.29).

The next stage is to leave a large enough cuff of tissue attached to the posterior femur for subsequent closure. Failure to do this will require the surgeon to drill holes in the back of the greater trochanter later in order to obtain a secure closure of the external rotators and capsule.

The quadratus femoris (QF) is divided from the femur in one layer with the posterior capsule and care is taken to leave

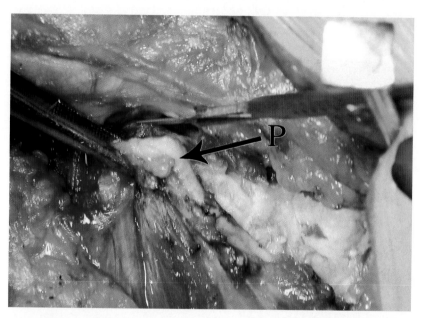

FIG. 19.28.

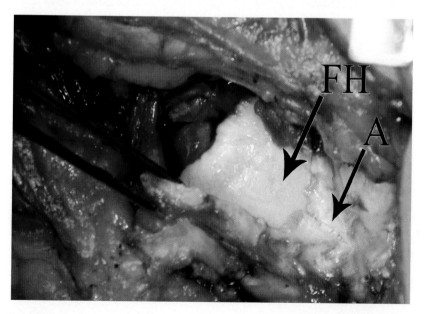

FIG. 19.29.

a cuff of quadratus femoris attached to the posterior femur (Fig. 19.30). As the deeper parts of the quadratus femoris muscle are divided, the ascending branch of the medial circumflex femoral artery (MCFA) is cut and requires coagulation. It is interesting how variable the bleeding from the cut MCFA is. It is possible to do a posterior approach without cutting the MCFA, and I have done this. The incision in the quadratus femoris needs to be brought much more posteriorly and close to the region of the sciatic nerve. This preserves the integrity of MCFA but leaves a mass of muscle on the intertrochanteric region, which is in the way for femoral instrumentation. If there was a really good reason to pre-

serve this vessel, I would persist with this modified posterior approach, but it does not seem worth it. A full discussion relating to the blood supply of the femoral head can be seen in Chapter 9 and Chapter 10.

Here, forceps are used to show the cuff of soft tissue left on the femur, which is used for closure of the external rotators and capsule (Fig. 19.31).

Many surgeons use the technique of cutting to bone and staying on bone during their surgical approach to the hip joint. This is not good for hip resurfacing. As I cut the MCFA on every occasion, I try not to do any other vascular damage. In particular, I have become obsessional about leaving soft tissue remaining

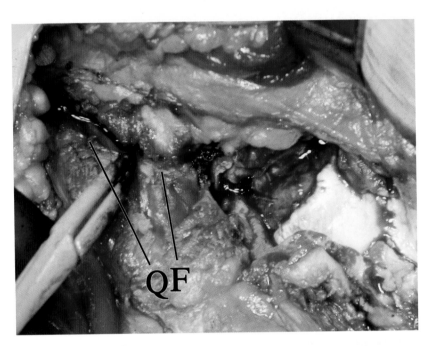

FIG. 19.30.

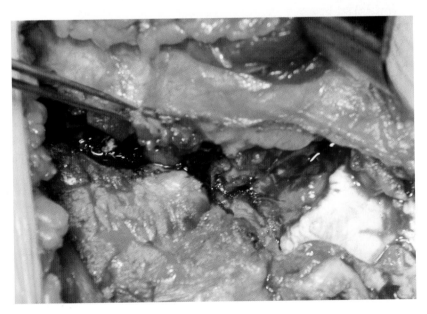

FIG. 19.31.

on the surface of the femoral neck. The importance of the retinacular vessels traveling in this soft tissue is shown in a beautiful piece of work from Prof. Sugano and his colleagues in Chapter 10. I am not able to see at my age the vessels in the retinaculum, but Prof. Sugano tells me that he can cannulate these vessels with the naked eye, without the aid of a microscope. This tends to indicate that these retinacular vessels are a significant size.

Here, forceps are used to show that during the dissection soft tissue is left attached to the femoral neck (Fig. 19.32).

The posterior capsule is grasped with heavy Kocher forceps and tension is placed on the posteroinferior capsule by pulling on the Kocher clamp. A radial incision is made in the posteroinferior capsule (Fig. 19.33). This allows the posterior capsule and attached quadratus femoris muscle to be retracted more posteriorly. This maneuver exposes the posterior wall of the acetabulum including any osteophyte. I perform this step in all my hip arthroplasty patients, but the exercise needs to be exaggerated in patients with developmental dysplasia. In these patients, the femoral head is translated anteriorly, the anterior acetabular wall is thin, and the posterior acetabular wall is both prominent and thickened.

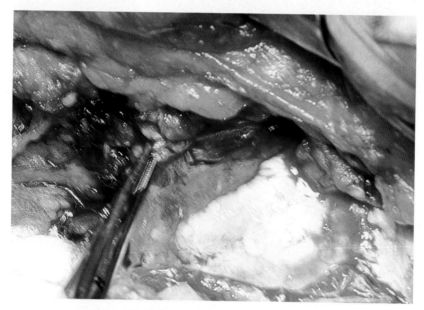

Fig. 19.32.

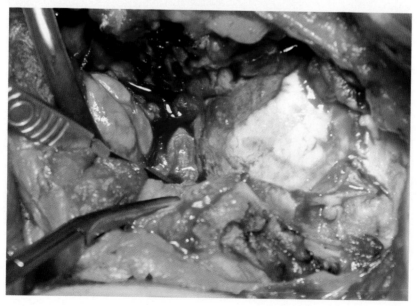

Fig. 19.33.

A retractor pin is inserted into the ischium 1.0 to 1.5 cm away from the acetabular edge (Fig. 19.34). In the DDH patient, I aim to insert the pin retractor 2 to 3 cm posteriorly to the hip joint. This gives room to define the anatomy and to preferentially ream the thickened posterior wall in the dysplastic acetabulum.

I am often asked whether the pin retractor can cause injury to the sciatic nerve, and I have never seen this occur to date.

In this patient, I have exposed the femoral head, the posterior acetabular wall, the quadratus femoris muscle, the greater trochanteric bursa, and the sciatic nerve.

It can be seen that the pin in the ischium is separated from the sciatic nerve (SN) by capsule, quadratus femoris muscle (QF), and greater trochanteric bursa (TB) (Fig. 19.35).

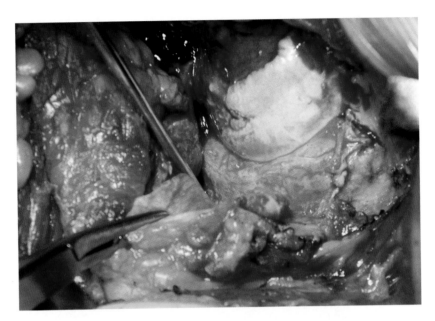

Fig. 19.34.

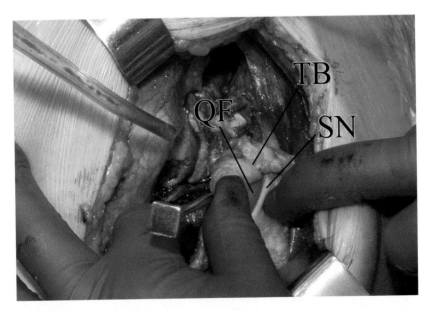

Fig. 19.35.

The superior hip capsule is divided at the edge of the acetabulum by sharp dissection (Fig. 19.36).

The hip is now ready to dislocate in most osteoarthritic patients. If the patient has protrusio acetabulae, then great care should be taken at this stage, and it is wise in such patients to excise the posterior acetabular wall osteophyte. This is done using an osteotome. The osteophyte is grasped with a rongeur, and any connecting soft tissue is divided by sharp dissection. In the protrusio patient, a trial dislocation using minimum rotational force is employed. If the aim is to carry out a hip resurfacing, then enough exposure must be made to allow

dislocation, but of course if a total hip replacement is being performed, then recourse can be made to division of the femoral neck in situ and removal of the femoral head either whole or piecemeal. In either case, care must be taken not to fracture the shaft of the femur by forceful rotational dislocation of a trapped femoral head.

In 99% of patients, the surgeon is able to dislocate the femoral head from the acetabulum by flexion and internal rotation of the hip without having to excise posterior wall osteophyte and without risking fracture of the shaft of the femur (Fig. 19.37).

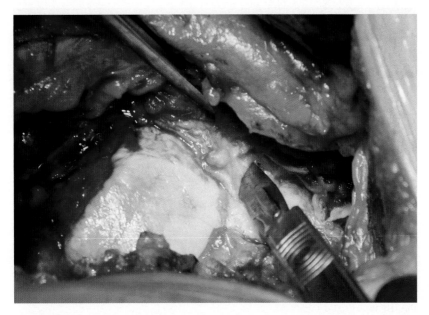

FIG. 19.36.

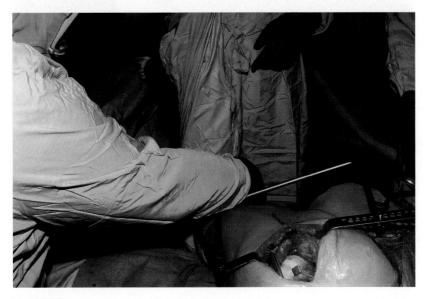

FIG. 19.37.

With the hip dislocated and the tibia vertical, it can be seen that the femoral head is still in the wound. In this position, the femoral head is almost impossible to resurface (Fig 19.38). This is another trap for the learner surgeon. He will be tempted to extend the wound posteriorly, and he will be tempted to split the fibers of gluteus maximus more proximally. This is not a good idea because proximal splitting of the fibers of gluteus maximus will in most instances lead to damage to the inferior gluteal nerve supply to gluteus maximus with resultant atrophy. The learner surgeon will put levers under the front of the femoral neck in an attempt to deliver the femoral head into the wound with undesirable soft tissue trauma. When I moved from traditional large-incision surgery to small-incision surgery, I fell into the trap of making my incisions too small initially. This required the use of heavy retraction, and it was very noticeable that those patients complained of severe pain in the postoperative period, although the pain was controlled by our local anesthetic cocktail injections in the first 12 hours. I have now learned that a balance needs to be struck between reducing the length of the incision on the one hand and on the other hand minimizing the amount of trauma to the muscle, fat, and skin.

Electrocautery of bleeding vessels in the posterior intertrochanteric region of the femur is undertaken (Fig. 19.39).

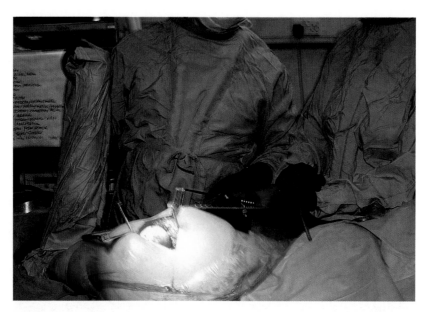

Fig. 19.38.

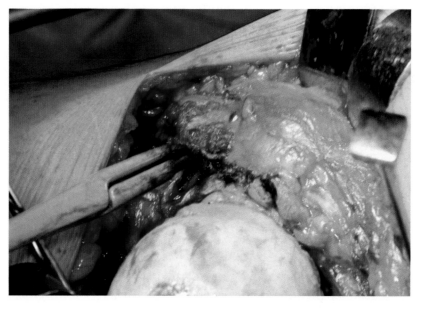

Fig. 19.39.

The next maneuver is to position the hip so that the anterior hip capsule can be divided. The first assistant fully extends the hip so that the knee is in the midline longitudinal axis of the patient (Fig 19.40).

The first assistant then forcibly internally rotates the hip delivering the femoral head into the superficial aspect of the wound thus allowing the surgeon to gain access to the anterior aspect of the hip capsule (Fig. 19.41). This maneuver will deliver the femoral head upwards enough to give the surgeon clear site and access to the anterior hip capsule. I frequently observe other surgeons tolerating an underfed, sleepy assistant failing to help at this critical stage. The procedure is all the more difficult in large, muscular men, and the muscle strength of the first assistant must match the muscle strength of the patient.

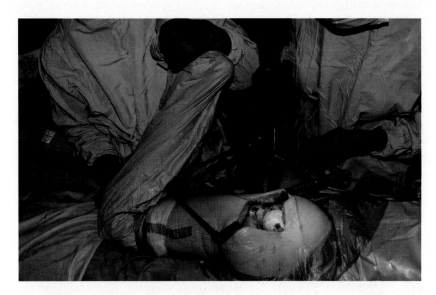

Fig. 19.40.

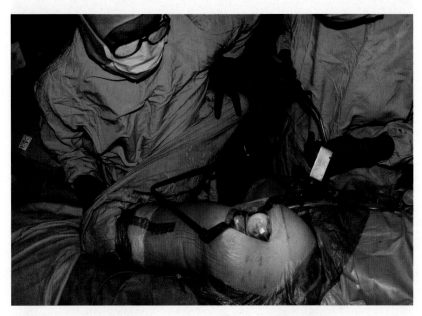

Fig. 19.41.

The surgeon identifies the upper border of the psoas tendon and, using Muller scissors, cuts the inferior aspect of the anterior hip capsule from inferior to superior. Care is taken not to divide any of the fibers of psoas (PT) (Fig. 19.42). It used to be taught, particularly by the Exeter group of surgeons, that division of the psoas tendon carried no penalty. This is not so. These young, active patients having a hip resurfacing will notice a functional deficit if their psoas tendon is divided. Active flexion of the hip beyond 90 degrees is impaired if the psoas is divided. Patients with a divided psoas tendon can complain that they have difficulty flexing their hip up enough to get their foot on and off car pedals. I therefore strive not to divide the psoas tendon, but there are some occasions where it just has to be done. In a patient with a previous intertrochanteric osteotomy, the psoas tendon can be embedded in a mass of scar tissue, and in order to mobilize the femur, all of the scar tissue and the psoas tendon need to be divided.

This division of the inferior aspect of the hip capsule is carried proximally as far as possible (arrows, Fig. 19.43).

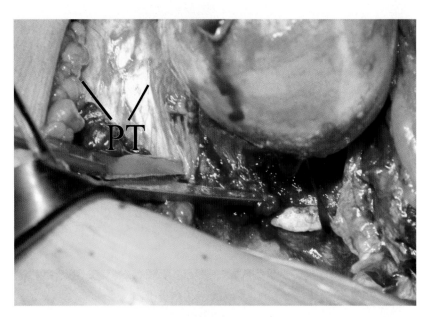

Fɪɢ. 19.42.

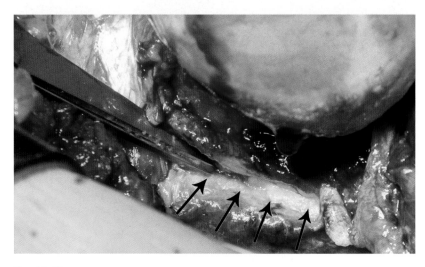

Fɪɢ. 19.43.

The first assistant now flexes the hip to 45 degrees and again forcibly internally rotates the hip (Fig. 19.44). This part of the procedure is very easy provided the first assistant is assisting. It is division of the inferior part of the anterior hip capsule that presents the greatest difficulty. However, if the inferior part of the anterior hip capsule is not divided first, then it is very difficult, and usually impossible, to get the hip into the position shown. I achieve this position in more than 99% of my resurfacing procedures. If this position is not achieved at this stage, then the surgeon needs to go back and re-do properly the steps that have been missed.

This delivers the superior aspect of the anterior hip capsule into vision for the surgeon. The superior part of the anterior hip capsule is divided from superior to inferior to connect with the previous incision in the inferior aspect of the anterior hip capsule (PI) (Fig. 19.45). The point of division for the anterior hip capsule is neither up against the femur nor against the acetabulum. A point half way between the edge of the acetabulum and the femur is chosen as a convenient division area for the anterior hip capsule. I am frequently asked if I have ever injured the femoral vessels during anterior capsule division, and the answer is not yet. When the leg is in this rotated position, the femoral vessels are a safe distance away. This can be confirmed during cadaveric dissection.

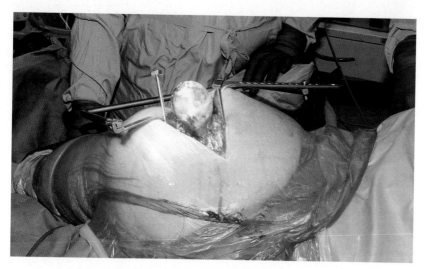

FIG. 19.44.

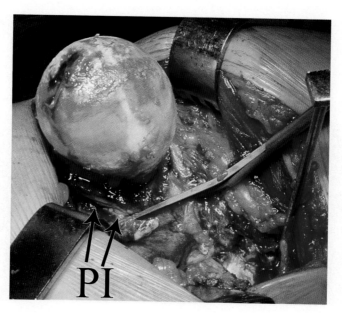

FIG. 19.45.

It should now be confirmed by direct vision and palpation with a finger that all of the anterior capsule has been divided (arrows, Fig. 19.46).

If osteophytes are present, then these should be trimmed from the femoral head-neck junction taking care not to tear soft tissue off the femoral neck (Fig. 19.47). As has already been alluded to, the soft tissue on the surface of the femoral neck contains vital retinacular vessels that supply nourishment to the femoral head. It is not desirable to remove the soft tissue from the femoral neck and sacrifice these vessels. However, it is also important to get clear visualization of the femoral neck with its overlying soft tissue so that accurate placement of the femoral component of the BHR can be obtained.

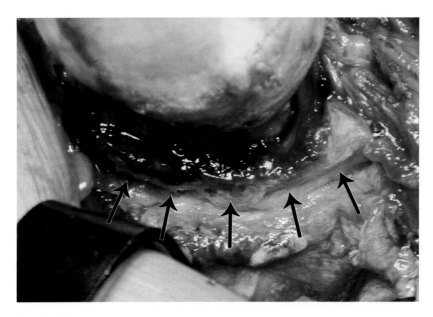

FIG. 19.46.

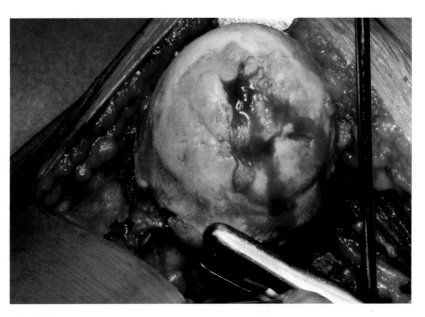

FIG. 19.47.

Special attention is directed toward the anterosuperior femoral neck because it is common to have osteophyte plastered on the anterosuperior femoral neck thus thickening the dimension of the femoral neck plus osteophyte. This anterosuperior osteophyte must be excised from the surface of the femoral neck otherwise this will force the surgeon into using a femoral component that is too large. That in turn means that excessive reaming of the acetabulum has to be performed to insert a hip resurfacing (Fig. 19.48). The learner hip surgeon will be tempted to stay away from the femoral neck with both instruments and the periphery of the femoral component. This is not a good policy, and it is regarded as very important in hip resurfacing not to overream the acetabulum. In my hip surgery practice, I use the same BHR acetabular components for both my total hip replacements and my resurfacings. I find no difference in the amount I have to ream the acetabulum between my total hip patients and my resurfacings. I would prefer to carry out a total hip replacement rather than overream the acetabulum in a young patient.

When the osteophyte has been cleared off the anterosuperior femoral neck, the maximum neck dimension is measured with a caliper (Fig. 19.49).

We perform four measurements of neck and head dimensions and record these for research purposes. In Chapter 11, some of these measurements are used to demonstrate conservation

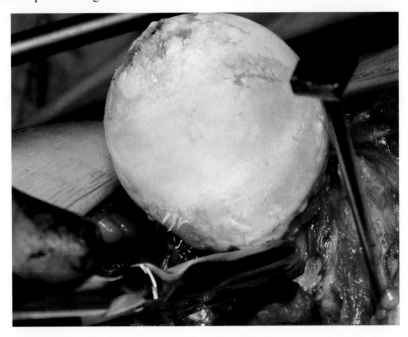

Fig. 19.48.

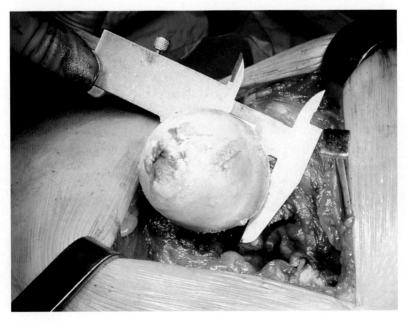

Fig. 19.49.

of acetabular bone stock. Essentially, the maximum neck dimension governs the smallest femoral component that can be applied to that particular patient without damaging the femoral neck. In normal anatomy, it is usually possible to place a femoral component in any given patient smaller than the actual size that eventually gets used. The minimum head dimension governs the support offered by the femoral head to the femoral component, but as will be seen in Chapter 25, this is a much too simplified view of the problem. In the patient with slipped epiphysis, the component has to be placed eccentrically on the femoral head, and the minimum head dimension in these circumstances becomes largely irrelevant. The maximum head dimension is a very useful measurement, and even for routine clinical practice, it is sensible to measure the maximum head dimension having dislocated the hip. Thought of in the simplest possible way, if the femoral head fits into the acetabular cavity, then so too would a similar size of acetabular cup. It is seen in Chapter 11 that in a large series of BHR procedures, the outer diameter of the cup used is on average the same size as the maximum head diameter.

The minimum neck dimension (Fig. 19.50) is also measured.

The maximum head dimension and the minimum head dimension are also measured (Fig. 19.51).

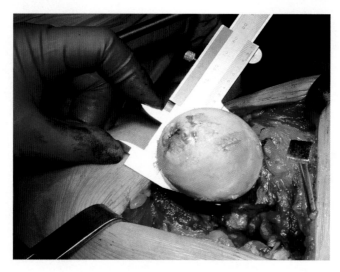

Fig. 19.50.

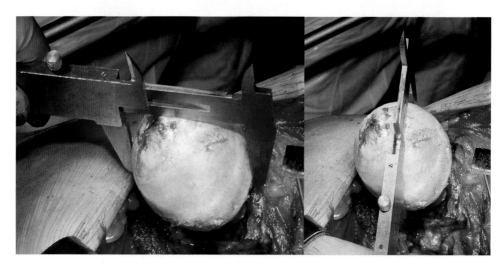

Fig. 19.51.

The next task is to place a head-neck template over the femoral neck (Fig. 19.52).

The surgeon needs to know which is the smallest head-neck template size that can be made to clear the femoral neck even if this is tight to apply. Experience has shown that if a given size of head-neck template can be positioned over the neck, then the corresponding femoral head size can be placed, provided there is accurate placement of the guide wire.

The surgeon must then determine the maximum size of head-neck template that can be applied to the femoral head while still obtaining peripheral head support. All this gives the surgeon a clear knowledge of the smallest and largest femoral components that can be applied to the patient (Fig. 19.53).

In only the exceptional cases does the femoral neck dimension govern the size of components used. Usually, a bigger component needs to be employed in order that the corresponding acetabular component gains a sufficiently good fix in the acetabulum. This means that in the normal case, I allow the acetabulum to dictate the size of components used. I do not prepare the femoral head first except in complex anatomy like Perthes disease, where the mushroom-shape femoral head can be enormous. I have all the information recorded relating to the smallest size of femoral component I could use without damaging the femoral neck and the largest size of femoral component I could use without running out of peripheral femoral head support for the femoral component.

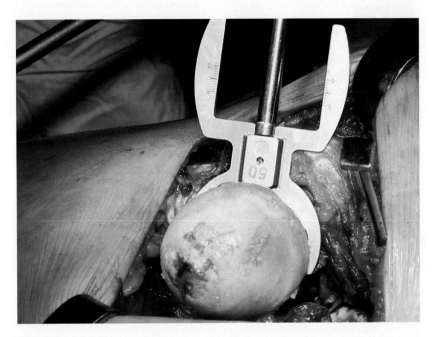

FIG. 19.52.

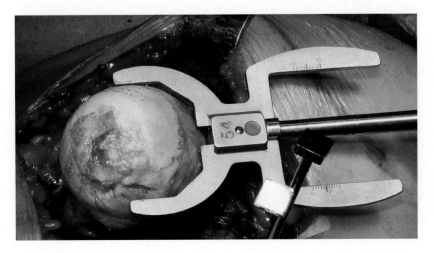

FIG. 19.53.

For the surgeons new to the BHR system, it is helpful at this stage to glance at the chart (Fig. 19.54). At the time of writing, this chart is used in the rest of the world *outside* the United States. At the time of writing, only 4-mm-increment femoral heads are available in the United States. I have had access to 2-mm-increment femoral heads for some years now, and these are useful in borderline cases with a broad femoral neck where a 2-mm-smaller femoral component would not notch but a 4-mm-smaller femoral component would notch the femoral neck. Hopefully, 2-mm-increment femoral components will soon be available in the United States.

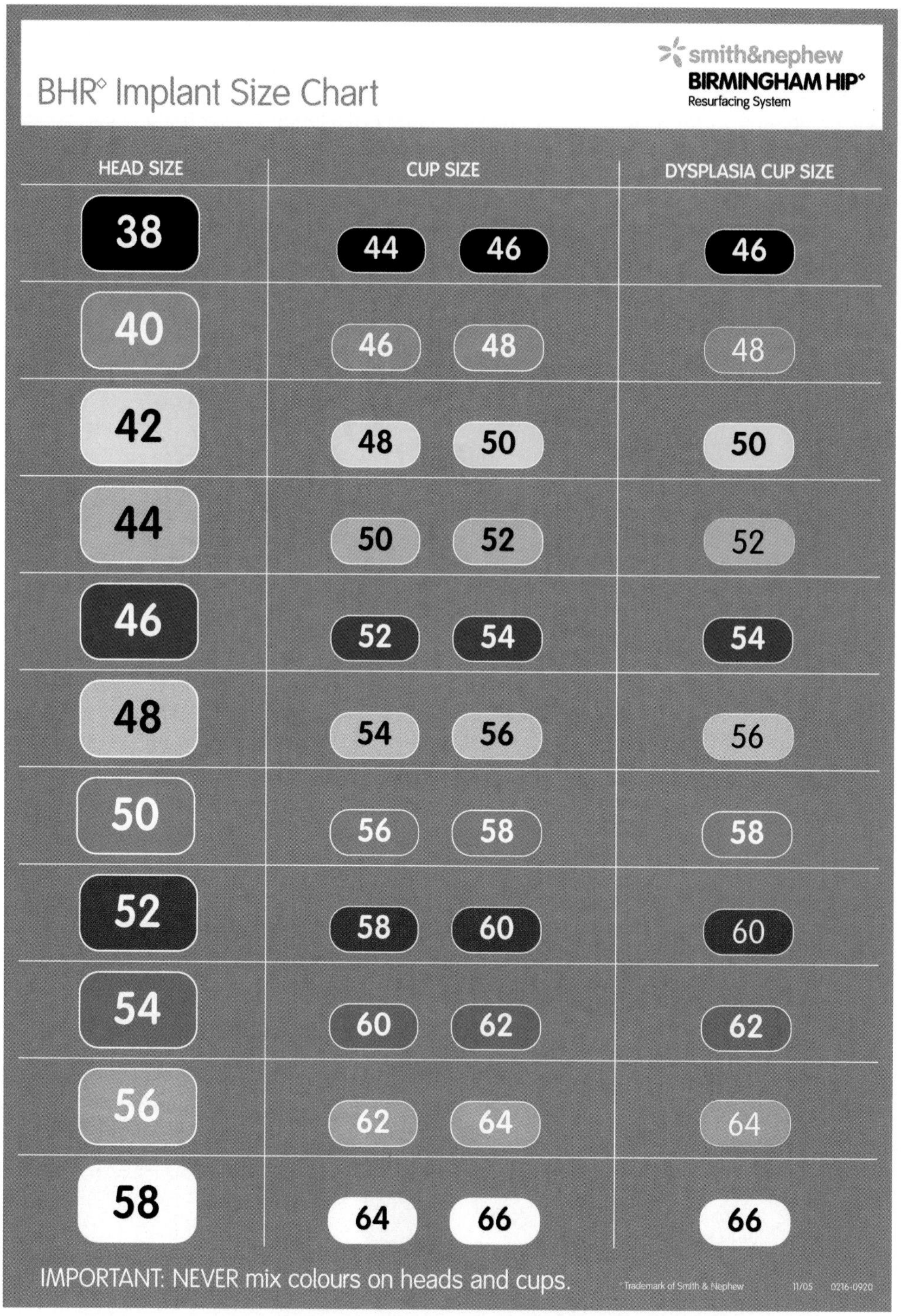

FIG. 19.54.

A large hook is placed around the femoral neck, and the second assistant displaces the femoral head and neck in an anterosuperior direction (Fig. 19.55). The details of the hook used are very important. The hook on my retractors is large and has a blunt tip. There are many designs of unsuitable hooks available, and the unsuitability relates to the radius of curvature of hook and the sharpness of tip. If a small radius of curvature hook is used, particularly if it has a sharp tip, then the anterior femoral neck will be damaged by the hook. I have confirmed this in patients having a total hip replacement. Given that fracture of the femoral neck is a major issue in hip resurfacing arthroplasty, it seems casual to go damaging the anterior femoral neck when selection of a better hook design would prevent this problem. When I used to do extensile approaches for hip resurfacing, the next step was not very important, but with a smaller incision, the next step does become very important indeed. The idea of the hook and the attached assistant is to displace the head and femoral neck forwards thus giving the surgeon a view of the anterosuperior acetabulum.

The anterosuperior acetabular labrum is then grasped with heavy Kocher forceps (Fig. 19.56).

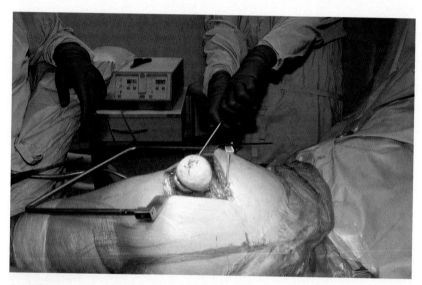

Fɪɢ. 19.55.

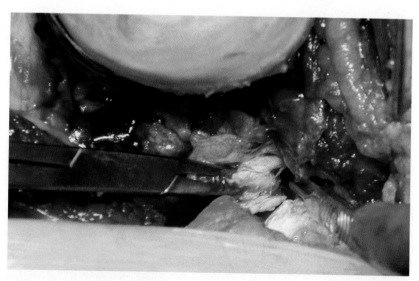

Fɪɢ. 19.56.

The anterosuperior labrum is then excised giving clear sight of the anterosuperior acetabular edge (AE) (Fig. 19.57). The surgeon must take care at this stage because this tissue is preferentially removed with a knife. Either the knife should be directed from outside the acetabulum to inside or the blade of the knife can be guided by the acetabular cavity with a reciprocating motion cutting the attachment of the labrum. In this area, the femoral vessels are close.

Using the Muller scissors and keeping the tips of these scissors on bone, the capsule, muscle, and reflected head of rectus femoris are slowly divided from the anterosuperior acetabulum (ASA). The tips of the scissors must never leave contact with the bone as cutting into the soft tissues in this area could, of course, cut the femoral vessels (Fig. 19.58). The anterior superior acetabular edge (arrows) can clearly be seen where a segment of the anterosuperior labrum has been excised. On either side of the arrows can be seen the remaining, intact acetabular labrum. This procedure of snipping around the anterosuperior acetabular edge is widely used in revision hip surgery to mobilize the femur and get sufficient anterior displacement of the femur to perform the acetabular revision.

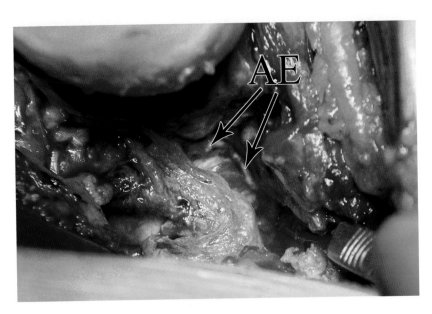

Fig. 19.57.

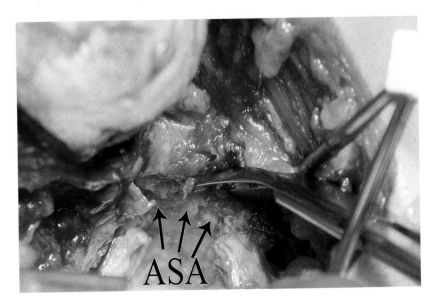

Fig. 19.58.

A Hohmann retractor with a sturdy tip is driven into the bone half way between the anterior-inferior iliac spine and the edge of the acetabulum (Fig. 19.59). Many years ago, I used to place this retractor over the upper part of the anterior acetabular edge, but I have stopped doing this. In some muscular men with very stiff hips, the force required to displace the femoral head out of the way can fracture the anterior acetabular wall if a retractor is placed over it.

I therefore drive the tip of the Hohmann retractor into the ilium at least 1 cm away from the acetabular edge to avoid fracture (Fig. 19.60).

The surgeon should check that the tip of the Hohmann is of sufficient strength not to fracture under heavy retraction. I have had a fine-tipped Hohmann retractor fracture off during this procedure, and it is near impossible to remove the fractured tip from the bone.

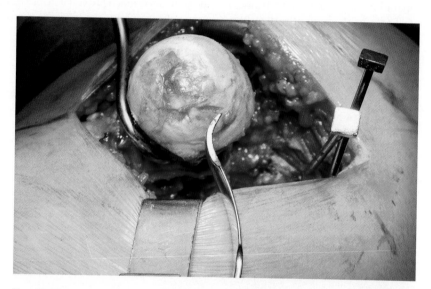

FIG. 19.59.

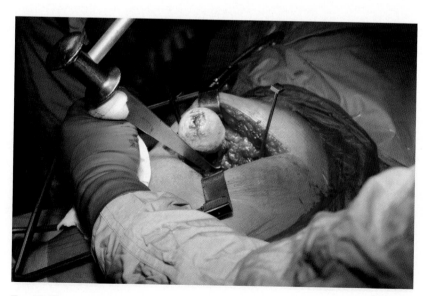

FIG. 19.60.

The surgeon takes the patient's foot in one hand and the Hohmann retractor in the other, and by slowly externally rotating the leg and applying pressure on the retractor, the femoral head is prolapsed under the abductor muscles (AB) (Figs. 19.61–19.63). If the previous steps of the procedure have been carried out as shown, then prolapsing the femoral head under the abductor muscles is easy. If the femoral head will not prolapse, then either you have an enormous Perthes-size femoral head or vital steps in the exposure have been missed. When the surgeon lets go of the foot, the leg is allowed to adopt its own comfortable position. This position invariably is just off the front edge of the operating table. A sterile covered pillow (Fig. 19.61) therefore is placed between the operating table and an instrument trolley so that the tibia and foot of the patient rest on this

pillow and so that the leg does not fall off the front of the operating table.

The surgeon must judge how easy or difficult femoral head displacement is in each particular patient. In stiff, heavy muscled men, the second assistant will have to work hard to give the surgeon a good view of the acetabulum (Fig. 19.63). However, patients such as slim ladies, patients with DDH who have not had previous surgery, and patients with avascular necrosis of the femoral head tend to have much more mobile hips, and the second assistant needs controlling so that they do not pull excessively in a patient with a mobile hip. In such a patient, if a strong second assistant pulls hard, then the femoral head is displaced too proximally, and injury to the femoral nerve can occur. In addition, if too much proximal displacement of the femoral head occurs, then the inferior part of the exposure is compromised.

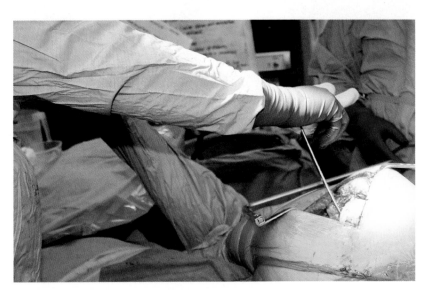

FIG. 19.61.

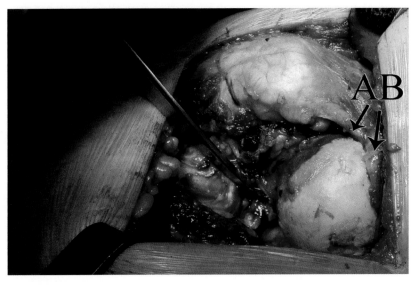

FIG. 19.62.

It can be seen that the femoral head will displace over the anterosuperior acetabulum allowing full access to the periphery of the acetabulum for exposure, preparation, and insertion of the acetabular cup. The anteroinferior capsule is always tight when the femoral head and neck are displaced upwards and forwards, and a second radial cut in the capsule is performed anteroinferiorly. This allows a retractor to be placed over the front of the acetabulum giving a wider exposure and better view for the surgeon. This radial cut in the anteroinferior capsule (arrows) is made over the position of the psoas tendon so that if inadvertent penetration occurs, only the psoas tendon will be damaged and not the femoral vessels (Fig. 19.64).

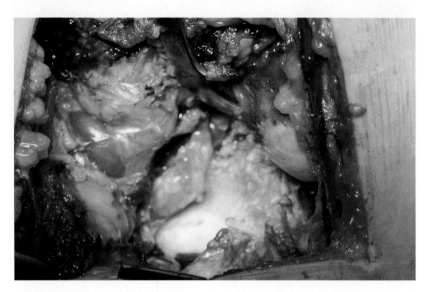

Fig. 19.63.

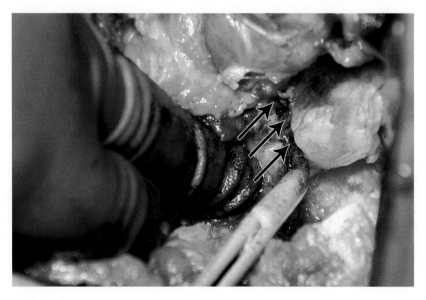

Fig. 19.64.

An inferior Hohmann (H) retractor is placed below the transverse ligament and below the tear-drop and hooked onto the Charnley frame (Fig. 19.65).

A small retractor (R) is placed close to bone over the anterior acetabular wall to give a final full view of the acetabulum for preparation and cup insertion.

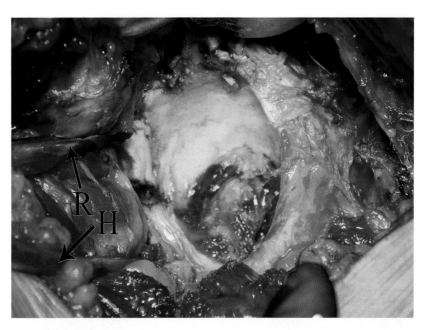

FIG. 19.65.

20
Acetabular Preparation and Insertion of the Standard Birmingham Hip Resurfacing Cup

Derek J.W. McMinn

Whether the surgeon is performing a total hip replacement or a hip resurfacing, through either a traditional extensile approach or a mini incision surgery (MIS) approach, then the acetabular anatomy must be seen. I refuse to allow trainee surgeons to proceed with reaming the acetabulum until they can show me a 360-degree view of the acetabular walls, the tear drop, and the true floor of the acetabulum.

The acetabular labrum is fully excised and the ligamentum teres remnant is excised also (Fig. 20.1). In the position that the scalpel has reached in this figure, it is common to encounter a posterior wall acetabular osteophyte preventing distal excision of the posterior wall acetabular labrum.

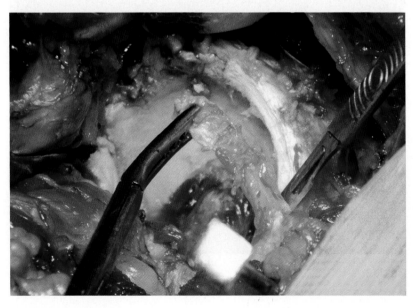

Fig. 20.1.

If osteophyte is present on the posterior acetabular wall, this is divided with an osteotome (Fig. 20.2).

How this osteophyte is excised is a matter of personal preference of the surgeon, and certainly it can just be removed with a rongeur, but I find it easier to divide the osteophyte from the acetabular wall with an osteotome and then use a rongeur.

This is the time when the divided osteophyte is grasped with a rongeur, but usually soft tissue connection prevents the osteophyte from being removed (Fig. 20.3). The soft tissue connection is divided with a knife or electrocautery to allow osteophyte removal. Osteophyte can be present on the anterior acetabular wall, although these are thinner osteophytes and they can easily be removed with a rongeur without using an osteotome. However, the rongeur tips must be sharp, because if a blunt rongeur is used, then removal of anterior osteophyte can break into the anterior acetabular wall creating a defect.

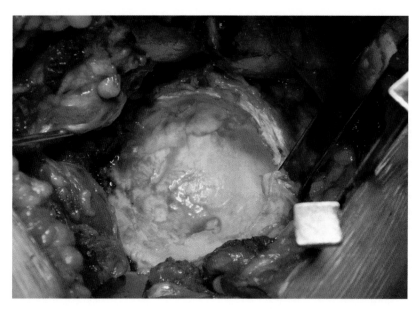

Fɪɢ. 20.2.

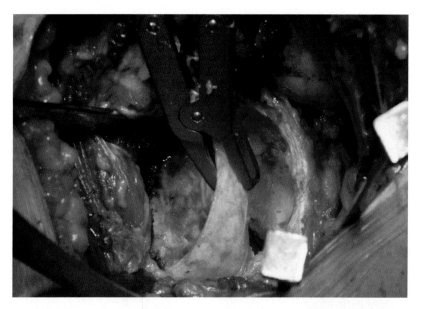

Fɪɢ. 20.3.

Osteophyte in the acetabular floor, if present, is excised using an osteotome (Fig. 20.4). The normal horseshoe shape of the fovea is re-created using the osteotome.

Osteophyte overlying the transverse ligament is divided with an osteotome. Figure 20.5 shows the stage where the acetabular floor osteophyte has been divided, the horseshoe shape of the fovea has been re-created, and the osteophyte over the transverse ligament has been divided.

The next stage is to grasp the divided osteophyte with a rongeur and remove it. This works well for the osteophyte in the acetabular floor, but osteophyte that overlies the transverse ligament usually needs division of connecting soft tissue by sharp dissection or electrocautery to allow removal. At this stage, the inferior Hohmann retractor often falls out as it was taking purchase on the inferior osteophyte rather than deep to the transverse ligament and deep to the tear drop. Replacement of the Hohmann retractor is now performed.

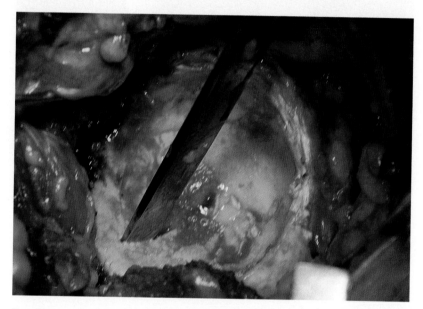

Fig. 20.4.

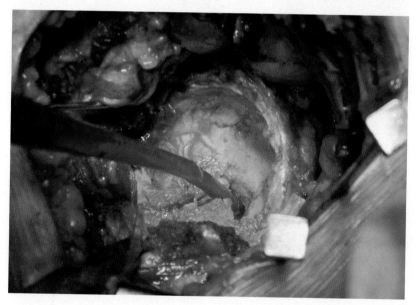

Fig. 20.5.

Having removed the osteophyte from the acetabular floor, the surgeon now has to clear the fovea of all soft tissue. This can be satisfactorily accomplished using a rongeur (Fig. 20.6) or curettes. It is common for bleeding to occur at this stage as acetabular vessels passing on the surface of the tear drop deep to the transverse ligament are torn. A check is made at this stage to ensure that the transverse ligament has been excised. Some surgeons retain the transverse ligament as a guide to acetabular component placement. I have found the transverse ligament to be totally unreliable as a guide to acetabular component placement.

When all soft tissue from the fovea has been removed and when the transverse ligament has been removed, then bleeding acetabular vessels are coagulated where they enter the acetabulum over the tear drop (Fig. 20.7).

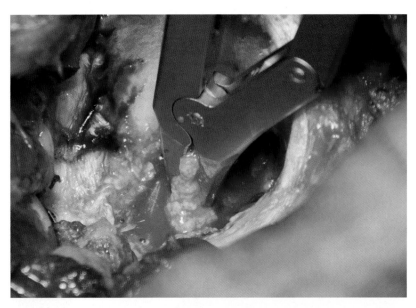

Fig. 20.6.

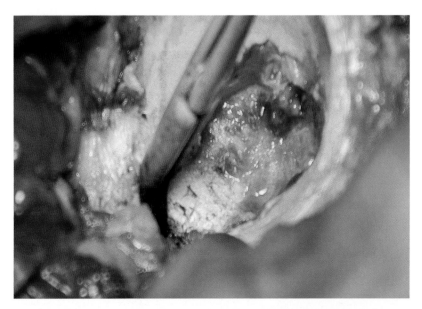

Fig. 20.7.

There are many ways of reaming the acetabulum. I prefer to start with a small acetabular reamer, reaming in the true acetabulum to reach the acetabular floor (Fig. 20.8).

For an averaged-size man, I start reaming with a size 45-mm reamer. The reamer is constantly inserted and removed until the surgeon is confident that the acetabular floor has been reached. It is never satisfactory to place the acetabular reamer in the acetabulum and pull the trigger of the power unit allowing the reamer to find its own place of reaming. The surgeon with his second hand should control exactly the position that the acetabular reamer removes bone from the acetabulum. In the average osteoarthritic hip, one is attempting to bias the reamer in an anterosuperior direction so that when final reaming is reached, satisfactory support for the component will occur. As we shall see later, the complete opposite is true in DDH.

I then ream up in 2-mm increments until we come close to the final acetabular reaming, and for the last three reamers I increase in 1-mm increments. In the early stages of reaming, the aim is to center the reamed acetabulum to gain maximum bony support; one is constantly having to alter the bias of the reamer to get the best acetabular support possible. Commonly, one is biasing the reamer toward the anterosuperior acetabulum where it has been eroded away by the arthritic process (Fig. 20.9).

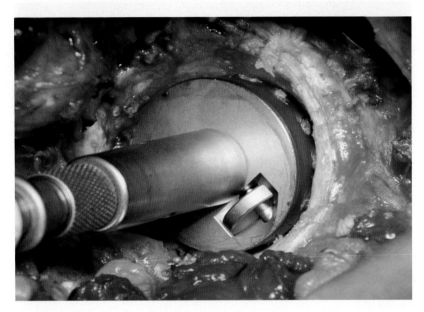

FIG. 20.8.

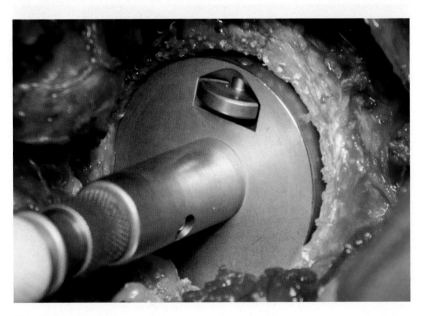

FIG. 20.9.

The reamed surface of the fully prepared acetabulum is a mixture of cancellous and cortical bone (Fig. 20.10). It should never be the aim of the surgeon to keep on reaming the acetabulum until cancellous bone is exposed in all areas of the acetabulum, otherwise severe acetabular overreaming will have occurred.

It must be clearly ascertained, however, that the areas of cortical bone do not have any overlying articular cartilage or any soft tissue remaining on the reamed surface.

It is my practice to curette over the area of cortical bone in the acetabulum and make certain that all articular cartilage is removed. The most important time to carry out this maneuver is in a patient with mild protrusio. In these patients, the acetabular eburnation is posterior, and when the acetabulum is reamed, almost routinely, acetabular cartilage remains intact in the anterosuperior acetabulum. I have inserted hydroxyapatite-coated cups over the past 15 years, and if the implant is stable, any small radiolucency at the interface caused by a gap between the implant and bone will fill in. However, if that radiographic gap is caused by remaining articular cartilage, it has been my experience that the radiographic gap will never fill in (Fig. 20.11).

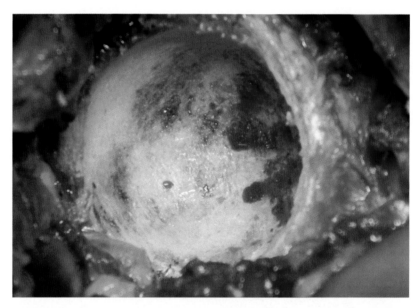

Fig. 20.10.

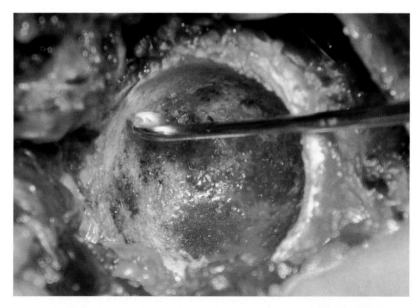

Fig. 20.11.

A trial acetabular cup is then placed in the acetabulum and impacted into position (Fig. 20.12).

For the Birmingham Hip Resurfacing (BHR), I normally have a 2-mm press-fit on the acetabular component by underreaming 2 mm for any given cup size. The exceptions to this are (1) in patients, usually women, with very small sclerotic acetabulae where the reamed acetabulum can be fractured with a 2-mm press-fit. Instead in these patients, I underream by 1 mm. (2) In some very large men, soft cancellous bone is exposed in the reamed acetabulum, and in those patients I underream by 3 mm. However, in the normal arthritic hip, I underream by 2 mm. It must be noted that the trial cup for each cup size is 1 mm smaller than the definitive implant, so in a typical male patient where a 56-mm acetabular cup is being inserted, the trial is 55-mm diameter and the reaming is to 54-mm diameter. The extent of press-fit achieved in any situation is a reflection on how hard and noncompliant the acetabular bone stock is and the nature of the reamers used (Fig. 20.13). If the acetabular reamers are slightly blunt, then the tips of the reamers are worn off and the reamed cavity will be undersized. This can all be detected at the trial cup stage. The trial cup should be firmly enough fixed in the reamed acetabulum

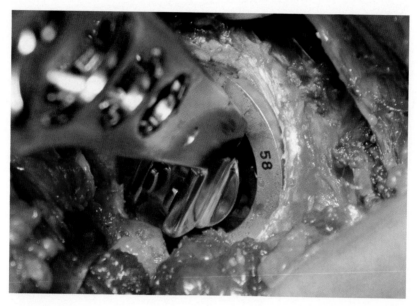

FIG. 20.12.

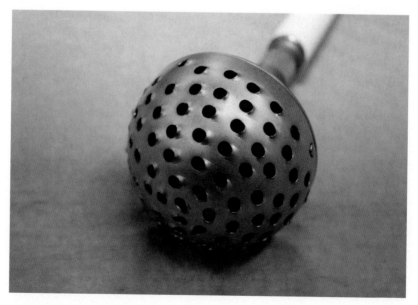

FIG. 20.13.

that the position of the introducer is held without any finger pressure (Fig. 20.14). The alignment of the cup in the reamed acetabulum should be changeable by moderate pressure from the surgeon. If the surgeon has to hammer hard to get the trial acetabular cup in, and, if when in position the trial cup is very difficult to move in position, the press-fit of the definitive implant will be too tight. Almost certainly, in these circumstances, the reason for the excessive press-fit is acetabular underreaming as a result of blunt acetabular reamers. The acetabulum needs to be reamed in 1-mm increments until the desired amount of fix of the trial component is achieved.

When the surgeon is confident about the fix of the trial acetabular component in the reamed acetabulum, the definitive implant is opened. Any soft tissue at the periphery of the acetabulum, such as labrum, that could prolapse between the reamed acetabulum and the new cup should be removed with a rongeur (Fig. 20.15). The surgeon should also try introducing the cup trial before offering up the definitive implant. This will ensure that suitable retraction is in place so that no soft tissue can catch and become prolapsed between the acetabular cup implant and the bony acetabulum.

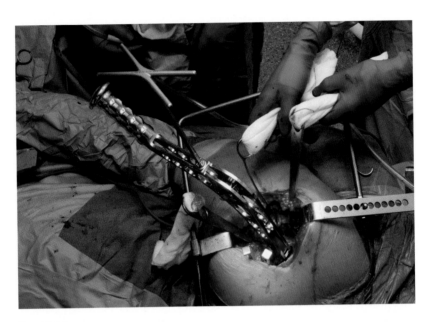

FIG. 20.14.

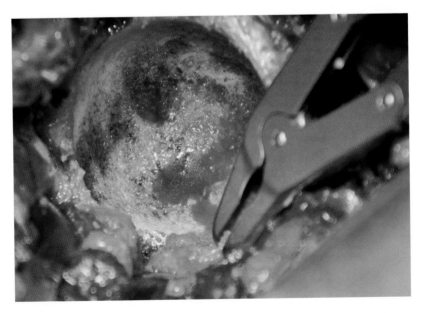

FIG. 20.15.

With regard to acetabular cysts, there are very different practices by different surgeons across the world. Some surgeons ignore acetabular cysts, claiming that they do not matter and further claiming that they fill in with bone. It is certainly a puzzle that one is faced with sometimes in postoperative x-rays, knowing whether a cystic lesion is an acetabular cyst that was there from the time of surgery or whether the cystic lesion represents new osteolysis. My practice has been to meticulously curette cysts in the acetabulum even if they are small (Fig. 20.16). With large acetabular cysts, I aim not only to curette the cyst but also to remove the cyst wall lining from the bone so that bleeding bone is exposed.

I then bone graft the cyst with cancellous bone acetabular reamings (Fig. 20.17). Despite all this curetting and grafting, it is disappointing sometimes to see that as one follows postoperative x-rays, a grafted bone cyst sometimes fails to ossify and returns to being a cyst.

The acetabular cup is attached to the introducer and offered up to the acetabulum with the correct rotational alignment. This involves rotating the acetabular components such that the antirotation flanges cut into the ischium and the pubis. Under no circumstances should the acetabular component be turned upside down so that the antirotation flanges are superior. Any peripheral soft tissue from

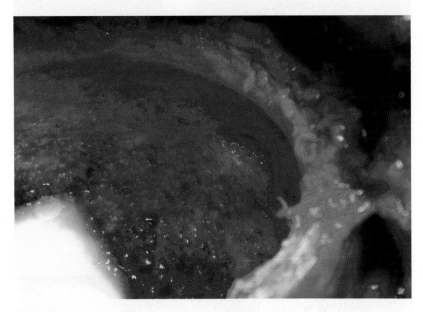

FIG. 20.16.

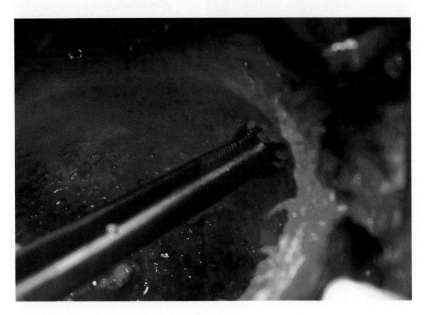

FIG. 20.17.

D.J.W. McMinn

the acetabulum is retracted so that the new cup is cleanly inserted into reamed acetabular bone without any interposing soft tissue (Fig. 20.18).

The acetabular component is impacted using a heavy mallet. There are two ways of detecting when the acetabular component is fully seated. A change in sound can be heard as soon as the acetabular component hits the floor of the acetabulum. Alternatively, a careful watch should be made at the cup-acetabular interface with each hammer blow, and when the implant fails to progress with subsequent hammer blows, then seating is completed. Anteversion is checked with an external alignment guide (Fig. 20.19). The cross-bar marked "Left" in this patient should point along the trunk of the patient to give 20 degrees of anteversion.

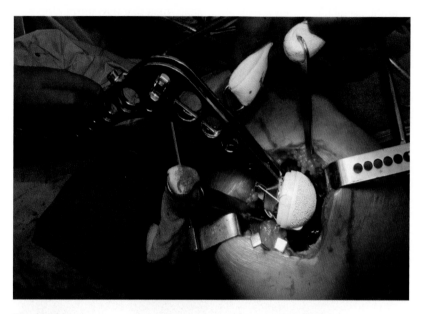

FIG. 20.18.

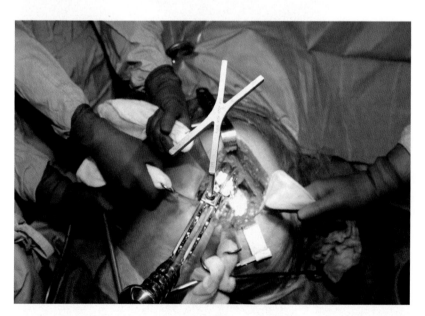

FIG. 20.19.

One is aiming for 40 degrees of inclination and 20 degrees of anteversion. It should be noted that the acetabular wall inclination is approximately 55 degrees, and if the acetabular walls are used to line up the cup edges, the acetabular component will be inserted with a much too high inclination angle. Inclination is estimated by comparison of the cross-bars on the alignment guide with the floor (Fig. 20.20).

With both the straight acetabular introducer and the offset acetabular introducer, as cup impaction proceeds, the cables have a tendency to become stretched, and the surgeon needs to keep tightening the introducer mechanism so that sufficient tension is placed in the cables to get good fixation of the cup on the introducer (Fig. 20.21). This allows the surgeon to test the quality of the acetabular fixation by attempting to move the whole patient from side to side using the introducer handle.

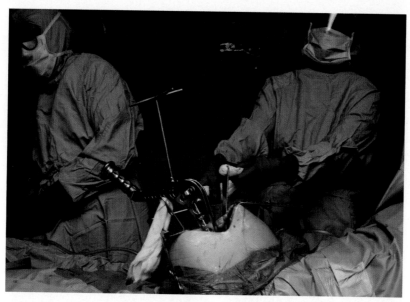

FIG. 20.20.

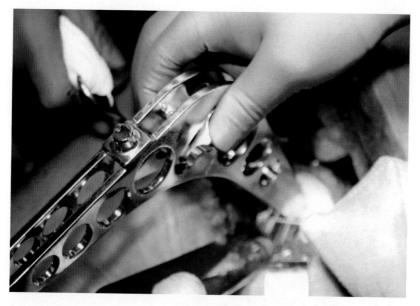

FIG. 20.21.

When the acetabular implant is satisfactorily aligned with respect to inclination and anteversion, and when the implant is securely fixed and fully bottomed-out, the introducer is removed and the polyethylene impactor cap retracted (Fig. 20.22).

A visual check is made all around the edge of the acetabular component to assess position of the component and to assess anterior bony coverage of the acetabular component. Except in the rare cases of anterior acetabular wall dysplasia, the anterior edge of the acetabular component should be fully covered by anterior bone. If the surgeon is unhappy with the acetabular cup position, then the introducer is reattached. The acetabular component position can be altered by either extracting the cup with reinsertion or by a combination of side pressure on the introducer handle and hammering, attempt to alter the acetabular component alignment.

When the surgeon is satisfied with component position, the acetabular cables are cut, and the impactor cap with the cut cables is removed (Fig. 20.23).

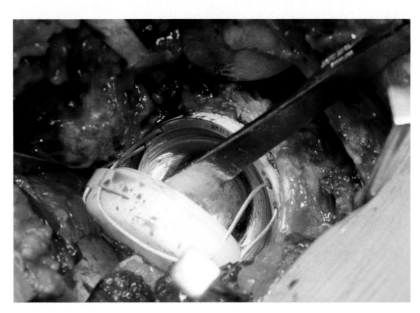

Fig. 20.22.

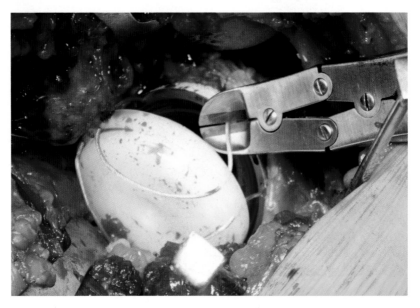

Fig. 20.23.

A check should be made by the scrub nurse or the surgeon that the cables have not been damaged during the process of cable extraction from the cup edge. We know of two instances where the plastic coating on the cables has been stripped off from the underlying metal during the process of cable removal, and a specific check should be made to ensure that this has not happened (Fig. 20.24).

Having removed the impactor cap and cables, now would not be a good time for the surgeon to decide that he did not like the cup position. However, if that unfortunate circumstance does happen, then there is a disposable extractor kit available, but it does involve threading the wormholes in the cup edge. It is much more preferable to check that the cup is in a good position before cutting the cables.

Protruding osteophyte is trimmed off around the acetabular component to prevent impingement (Fig. 20.25).

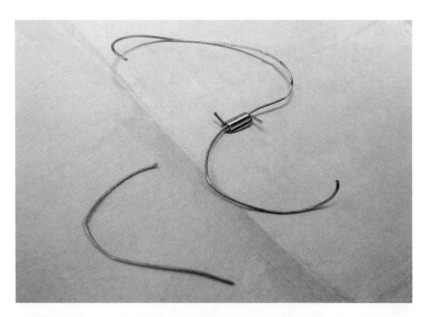

FIG. 20.24.

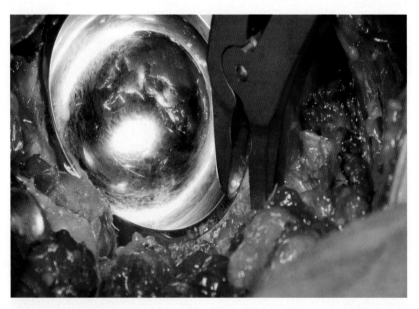

FIG. 20.25.

Posterior osteophytes can usually be excised with a rongeur. If the osteophyte is very sclerotic, then initial division with an osteotome is required.

With respect to the anterior acetabular wall, trimming of osteophyte in this area should be done carefully. At the end of trimming of osteophytes, there should be 2 mm of bone protruding beyond the metal edge of the cup so that the psoas tendon is not exposed to the acetabular cup edge (Fig. 20.26). As mentioned previously, only a sharp rongeur should be used when removing anterior osteophyte. If a blunt rongeur is used, then the surgeon has to lever the instrument to remove bone. This can cause removal of not only osteophyte but also important bone stock in the anterior acetabular wall. An attempt is made to leave the trimmed anterior wall osteophyte smooth to again prevent psoas irritation.

It is our practice to inject the first dose of Naropin (ropivacaine), Adrenalin (epinephrine), and Toradol (ketorolac) into the raw tissues around the acetabulum at this point. (Fig. 20.27) (See chapter 16).

Acetabular component insertion is now complete.

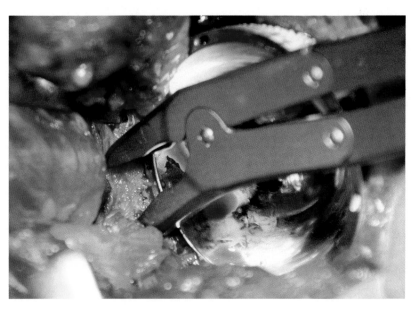

FIG. 20.26.

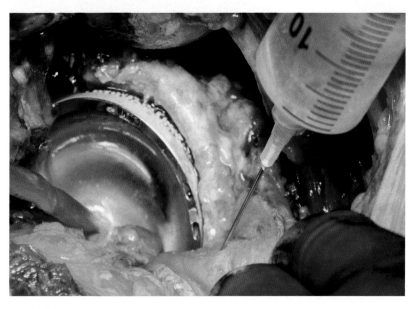

FIG. 20.27.

21
Acetabular Preparation and Insertion of the Dysplasia Birmingham Hip Resurfacing Cup

Derek J.W. McMinn

This chapter concerns the dysplasia cup, which has been available for the past 10 years with the Birmingham Hip Resurfacing (BHR). There are many ways of dealing with the deficient acetabulum, including medialization of the acetabular component, use of a high hip center aiming to get better fixation for the acetabular component higher in the pelvis, and use of structural bone graft. In addition, many techniques of cages and constrained morcellized graft can also be used. These are discussed in Chapter 25. For patients with minor dysplasia, we use the techniques of medialization of the acetabular component and mild elevation of the hip joint center. Before the dysplasia cup was available, I used structural bone graft to support the acetabular component of the McMinn resurfacing cup in severe DDH. Since the advent of the dysplasia cup, I have not used a single structural bone graft in the acetabulum. This is not an easy implant to perform, but then severe acetabular dysplasia is not an easy diagnosis to deal with well. Many of these patients are very young and deserve our best efforts to achieve a good bony reconstruction of their acetabulum and a good functional outcome.

The dysplasia BHR cup is used most often in patients with developmental dysplasia (Fig. 21.1). In most of our patients with mild acetabular dysplasia, the dysplasia cup is not necessary as the techniques mentioned above can deal satisfactorily with the bony insufficiency.

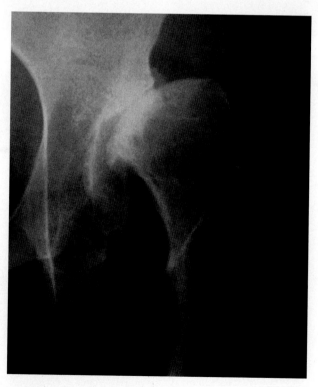

Fig. 21.1.

Other indications include destructive arthritis with a wandering acetabulum (Fig. 21.2) or an old acetabular fracture that has healed with proximal migration of the femoral head.

With developmental dysplasia, there are several points that need special attention in the surgical exposure. First, it is sensible to perform a more extensile exposure so that a clear appreciation of the acetabular abnormality can be obtained.

With DDH and acetabular rotation, the ischium is often very prominent and the sciatic nerve can be tented over the prominent ischium making it vulnerable to injury (Fig. 21.3). When the surgeon sees the prominent ischium outlined in this figure, then he knows that significant acetabular anteversion is present. In order to see and feel the sciatic nerve in this case, I have divided the greater trochanteric bursa over the sciatic nerve.

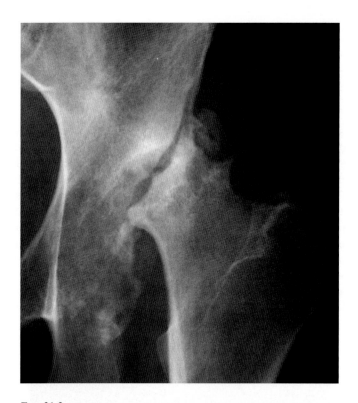

Fig. 21.2.

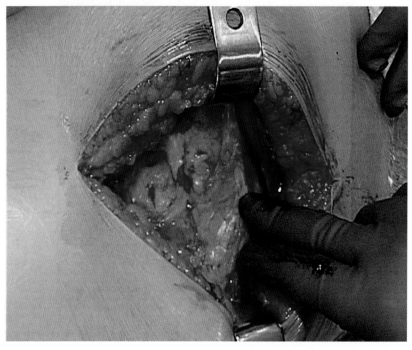

Fig. 21.3.

Because the leg is usually lengthened with DDH, it is wise for the surgeon to palpate the sciatic nerve before any hip reconstruction is performed so that an assessment of the tension in the sciatic nerve after hip reconstruction can be made (Fig. 21.4).

It is important to assess leg length intraoperatively against the preoperative plan. Many intraoperative devices are in use, and any number of these are satisfactory. We use a very simple technique that is demonstrated in the accompanying DVD.

In the posterior surgical approach in a patient with DDH, it should be borne in mind that commonly the posterior acetabular wall is thickened and will require thinning, and the anterior wall of the acetabulum is commonly thin and deficient. The posterior acetabular wall therefore needs to be reamed into, with the acetabular reamers being biased posteriorly. Good visualization of the posterior acetabular wall is required. To do this, the exposure of the posterior wall and the nail retractor insertion into the ischium need to be exaggerated compared with the normal osteoarthritic hip. In Fig. 21.5, the femoral head (FH), posterior acetabular wall (PAW), and the retractor pin (P) in the ischium are marked. It can be seen that I have cleared the capsule from the posterior acetabular wall out onto the ischium to give good visualization of the anatomy and to give plenty of access for thinning of the posterior acetabular wall during acetabular reaming. With a prominent ischium, it is also good to be able to slope the ischium onto the posterior edge of the cup after cup insertion to prevent impingement.

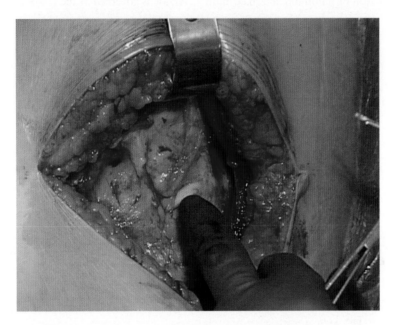

FIG. 21.4.

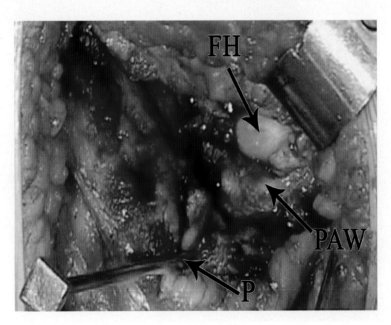

FIG. 21.5.

Femoral neck anteversion measurements up to 45 degrees can be accommodated by inserting the acetabular component with less anteversion than normal. It should be noted that femoral neck anteversion plus acetabular component anteversion should equal 45 degrees. I have inserted acetabular cups in DDH patients with as little as 0 degrees anteversion, but when the femoral neck anteversion is greater than 45 degrees, hip resurfacing needs to be combined with a subtrochanteric derotation osteotomy (Fig. 21.6). This patient had 60 degrees of femoral neck anteversion, and clearly this could not be accommodated by only reducing anteversion on the acetabular component. A dysplasia cup with bone grafting has been used, and the BHR procedure has been combined with a subtrochanteric derotation osteotomy. The exposure and determination of minimum and maximum femoral prosthetic size that can be used is the same as in a standard osteoarthritic case.

However, one aspect needs attention, and this relates to femoral neck anteversion. Excessive femoral neck anteversion is a common accompaniment to developmental dysplasia, and the surgeon must assess the degree of femoral neck anteversion early on in the operation (Fig. 21.7). An instrument is placed along the line of the femoral neck, and another instrument is placed at the back of the tibia. The angle between these two is used to give an assessment of femoral neck anteversion, and in the case shown, no excess femoral neck anteversion is present. The surgeon must know the anteversion number on the femoral neck before turning to the acetabular component preparation and insertion because, as has already been mentioned, the acetabular component anteversion is governed by the femoral neck anteversion.

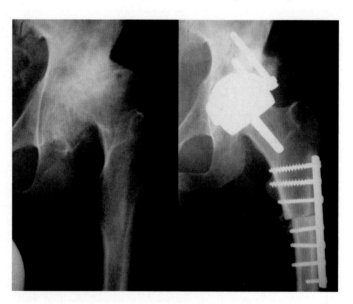

Fig. 21.6.

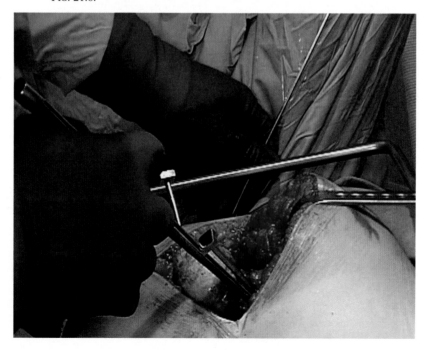

Fig. 21.7.

The femoral head is displaced anterosuperiorly in the normal way, and the acetabular labrum is excised (Fig. 21.8).

In this patient with a destructive arthritis and a wandering acetabulum, it is exceedingly important to establish the normal acetabular anatomy. Here, a large amount of poste- rior osteophyte is being divided from the rest of the posterior acetabular wall. This divided-off osteophyte requires grasping with a rongeur and division of connecting soft tissue to allow removal of the osteophyte (Fig. 21.9).

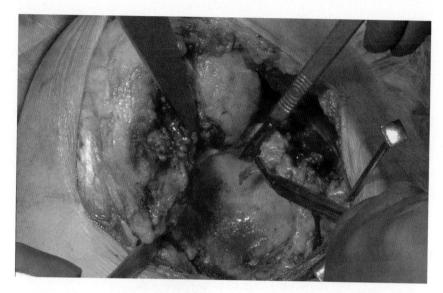

FIG. 21.8.

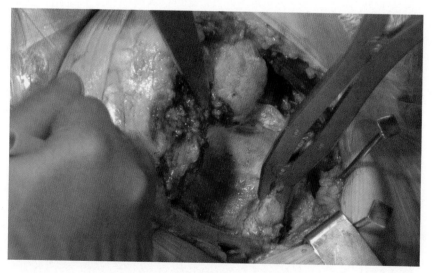

FIG. 21.9.

The osteophyte bone in the acetabular floor is being excised in order to reach the true acetabular floor (Fig. 21.10). With a destructive arthritis, the anterior acetabular wall is usually not deficient, and the posterior acetabular wall is usually not thickened. This makes acetabular reaming relatively easy compared with the situation in DDH. In DDH, the true acetabulum is tiny from front to back, and the deficient anterior acetabular wall must be preserved.

When the acetabular floor osteophyte and the inferior osteophyte have been removed in dysplasia patients, it is sometimes the case that the inferior acetabular retractor has to be repositioned because the initial purchase of this retractor was in fact on osteophyte, and what needs to be achieved is purchase under the acetabular tear-drop (Fig. 21.11).

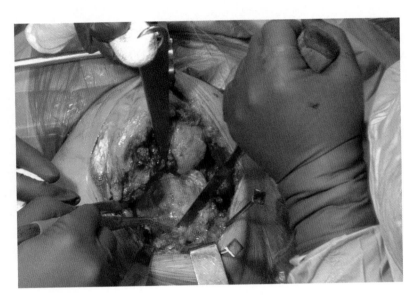

Fɪɢ. 21.10.

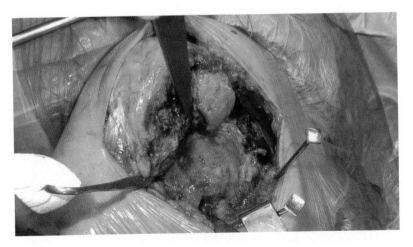

Fɪɢ. 21.11.

In the deficient acetabulum, it is sensible to remove all osteo-phyte giving oneself the maximum information possible in order to get good component placement. If available, an acetabular positioning system or navigation is desirable (see Chapter 24).

In dysplasia patients, I prefer to start reaming with a small (e.g., 40 mm) acetabular reamer. Reaming is always begun in the true acetabulum. In DDH, the acetabular reamer must be biased posteriorly to preserve the deficient anterior acetabu-lar wall. The second hand of the surgeon, therefore, is vital in controlling the anteroposterior position that the acetabular reamer adopts (Fig. 21.12). In this shot, it can be seen that my right hand is available to bias the acetabular reamer in a posterior direction.

Reaming is gradually increased in 2-mm intervals (Fig. 21.13).

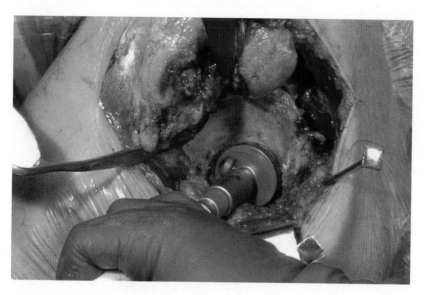

Fig. 21.12.

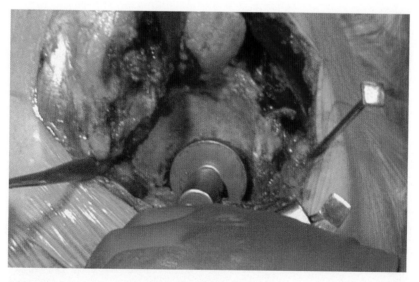

Fig. 21.13.

As the reaming increases, a careful look at the acetabulum after each reaming is mandatory. In Fig. 21.14, we can see the unwelcome appearance of a very large acetabular cyst in the anterosuperior true acetabular roof (C). Above the reamed area can be seen the false acetabulum (F).

The surgeon knows from his femoral neck dimensions the minimum size of femoral component that can be inserted in the dysplasia patient and therefore knows the minimum size of acetabular component that has to be inserted to carry out a resurfacing procedure. It is the front-to-back dimension that governs how much acetabular reaming can safely be performed in the dysplasia patient. If reaming cannot be increased because of the risk of anterior or posterior wall acetabular damage, then the surgeon and his patient must accept that a total hip replacement will have to be performed. It is unacceptable to overream the acetabulum in any hip arthroplasty procedure, but, in particular, it is unacceptable when dealing with young patients. Now the last reamer that can be safely used without sacrificing anterior or posterior acetabular wall bone stock is in position (Fig. 21.15).

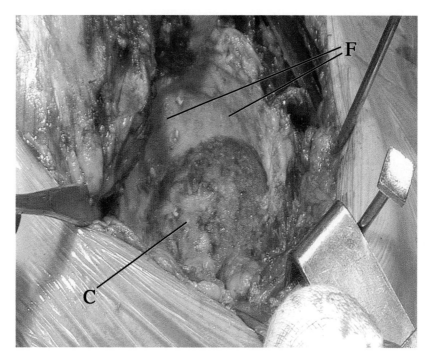

Fig. 21.14.

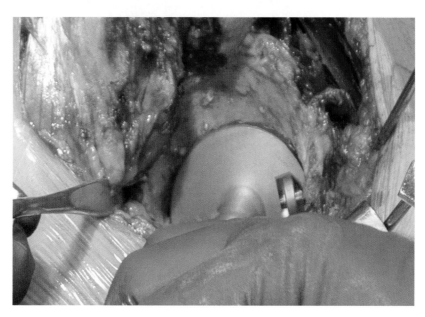

Fig. 21.15.

Here, one can see the trial acetabular component *in situ*. The position of the trial and therefore the definitive component is governed by the femoral side anatomy. The acetabular anteversion is adjusted so that it matches the femoral side anteversion with the total of both equaling 45 degrees. The inclination angle in the dysplasia patient should be made to match the femoral side anatomy also. It is common for excessive valgus of the femoral neck to be present, and in this situation a lower inclination of the acetabular cup should match this abnormal femoral anatomy. It is a big mistake to insert the acetabular component in a dysplasia patient with excessive inclination in the hope that this will gain superior bony support, because all that will happen is

that edge loading of the acetabular component will occur, with run-away wear of the components and premature failure. One is looking for good anteroposterior support for the trial component and, of course, wishing to see as much superior support as is available but not allowing the defective acetabular anatomy to govern the acetabular component inclination angle (Fig. 21.16).

In addition to anteversion, an assessment is being made of acetabular inclination, and with this system these measurements are gauged using the alignment bars on the acetabular component introducer. It can be seen that I am aiming to insert the acetabular component with less than 45 degrees of inclination in order to compensate for a slightly valgus femoral neck (Fig 21.17).

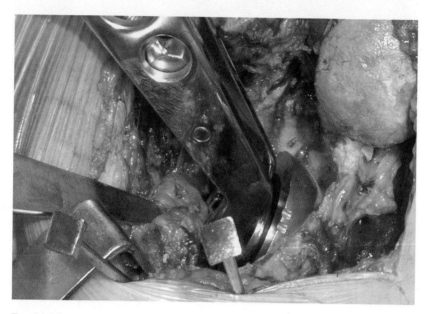

FIG. 21.16.

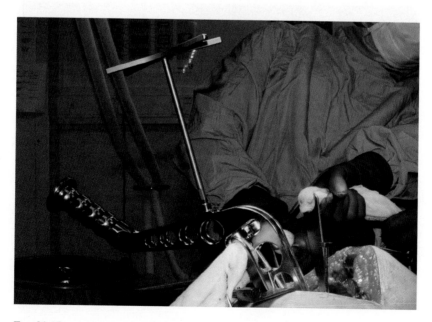

FIG. 21.17.

Now we have reached the stage for preparing for the dysplasia cup insertion. The component size has been decided from the cup trial. It can be seen from the unsupported trial acetabular component that a regular acetabular cup in this patient would not be a sensible option, and it was decided to use a dysplasia cup. The cyst in the acetabular roof is being curetted (Fig. 21.18). When there is debate about whether to use a standard acetabular component or a dysplasia component with screws, not only is the amount of unsupported acetabular component important but the quality of the bone that does exist also matters. When a large cyst is present, this just makes up the surgeon's mind to have supplementary screw fixation with the dysplasia cup.

The false acetabulum is now being cleared of all soft tissue. I find that tooth curettes are particularly useful for this task. Burrs can also be used and rongeurs are sometimes useful (Fig. 21.19). Unlike the poor bone in the roof of this patient's acetabulum, the quality of bone in the false acetabulum is excellent. This is also the case in the DDH patient where load transfer through the false acetabulum gives sclerosis and an excellent fixation for the dysplasia screws.

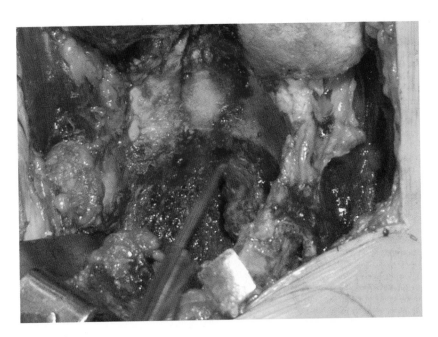

FIG. 21.18.

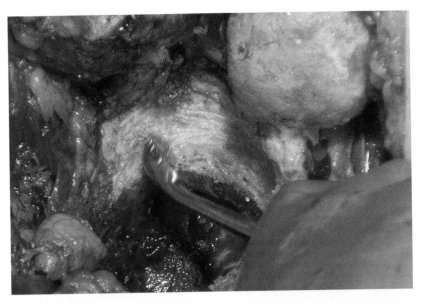

FIG. 21.19.

Because load is transferred through the false acetabulum, the true acetabulum is relatively stress shielded and osteopenic. This makes screw fixation into the acetabular roof using a standard total hip replacement (THR) cup shell rather precarious. The acetabular roof cyst is now being bone grafted with reamings (Fig. 21.20).

Now the dysplasia BHR cup is being inserted. It is very important to understand that the acetabular defect in DDH is anterosuperior and the false acetabulum is an anterosuperior structure. The acetabular component, therefore, on the introducer must be rotated so that the lugs are inserted in line with the anterosuperior false acetabulum (Fig. 21.21).

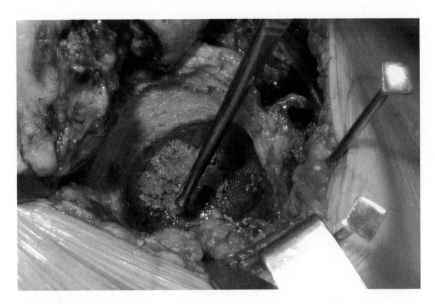

FIG. 21.20.

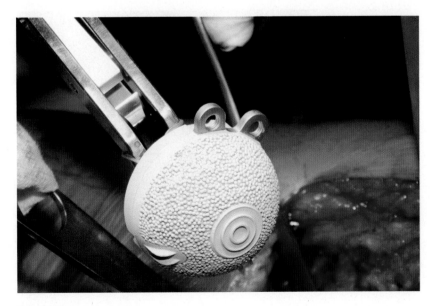

FIG. 21.21.

The false acetabulum is the area where plentiful bone allows good fixation of the dysplasia screws that will stabilize this implant. This picture shows satisfactory anterior rotation of the acetabular component on the introducer (Fig. 21.22). This anterior rotation of the acetabular lugs is necessary to gain support in the good-quality bone of the false acetabulum with the dysplasia screws. In addition, if the acetabular lugs are not rotated toward the false acetabulum, the posterior screw will miss the bone of the false acetabulum and end up getting no purchase or an unsatisfactory purchase on the thin acetabular edge bone.

The acetabular component is impacted until fully seated and with alignment in the desired anteversion and inclination angles, given the femoral anatomy in that particular patient.

When the cup has been inserted satisfactorily, the cup introducer is removed. Again one can see that the lugs of the implant have been rotated anterosuperiorly so that the screws will be inserted into the false acetabulum (Fig. 21.23). A final check of component alignment is carried out and the cup introducer is removed. The impactor cap is retracted, and a visual check of satisfactory cup placement undertaken. Do *not* cut the cables.

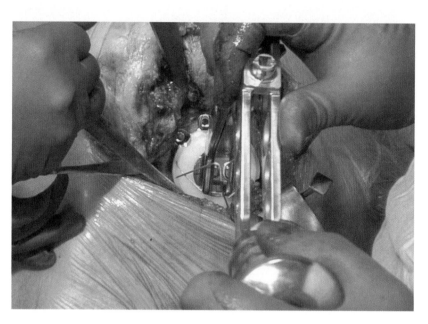

FIG. 21.22.

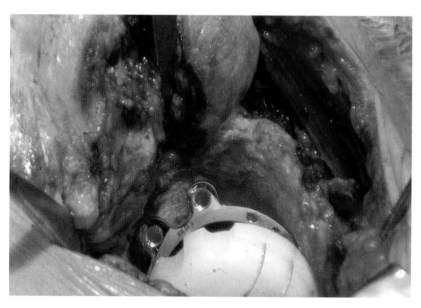

FIG. 21.23.

It is now time to insert the two acetabular screws. A drill guide is inserted into the posterior lug. It is important to always drill the posterior lug first, because if bone is going to be missed, then it will always be missed with the posterior drill hole. If the drilling misses bone, then the acetabular component must be removed and the lugs rotated more anteriorly so that the screws hit the bone of the false acetabulum. It is thus important that the cables are not cut, so that acetabular component extraction and reinsertion can occur. Here, the first drill is inserted through the drill guide drilling into the false acetabulum (Fig. 21.24).

A drill guide is inserted into the posterior acetabular threaded lug (Fig. 21.25). This lug is drilled, and care must be taken not to break the drill in the patient's bone. Because the drill is often hitting the false acetabulum at an angle, the drilling must be done carefully and slowly with regular withdrawal of the drill and constant irrigation.

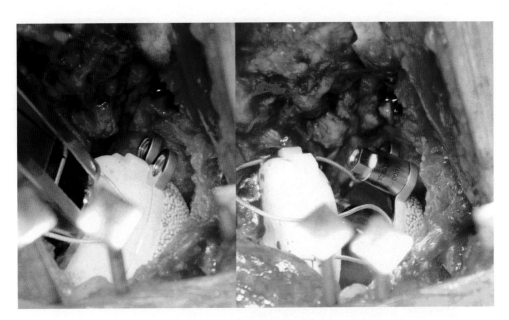

FIG. 21.24.

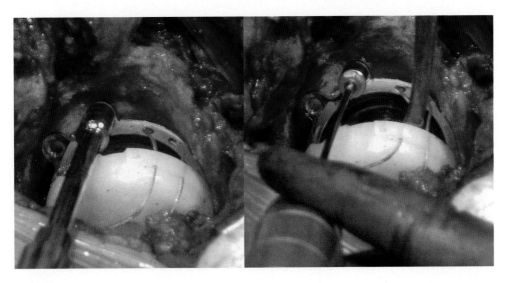

FIG. 21.25.

It is important to have a satisfactory exposure so that straight-line access to the drill guide can be obtained. Pressure from the wound edge on the power unit or the drill itself may cause malalignment and fracture of the drill (Fig. 21.26).

Happily, the drill did indeed enter good-quality bone in the false acetabulum. If the drill misses the bone posteriorly, then the cup needs to be extracted and reinserted with the lugs rotated more anteriorly.

The depth from the cup face to the extent of the posterior acetabular drill hole is now measured with a depth gauge. It is sometimes found that the distance is 70 or 80 mm. It is not necessary to insert an excessively long screw, and generally I insert a screw length in the posterior lug hole double the distance of the acetabular defect. The acetabular defect is measured from the edge of the acetabular component to the depth of the false acetabulum (Fig. 21.27).

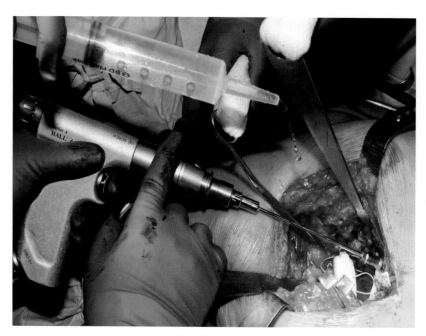

Fig. 21.26.

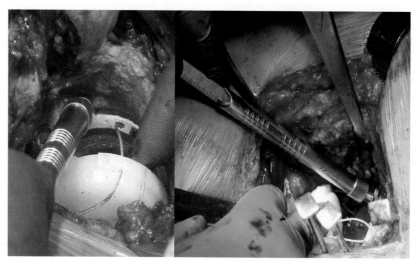

Fig. 21.27.

The posterior drill hole is now being overdrilled with a second drill to bring the size of this hole up to the core diameter of the screw that will be inserted (Fig. 21.28). Again, it is important to have straight-line access for the use of this drill. Deviation from the straight line can again fracture the drill because one has inserted the drill into such good-quality bone in the false acetabulum.

I am often asked by surgeons why we do not use cancellous screws and, of course, cancellous screws are a great invention for use in cancellous bone. What we deal with in the false acetabulum is not cancellous bone; this is more akin to hard cortical bone quality. In addition, a cortical thread for this dysplasia screw allows locking of the screw in the lug.

A screw of appropriate length is opened and threaded through the lug. The surgeon then must be careful and keep turning the screw until the tip of this self-tapping screw touches the bone in the posterior drill hole in the false acetabulum. This is the danger time (Fig. 21.29).

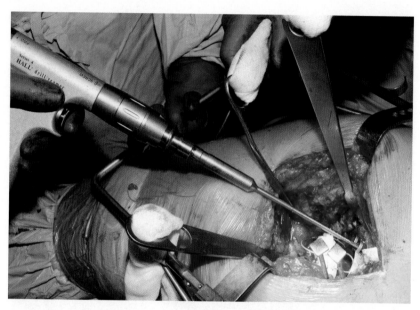

FIG. 21.28.

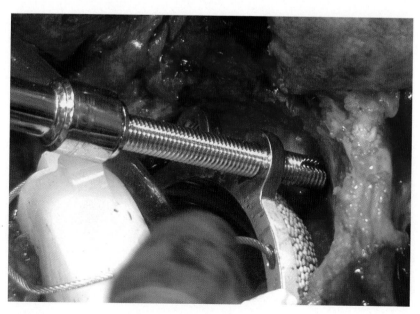

FIG. 21.29.

It is now most important not to just keep turning the screw-driver, because the advancement of the screw will merely push the acetabular component out of the bony acetabulum. Instead, the surgeon must apply strong longitudinal compression to the screwdriver and turn slowly so that the self-tapping threads grip into the bone (Fig. 21.30). A careful watch must be maintained at the cup-bone interface to be certain that the acetabular component is not being pushed out of the acetabulum. If the acetabulum gets pushed out by the advancing screw, then the surgeon has no alternative but to start the procedure from scratch only this time to make a determined effort to lock the dysplasia screw in the sclerotic bone of the false acetabulum.

When the screw achieves a good grip in the bone, it becomes very difficult to turn this with a screwdriver. However, the surgeon should persist for a few turns more with the screwdriver, if at all possible. When screw turning becomes tough, I change the screwdriver to "power reaming" setting on a power unit at this stage and insert the screw by power. It is important to irrigate the lug and the screw as the screw is inserted. Surgeons are regularly amazed at how strong a fix this screw obtains in the sclerotic bone of the false acetabulum (Fig. 21.31).

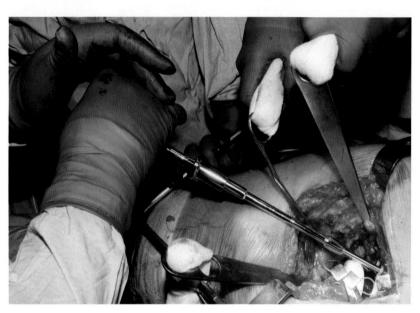

Fɪɢ. 21.30.

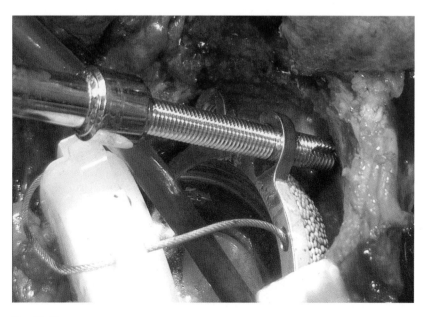

Fɪɢ. 21.31.

When the screw is fully seated on the lug face, then this is the stage at which a T-handle is attached and final locking of the screw is obtained. From here on in, the procedure is relatively easy because now the acetabular component cannot come out of the bony acetabulum with insertion of the anterior screw (Fig. 21.32).

The T-handle spanner is now used to fully tighten the dysplasia screw onto the face of the threaded lug hole (Fig. 21.33). There is a temptation having got such a good purchase with the first screw to not bother inserting the second screw, but this is a mistake. The mechanical advantage obtained with the second screw is enormous and well worth the minor effort of inserting the anterior screw, which is nowhere near as difficult as inserting the posterior screw (see Chapter 25).

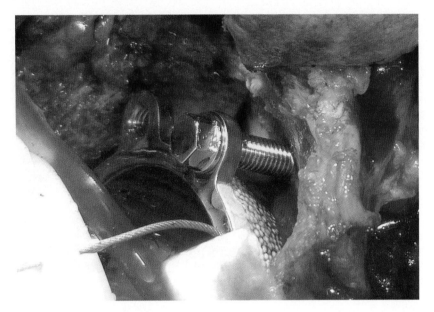

FIG. 21.32.

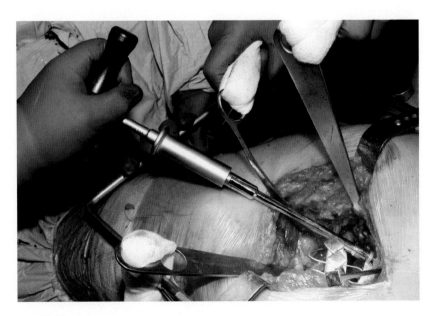

FIG. 21.33.

The drill guide is placed in the anterior lug, and the anterior drill hole is made into the false acetabulum. At this point, one must take great care not to plunge the drill into the pelvis because injury to the iliac vessels at this position can occur (Fig. 21.34).

The drill guide is removed, and the screw length to be used assessed carefully with a depth gauge. Under no circumstances must the self-tapping screw protrude into the pelvis as again this risks vascular injury. The diameter of the hole is enlarged up with a second drill, as before (Fig. 21.35).

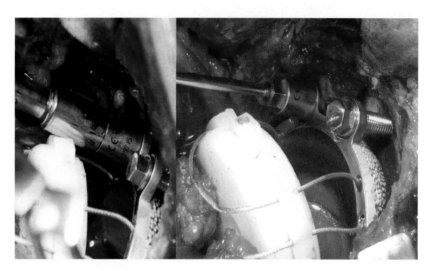

Fig. 21.34.

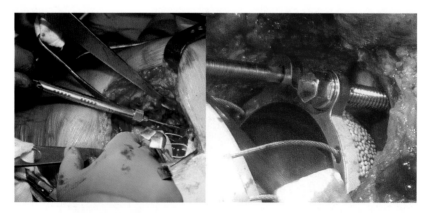

Fig. 21.35.

I hear surgeons who watch me inserting the dysplasia cup saying that they would not have bothered using the dysplasia cup in the particular case I am demonstrating to them. However, they are used to putting in a total hip shell, and if the primary fix of the shell is not what they first hoped for, then screws can be inserted through the acetabular component. No such luxury exists for the resurfacing surgeon who has to decide at the cup trial stage whether to use the dysplasia cup or the standard cup.

The anterior screw is inserted and tightened in exactly the same way as the posterior screw (Fig. 21.36).

Final tightening with a T-handle is again used. When the two screws have been inserted and the surgeon is happy with the final position achieved, then it is safe to cut the cables and remove the impactor cap (Fig. 21.37). There should be no surprises with the acetabular component position at this stage because the acetabular component position has already been checked before the screws were inserted. If the screws have been inserted correctly, then these, of course, do not change the alignment or position of the acetabular component.

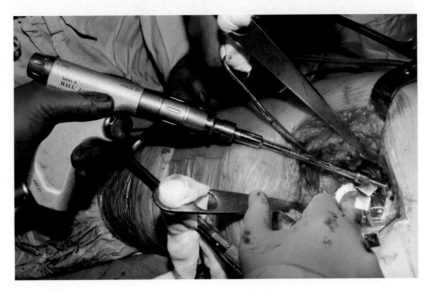

FIG. 21.36.

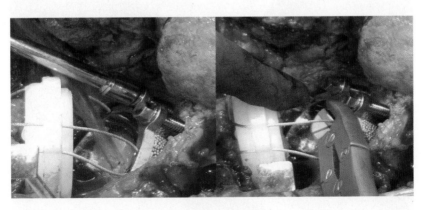

FIG. 21.37.

At this stage, it is important to excise osteophyte around the acetabular edge. The biggest trouble is encountered posteriorly in DDH. In a destructive arthritis, as in this patient, there is no problem trimming osteophyte around the posterior acetabular component edge using a rongeur, but in DDH the ischium is often very prominent, and it is not possible to excise the posterior acetabulum/posterior acetabular osteophyte level with the posterior acetabular component, without risking pelvic dis-

continuity by division through the ischium. In a severe DDH, therefore, one is often left with a situation where one has to satisfy oneself by excising the posterior acetabulum onto the superficial face of the ischium creating enough space for hip movement without impingement (Fig. 21.38).

Anteriorly, it is important to remove osteophyte to prevent impingement (Fig. 21.39). Again, like the normal acetabulum, it is also important to retain 2 mm of bone protruding

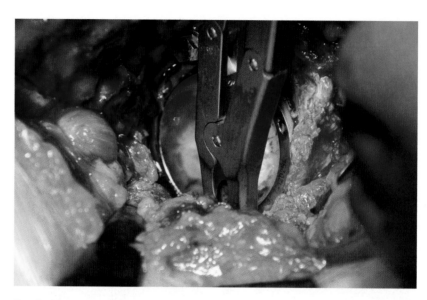

Fig. 21.38.

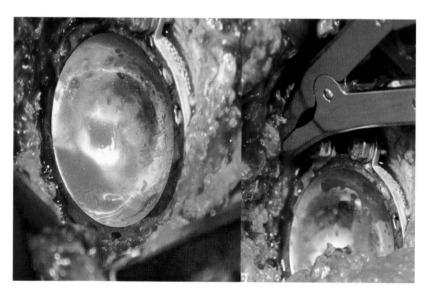

Fig. 21.39.

beyond the margin of the anterior acetabular component (Fig. 21.40).

In this patient, it can be seen that a very nice 2-mm rim of bone is protruding beyond the anterior metallic acetabular component wall. In the DDH patient, one can sometimes have a totally deficient anterior wall, and the anterior aspect of this component, or any other acetabular component, cannot be covered by bone. For this reason, it is sensible to have a smooth edge to the metallic acetabular component so that if psoas does rub on the cup in these circumstances, psoas irritation and damage does not occur. (See Chapter 6 to view the trouble one of my patients encountered having had a Durom resurfacing elsewhere. The acetabular component was left protruding from the anterior bony support, and he had 7 months of agony after his surgery with gross psoas irritation. Interestingly, after revision surgery, the pain from his psoas irritation disappeared instantly.)

More superiorly, one is attempting to remove bone but at the same time retaining bony cover over the anterior dysplasia screw (Fig. 21.41).

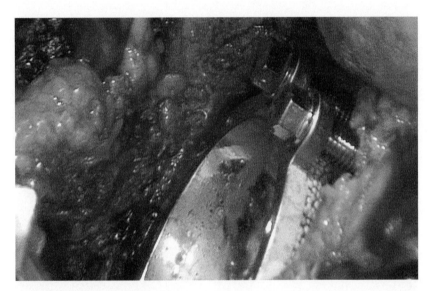

Fig. 21.40.

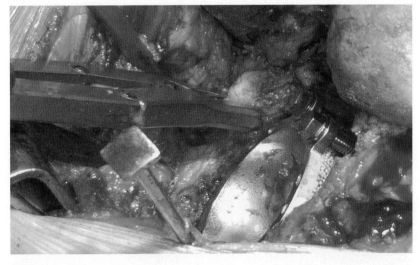

Fig. 21.41.

A final check for protruding osteophyte is made before moving onto the femoral component insertion.

The acetabular stage of this operation is finished for the moment, and one now proceeds to the femoral side of the operation either inserting a BHR, a BMHR (see Chapter 23), or a stemmed total hip replacement with a modular metal on metal bearing to match the inserted acetabular cup. It is not recommended to proceed with grafting the acetabular defect at this stage because of the risk of displacement of graft during the femoral procedure. Before finally leaving the acetabular component, we inject ropivacaine (Naropin), Adrenalin (epinephrine), and Toradol (ketorolac) (Fig. 21.42) (see chapter 16).

In this particular patient, the femoral head was too soft and too cystic to be able to carry out a BHR and instead a BMHR procedure was performed. The images from the femoral side of this man's hip arthroplasty are used in Chapter 23. When the femoral side procedure has been completed, a cover is placed over the prosthetic femoral head component, a hook placed around the neck so that the second assistant can displace the femoral head and neck anteriorly, and a Hohmann retractor is placed in the anterosuperior acetabulum to regain acetabular access (Fig. 21.43).

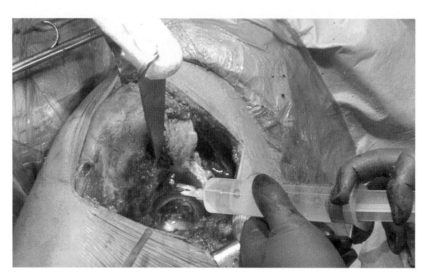

FIG. 21.42.

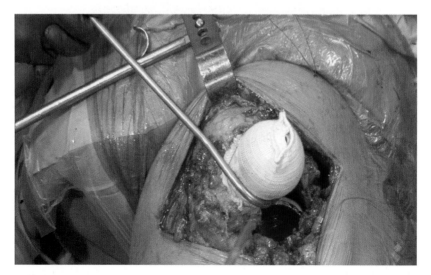

FIG. 21.43.

Having regained acetabular exposure, a final check is made that all soft tissue has been removed from the false acetabulum. It is a good idea at this stage to allow blood to well-up in the inferior aspect of the acetabular component (Fig. 21.44).

As will be seen later, Surgicel (Ethicon, Livingston, UK) is used to hold the morcellized acetabular graft in place, and blood is extremely useful to place on the Surgicel to make it sticky.

During the operation, all available bone graft is collected, and solid pieces of osteophyte are chipped-up by the scrub nurse for later grafting. Even with large acetabular defects, using the dysplasia cup, we have not had to resort to using allograft bone. The scrub nurse also ensures that any pieces of cartilage are removed from the acetabular reamings so that these too can be used for autograft (Fig. 21.45).

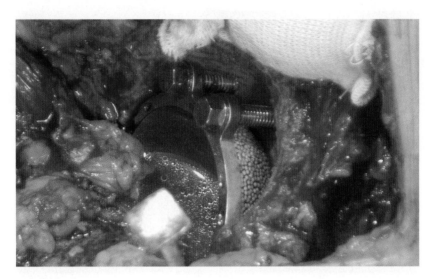

Fig. 21.44.

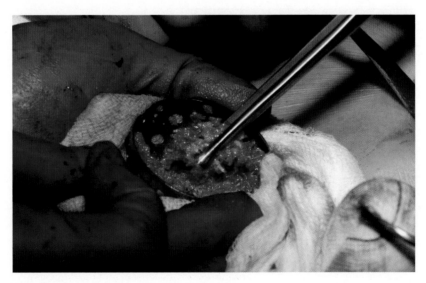

Fig. 21.45.

Packing of bone graft into the false acetabulum commences. As more graft is applied, it is impacted in position using a punch, a finger, or the special ends on the dedicated Innomed (Innomed Orthopaedic Instruments, Savannah, GA, USA) grafting forceps (Fig. 21.46).

This is a very easy bone grafting exercise, and when one compares this with the hard work of shaping and fixing a structural graft, life seems very comfortable for the resurfacing surgeon. Visitors often say to me that they regard this as a "Mickey Mouse" bone grafting exercise. Provided I am in a reasonable frame of mind, I remind them that the mechanical fixation of the acetabular component is achieved by the strong dysplasia screws. Compared with the mechanical support offered by a structural bone graft, these screws are in a different league. The morcellized autograft only has to encourage bone formation in the false acetabulum and has no mechanical support function in the early months. The biological activity from morcellized autograft is also in a different league to a dead piece of structural allograft. As can be seen in Chapter 25, my longest cohort of dysplasia cup patients out to 10 years follow-up have a zero cup failure rate.

Autografting proceeds (Fig. 21.47).

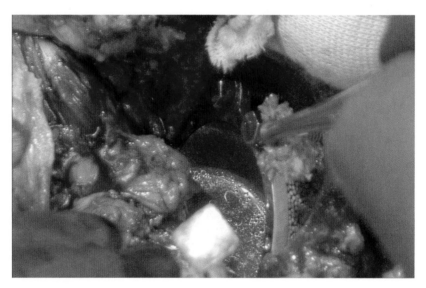

Fig. 21.46.

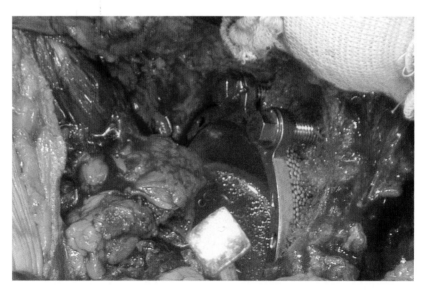

Fig. 21.47.

The false acetabulum is slowly filled with morcellized autograft and impacted thoroughly at each stage (Fig. 21.48). With large acetabular defects and when performing a resurfacing femoral component, we have resorted to grinding up the femoral head offcuts. Again, I have had the visitors object to this, but I question them as to how this differs fundamentally to grinding up an allograft fem- oral head. Furthermore, in my situation we are using the patient's own bone with a reduction in the overall cost of the procedure and also a reduction in the risks of transmitted disease.

In this patient, we ran short of acetabular reamings and now morcellized osteophyte is being used to fill the false acetabular defect (Fig. 21.49).

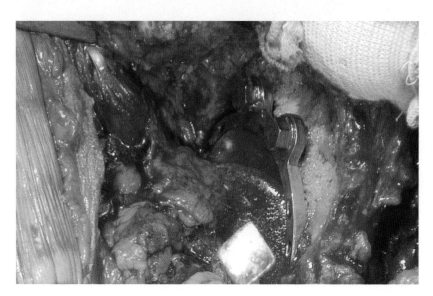

Fig. 21.48.

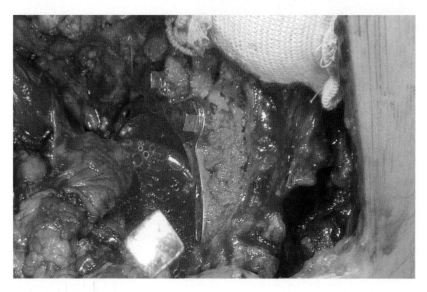

Fig. 21.49.

Finally, some good-quality acetabular reamings are applied as the most superficial layer of graft and thoroughly impacted with a punch and finger pressure (Fig. 21.50).

Surgicel is then placed over the graft. This will not stick in position unless blood is applied to the Surgicel, so the surgeon then dips his finger in the welled-up blood in the acetabular component, transferring this to the surface of the Surgicel, which then turns to a black color and becomes adherent to the bone graft (Fig. 21.51).

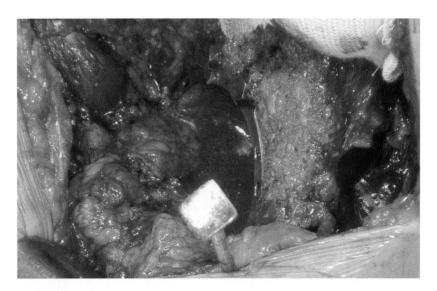

Fig. 21.50.

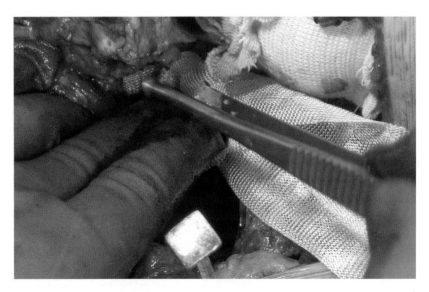

Fig. 21.51.

Surgicel can now be seen to cover all of the grafted, false acetabulum.

A PDS (Ethicon, Livingston, UK) suture is now inserted through the posterosuperior wormhole in the acetabular cup edge (Fig. 21.52).

The suture is placed through soft tissue above the false acetabulum and the knot tied holding the Surgicel in position.

It is important to remove the retractors carefully and displace the retracted femoral head component so that the Surgicel and the bone graft are not disturbed.

The acetabular part of the reconstruction is now complete, and reduction of the femoral head component into the acetabulum occurs (Fig. 21.53).

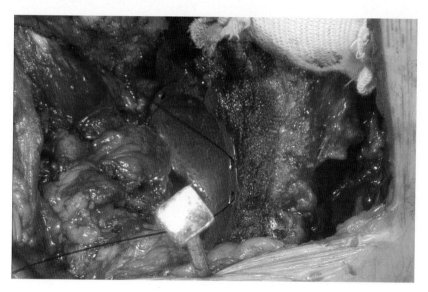

FIG. 21.52.

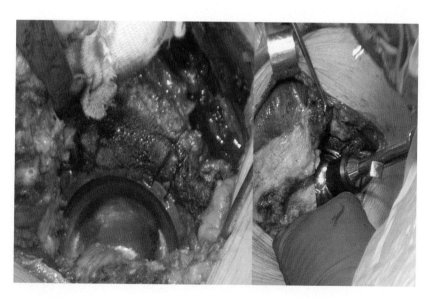

FIG. 21.53.

22
Implantation of the Femoral Component of the Birmingham Hip Resurfacing

Derek J.W. McMinn

Exposure for hip resurfacing is very much like the exposure one would make for revision of an acetabular component leaving the femoral component *in situ*. Hip surgeons will therefore not find the exposure particularly difficult in order to perform a Birmingham Hip Resurfacing (BHR). The acetabular component of the BHR is very similar to many other cementless acetabular components. Today, many surgeons are used to inserting cementless total hip shells without screws and therefore the acetabular component of the BHR is not a particular challenge for them. The femoral component of the BHR, however, is different from other procedures in hip surgery. It does take some training and some time in order to master this technique. To get sufficient exposure of the femoral head and neck to do this part of the operation, it is a requirement that all the steps in the surgical exposure are followed (see Chapter 19). If one is using a short incision, then the first assistant must assist the surgeon by moving the hip around to gain exposure of whatever particular aspect

of the femoral preparation is being performed. I now exclusively use the short-arm jig (Chapter 24) to facilitate correct guide-wire positioning, and although I have used a number of pin-less jigs in the past, I have not found these reliable. It is important to have templated the patient's x-ray prior to beginning the surgery (see Chapters 17 and 18).

In order to obtain the correct varus-valgus alignment of the femoral component, the templated distance from the tip of the lesser trochanter to the desired point on the intertrochanteric crest must now be transferred from the x-ray measurement into the operative field. In order to assist with this maneuver, a modified ruler has been made with the L extension abutting onto the lesser trochanter tip. I find it useful to mark the templated distance on the ruler part of this instrument so that no reading errors are made at surgery. It is important that the long arm of the L lies along the intertrochanteric crest and not at an angle to it. When the pin insertion point has been identified, this is marked using electrocautery (Fig. 22.1).

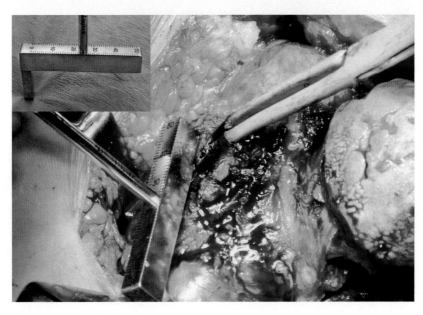

FIG. 22.1.

The guide pin is now placed through the short-arm jig aperture, and the pin is inserted into the previously marked point on the intertrochanteric crest. It is important that the guide pin and thus the jig are at right angles to the intertrochanteric crest and not angled either superiorly or inferiorly (Fig. 22.2). The guide pin now has a quick coupling attachment that makes connection and disconnection from the power unit easier for the surgeon.

The scrub nurse should hand the short-arm jig to the surgeon with all the locking nuts tightened so that parts of the jig do not fall onto the floor. When the guide pin has been inserted, then the two locking nuts (arrows, Fig. 22.3) should be released and the cannulated bar placed against the femoral head. The stylus is moved so that this touches on the femoral neck.

There are many ways of putting this jig together incorrectly, and these are detailed in Chapter 24. A configuration that renders the instrument unusable is annoying, but dropping part of the instrument on the floor is even more annoying. Practice with this instrument on dry bones and cadaveric workshops is a worthwhile exercise.

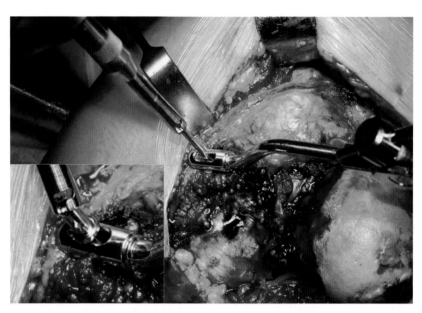

FIG. 22.2.

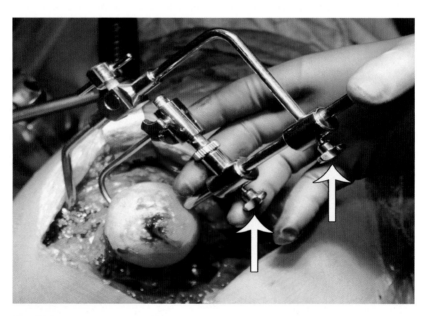

FIG. 22.3.

Having inserted the guide pin in the correct position, the varus-valgus alignment is now set. The surgeon does not have to worry any longer about varus-valgus alignment, and now attention is turned to obtaining the ideal lateral plane alignment. The release mechanism is now undone in the arm of the jig (arrow, Fig. 22.4) so that the correct lateral plane alignment can be achieved.

The biggest problem that surgeons have in the early stages with this jig is the "14 moving parts syndrome." The surgeon's grip on the instrument should be noted so that all parts of the instrument are under control. Again, practice in the dry bones situation is very helpful.

I find it useful to have the first assistant place a pick-up forceps on the front and back of the femoral neck to facilitate an estimation of the midlateral axis. In the situation shown (Fig. 22.5A), the lateral plane alignment is incorrect. If a guide wire was inserted in this position, then this would risk exit from the anterior aspect of the femoral neck. Similarly, the lateral plane alignment in Fig. 22.5B is also incorrect. If the guide wire was placed in this position, then this would risk exit from the posterior aspect of the femoral neck.

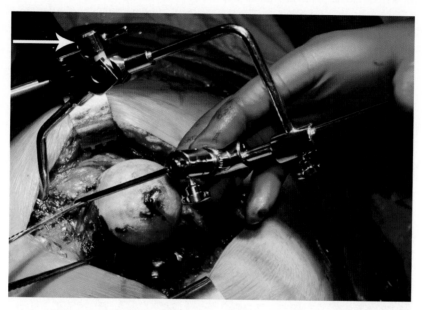

Fig. 22.4.

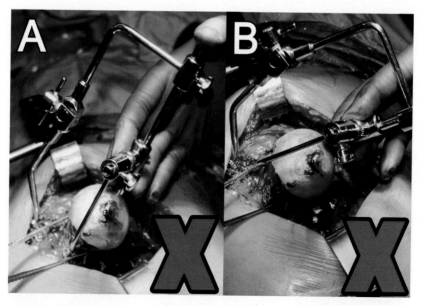

Fig. 22.5.

The correct lateral plane alignment is somewhere between these two extremes, and Fig. 22.6 shows a satisfactory lateral plane alignment, and with this alignment the guide wire should go down the center of the femoral neck when viewed in the lateral plane.

The first assistant is in the best place to judge when exactly the correct lateral plane alignment has been achieved. The surgeon can get a poor assessment of lateral plane alignment when viewing from his normal position. However, he can lean over and view the medial femoral neck or, if he has short legs like the author, he can walk around to the end of the operating table to judge exactly when the perfect lateral plane alignment has been achieved.

Surgeons ask me if an x-ray is necessary. With a guide wire in the femoral neck, the x-ray has the same deficiency as the surgeon, and if the femoral neck is not viewed exactly at right angles to its medial side, then a false impression of guide-wire position will be obtained.

When a satisfactory lateral plane alignment has been achieved, then the hinge of the jig is locked (Fig. 22.7).

By the previous maneuvers, correct varus-valgus alignment and correct lateral plane alignment of the guide wire and thus the component will be achieved. Now the ideal entry point for the guide wire must be ascertained. The following are the requirements for ideal guide wire positioning:

1. The stylus tip should pass comfortably around the femoral neck without touching the femoral neck at any point. This will ensure that when the cutter instruments are used, the femoral neck is not notched.

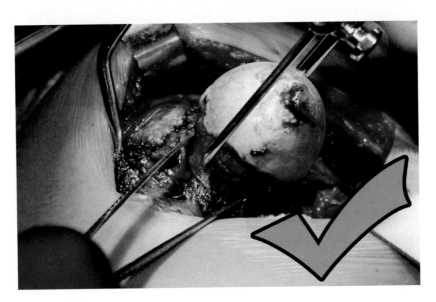

Fig. 22.6.

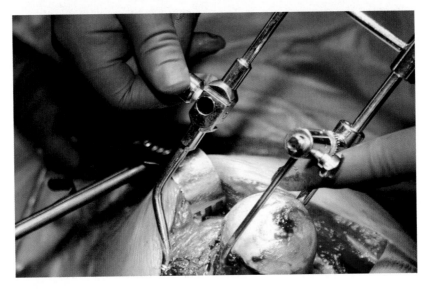

Fig. 22.7.

2. The anterosuperior head-neck offset after BHR component insertion should be maximized. This means that the anterosuperior offset after BHR should approximate to the normal head-neck anterosuperior offset. Furthermore when minor slipped capital femoral epiphysis (SCFE) morphology exists, it is the aim that after the BHR femoral head component insertion, the anterosuperior head-neck offset is improved upon the preoperative situation.

3. The stylus should touch the periphery of the femoral head all the way round. It is common and normal when preparing the femoral head for resurfacing to take very little bone off the periphery of the femoral head anterosuperiorly and much more bone off the femoral head posteroinferiorly. In severe SCFE, it is not possible for the stylus to clear the femoral neck all the way around and at the same time for the stylus to make contact with the periphery of the femoral head anterosuperiorly. This gap between the stylus and the anterosuperior head in severe SCFE would mean poor support for the femoral component and poor pressurization

for the cement. In this situation, it is now my practice to abandon the BHR at this stage and instead perform a BMHR (see chapter 23). However, in the vast majority of arthritic hips, a satisfactory guide-wire position can be achieved. To pick the ideal entry point, the surgeon starts by passing the stylus around the femoral neck (Fig. 22.8).

At the beginning of their experience, surgeons seem content when the stylus passes around the femoral neck without touching it. However, with more experience it will soon be realized that a much better job can be done with an even more accurate insertion point of the guide wire. The goal is to move the cannulated bar in an anterosuperior direction, millimeter by millimeter, all the while using the stylus tip to gauge how much anterosuperior offset one is achieving. The maximum movement of the cannulated rod in an anterosuperior direction is limited (1) when the stylus tip touches the posteroinferior femoral neck and (2) when the stylus tip starts to lose contact with the periphery of the femoral head anterosuperiorly (Fig. 22.9).

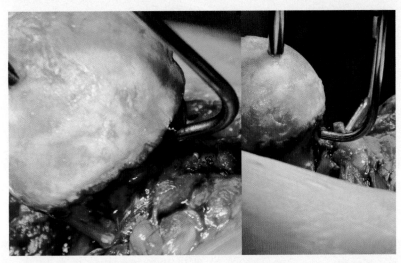

FIG. 22.8.

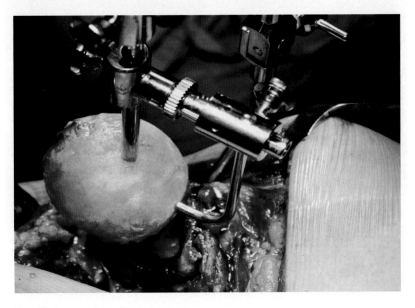

FIG. 22.9.

When the ideal entry point for the guide wire has been located, then the teeth on the cannulated bar are tapped into the superior femoral head and the guide wire is inserted (Fig. 22.10).

When the teeth on the cannulated bar are tapped into eburnated bone, then longitudinal pressure by the surgeons left finger and thumb on the cannulated bar hold a good position during guide-wire insertion. Trouble can arise if cartilage is present in this area of the femoral head. Even more trouble can occur if there is a loose osteochondral

fragment in avascular necrosis. It is often useful in these circumstances to remove the cartilage or an osteochondral flap with a saw or rongeur before attempting to tap the teeth of the guide bar into bone. This should be done before finalizing the jig position.

The cannulated bar is removed. This releases the couplings on the instrument to enable jig removal. The guide pin is removed, and the main body of the short-arm jig is then removed also (Fig. 22.11).

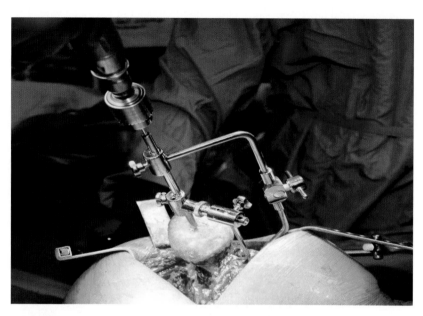

Fig. 22.10.

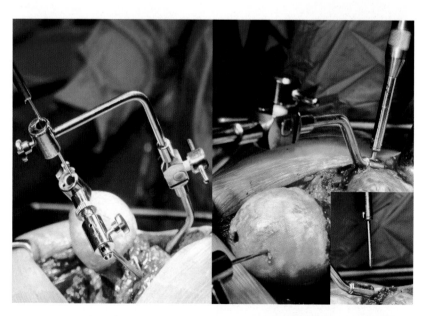

Fig. 22.11.

Now it is very important to check the final guide-wire position by reinsertion of the cannulated bar through the stylus part of the instrument. The surgeon then needs to pass the stylus tip around the femoral neck and touch on the periphery of the femoral head to ensure that he is entirely happy with the guide-wire position (Fig. 22.12). The stylus should not touch the femoral neck in any position, and the stylus should touch the periphery of the femoral head through 360 degrees.

These are the minimum requirements for guide-wire position, and as has already been mentioned, the aim is to achieve good anterosuperior head neck offset.

If the surgeon is not entirely happy with the guide-wire position, then two alternatives exist. Either the guide wire can be removed and the whole process of jigging correctly is started again, or the guide-wire repositioning instrument can be used (Fig. 22.13).

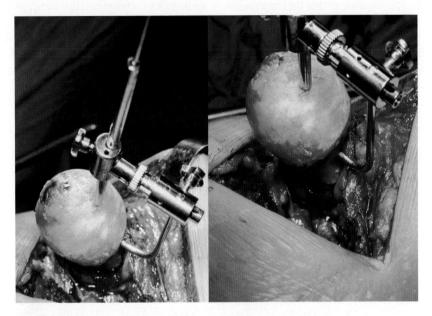

Fig. 22.12.

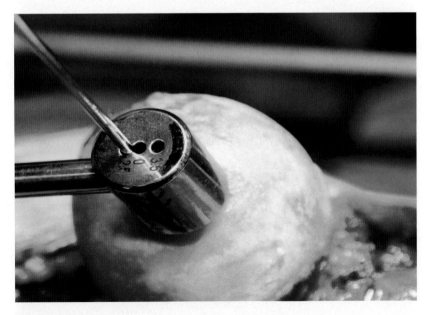

Fig. 22.13.

The efficiency of this instrument is governed by how inaccurately the initial guide wire was placed. If the guide-wire insertion point is several millimeters out, then this instrument is useful. However, the minimum distance that the guide wire can be moved is the thickness of the guide wire, and systems that use thicker guide wire than does the BHR will of necessity reposition the guide wire a greater distance from the center of the initial guide wire.

The next stage is for the assistant to retract the skin edge inferiorly with a Langenbeck-type retractor so that the surgeon can drill through the lesser trochanter into the canal of the femur. Drilling for only a few millimeters into the lesser trochanter is not satisfactory; the drilling must be carried right into the canal of the femur (Fig. 22.14). There is some scope for choosing the precise positioning of the cannula in the lesser trochanter.

This scope should be used to prevent side pressure from the skin edge causing kinking and damage to the cannula.

An arthroscopic irrigation cannula is placed through the drill hole in the lesser trochanter into the canal of the femur and attached by thick-walled tubing to a separate suction unit, which is set on maximum suction (Fig. 22.15). It is unsatisfactory to use cheap thin-walled irrigation tubing for suction because the tubing walls will collapse and sucking will cease. It is also important to turn the suction unit up to full suction (e.g., −600mm Hg). I always use a suction unit separate from the unit used at the surgery itself. When the suction is applied, if there is not an initial rush of blood through the tubing, then the surgeon knows that something is not working. It is of course pointless to go through the exercise of inserting a suction vent only to have it rendered useless.

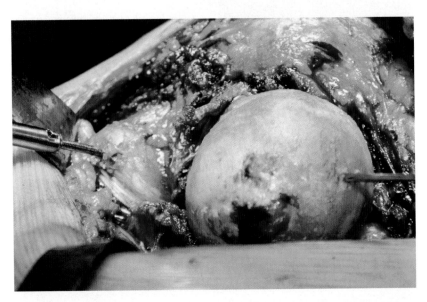

Fɪɢ. 22.14.

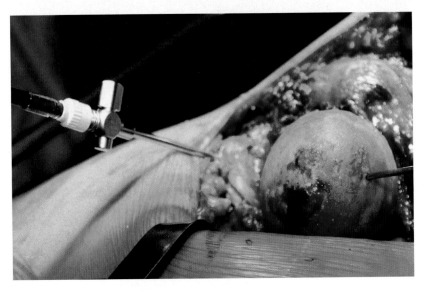

Fɪɢ. 22.15.

It is necessary to protect the soft tissues from being contaminated by bony reamings during the femoral preparation. I find it is satisfactory to use two swabs (sponges) with a complete swab being placed around the front of the femoral neck protecting the anterior soft tissues and a split swab being placed from the posterior direction and wrapped around the femoral neck base to protect the posterior superior and inferior soft tissues (Fig. 22.16).

It is very important that these swabs (sponges) are not caught up in the teeth of the cutting instruments. After placement of the swabs, I wet these with pulse lavage; this allows the swabs to be positioned away from the periphery of the femoral head (Fig. 22.17). As will be seen later, I use a head-neck template to further prevent swabs being caught in the cutter instruments.

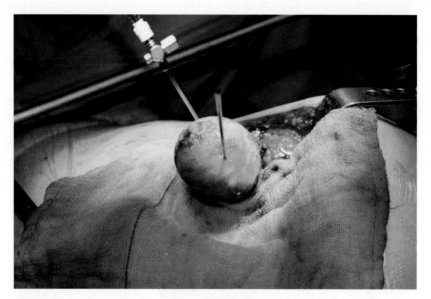

Fig. 22.16.

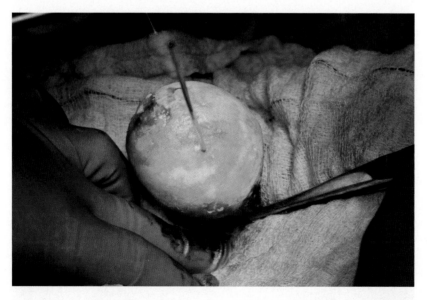

Fig. 22.17.

The guide wire is now overdrilled with the overdrilling instrument. This instrument should be used by drilling forwards and removing the drill repeatedly. At the same time, the second assistant irrigates the drill entry point (Fig. 22.18).

A guide bar is now placed in the drilled hole down the femoral head and neck (Fig. 22.19).

It is now too late to discover that the guide bar position is unsatisfactory, but this of course must be checked using the stylus as shown. The time to detect inaccuracy is at the guide-wire stage. If the guide wire is placed correctly, then the guide bar will be placed correctly, except in one circumstance. If there is sclerosis in the femoral head or neck for any reason (e.g., previous core decompression, previous pins in the femoral neck, etc.), then the sclerotic bone can deviate the guide wire. If there is any sclerosis on x-ray or a history of previous surgery, then great care must be taken at the guide-wire stage. What usually happens is that the guide wire goes in for a few centimeters perfectly well and then is deviated by hitting up against sclerotic bone. When it comes to the overdrilling stage, if the surgeon is careful, he should

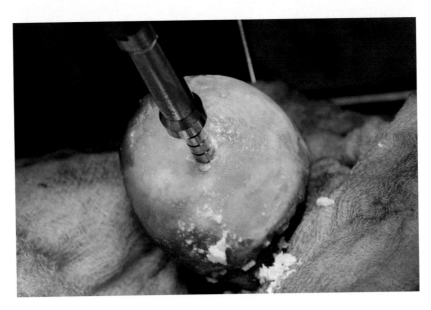

FIG. 22.18.

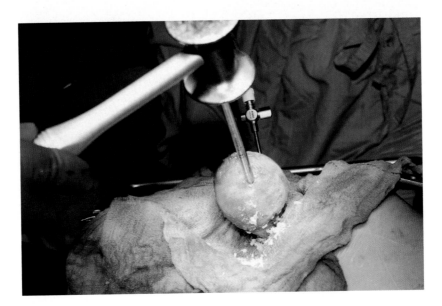

FIG. 22.19.

be able to detect by resistance when the alignment of the guide wire in the bone changes, and if this happens, then he should stop overdrilling and remove the guide wire. It is sometimes possible to use the few centimeters of track that has been drilled in the correct position to guide the more distal position of the drill freehand thus breaking through the sclerotic bone with the drill.

Correct positioning of the guide bar is confirmed using the stylus (Fig. 22.20).

When a satisfactory guide bar position has been confirmed, then the anti-notch device is inserted.

The stylus of the anti-notch device is advanced down the superior femoral neck to a safe position, where advancement of the peripheral cutter to that position will definitely not cause notching. At this position, an appropriate thickness of anti-notch plastic spacer is selected.

The anti-notch plastic spacer is placed over the guide bar onto the top of the femoral head, and this ensures that shoot-through of the peripheral cutter cannot occur (Fig. 22.21).

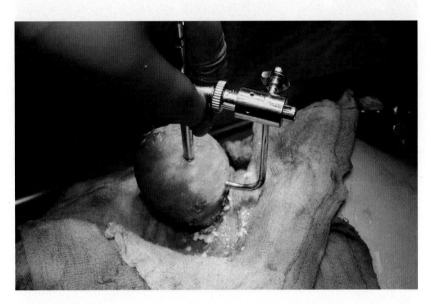

FIG. 22.20.

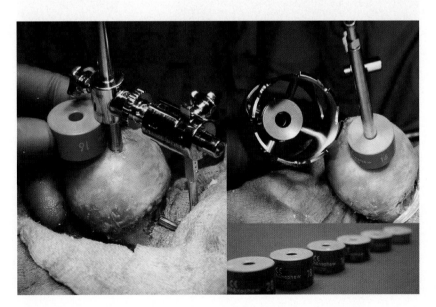

FIG. 22.21.

The peripheral femoral head cutter is then advanced on the ream setting until its advancement is halted by internal engagement of the anti-notch plastic spacer. During this peripheral cutting, I prefer to place a head-neck template on the femoral neck (which before the advent of the anti-notch device was our only protection against shoot-through and notching), but now I use it to retract the swabs (sponges) away from the femoral neck and prevent snarl up of the swabs in the teeth of the cutting instrument (Fig. 22.22).

If the peripheral cut is not complete and superior femoral neck safety is ensured, then the next thickness down of anti-notch spacer device is selected and the peripheral cutter advanced again (Fig. 22.23). If osteophyte is present at the medial head-neck junction and further advancement of the peripheral cutter cannot be safely achieved without risking superior femoral neck notching, then the medial intact bone is divided by placing a reciprocator saw blade down the saw track medially. Note that very little bone is being resected anterosuperiorly.

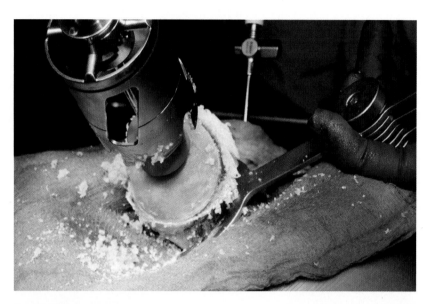

Fig. 22.22.

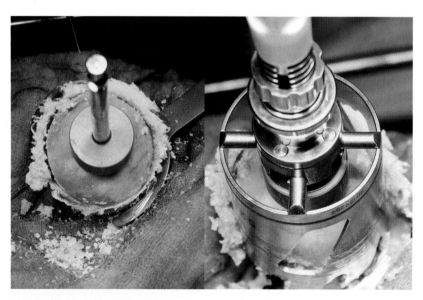

Fig. 22.23.

At this stage, the peripheral cut on the femoral head is almost complete (Fig. 22.24). This is tested by insertion of a periosteal elevator in the cut track. If the peripheral bone will easily crack off, then no further peripheral cutting is required. However, if the peripheral bone is still firmly attached, then further peripheral cutting is required.

The peripheral femoral head bone is now weakly attached. The peripheral ring of bone is cracked off using a periosteal elevator (Fig. 22.25A). Note that the resected thickness of

anterosuperior femoral head bone is much less than the thickness of the posteroinferior femoral head bone.

When the inferior and posteroinferior peripheral femoral bone is cracked off, this remains attached by soft tissue that has been carefully preserved on the surface of the femoral neck. This bone must not be pulled off. Instead, the connection between the peripheral femoral head bone and soft tissue should be released by sharp dissection, so that the minimum disturbance of soft tissue on the femoral neck occurs (Fig. 22.25B).

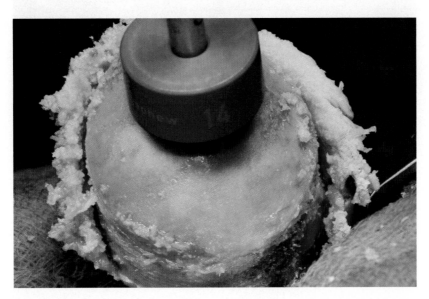

Fig. 22.24.

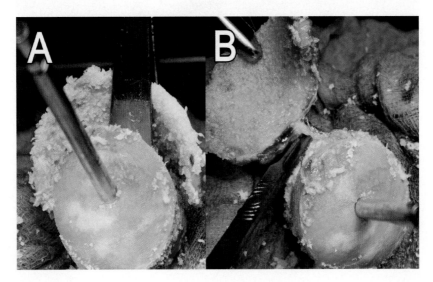

Fig. 22.25.

It is a mistake to grasp the detached peripheral femoral head ring with a rongeur and pull. This will strip a large amount of soft tissue from the bone on the medial side of the femoral neck destroying many retinacular vessels.

The surgeon then goes around the femoral head-neck junction with rongeur removing any protruding osteophyte (Fig. 22.26).

There are two ways to resect the summit of the femoral head. The first way is to use a method that I have used for the past 16½ years, and this employs a napkin ring. The medial cortical femoral head-neck junction is identified and marked with dissecting forceps. The inferior margin of the napkin ring is advanced to this point, and the locating nut is tightened (Fig. 22.27).

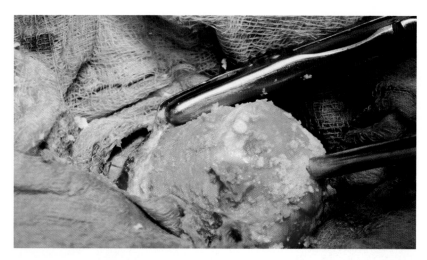

FIG. 22.26.

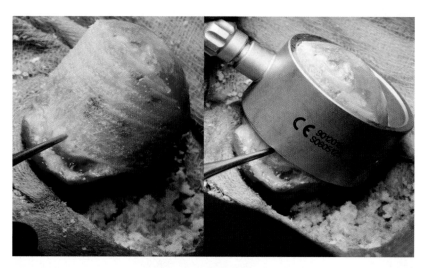

FIG. 22.27.

The summit of the femoral head is then resected using a reciprocating saw (Fig. 22.28A).

A final check is made with the head-neck template to ensure that the correct resection level has been achieved. If more bone needs removal, this is done with the face cutter instrument (Fig. 22.28B).

A more satisfactory method of performing this summit resection is shown in another patient. The head-neck template is advanced to the medial head-neck junction, and a mark is made at zero on the measurement scale of this instrument.

A face cutter instrument is then used to carefully resect the summit of the femoral head down to the marked point.

The demonstration in Fig. 22.29 is meant to show that resecting the summit of the head using either of the techniques gives the same outcome. Here, the summit has been partially resected using the napkin method and the saw blade is left in position for demonstration purposes. The head-neck template, zero mark, exactly coincides with the line of resection guided by the napkin ring. On the whole, the newer method with the face cutter is preferable as it guarantees that the resected bone is at right angles to the guide bar.

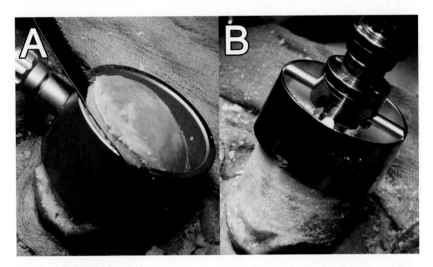

Fig. 22.28.

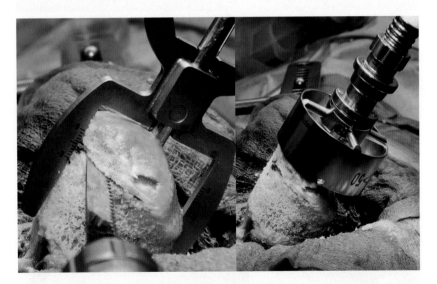

Fig. 22.29.

In a normal osteoarthritic hip, it is common to see an anterosuperior defect on the femoral head at the completion of summit head resection (Fig. 22.30A).

The chamfer cutter is then used over the guide bar until this instrument is fully seated. There is an internal stop in this instrument, and it is not possible to overresect bone with this chamfer cutter (Fig. 22.30B). The chamfer cutters on the old Midland Medical Technologies (MMT) instruments were not nearly so satisfactory as the new instruments. With the old instruments, the chamfer cutter tended to catch particularly in the junction between soft bone and hard bone. This could be overcome by performing chamfer cutting on the drill setting of the power unit and using very light touch to perform the chamfering in the method of wood planing. It was also necessary to use frequent irrigation. The new chamfer cutters are so sharp that they do not seem to catch in the junctional area between soft bone and hard bone and therefore can be used on either the ream or the drill setting of the power unit.

At the completion of chamfer cutting, the anterosuperior defect that was present at the end of the summit resection has now disappeared (Fig. 22.31A). This is the beauty of a chamfered cylinder design, first used by Sir John Charnley in the 1950s.

It can be seen that a cyst is being curetted at this stage (Fig. 22.31B).

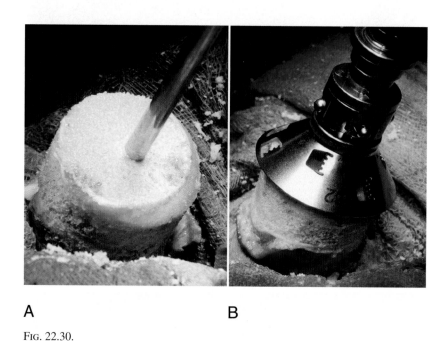

A   B

FIG. 22.30.

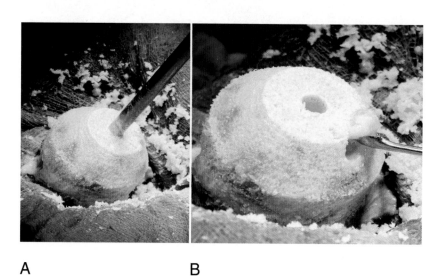

A   B

FIG. 22.31.

Keyholes are now drilled in the periphery of the femoral head but only drilled to the full depth in the region of the chamfer. This is the exact method of keyhole drilling that I have used on all my cemented femoral components since 1992 (Fig. 22.32).

I initially decided to make these keyholes for cement, first to assist with fixation, but the depth of the drill was chosen so that the cement plug tips would enter embryonic metaphyseal bone. If one was unlucky enough to get a small area of segmental avascular necrosis in embryonic epiphyseal bone, this would be underpinned by the cement plugs thus giving some protection against femoral loosening and/or femoral head collapse.

On the resected summit of the head, I only use the tip of the drill to break up the sclerotic surface of hard bone (Fig. 22.33).

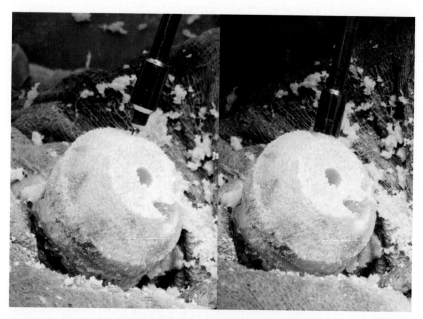

Fig. 22.32.

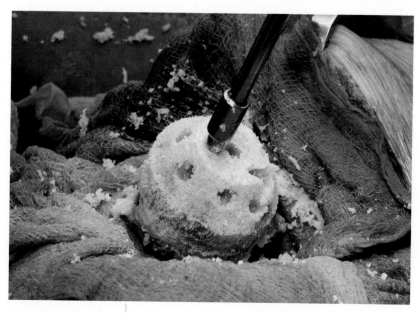

Fig. 22.33.

All loose bone is curetted from the head; any soft tissue or cysts are also cleared. I am often asked what I do about cysts in the femoral head. If the cysts are on the chamfered surface or the resected summit surface, then I merely curette the soft tissue from the cysts and allow these to fill with cement (Fig. 22.34). If cysts are present on the parallel sides of the prepared femoral head, then these in former years were curetted and autografted. Nowadays, I find myself accepting cysts in this area less and less, and I tend to move on and do a BMHR prosthesis (see Chapter 23).

The position in which the first assistant keeps the leg should be noted (Fig. 22.35). This gives satisfactory exposure of the femoral head and neck for the femoral side of the resurfacing operation. If the femoral head is stuck down in the wound and not delivered in a satisfactory manner, this can make life very difficult for the surgeon. The conditions that lead to this unsatisfactory state of affairs are (1) inadequate soft tissue release by the surgeon or (2) the conscious state of the assistant.

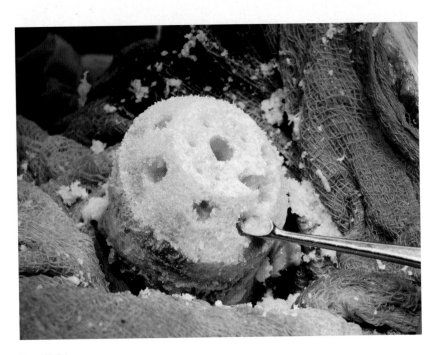

Fɪɢ. 22.34.

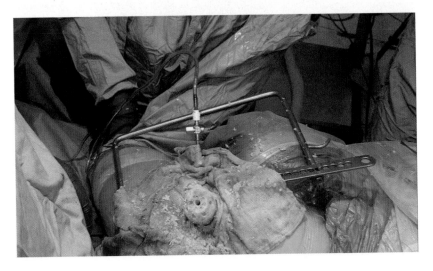

Fɪɢ. 22.35.

At this stage, the central hole in the femoral head and neck is enlarged from a parallel-sided hole to a taper by the use of a taper drill. I did not formerly perform this maneuver routinely, but now I do (Fig. 22.36).

Press-fitting the tapered stem of the BHR femoral component into a parallel-sided drill hole is perfectly satisfactory in normal bone. However, in sclerotic bone, the press fit is very tight and can cause incomplete seating of the femoral component with a requirement for heavy hammering. In order to prevent these difficulties, I now convert the parallel-sided drill hole in the femoral head and neck into a tapered drill hole in all cases. I wish to acknowledge that the work of my colleague Mr. Peter Howard,

FRCS, led to the introduction of the tapered drill as a standard feature in the BHR instrument set. I still get surgeons asking me why they cannot fully seat the femoral component of the BHR. The possibilities include (a) the summit resection being at an angle, preventing full seating of the femoral component, (b) the mark at the medial head-neck junction having been made in the wrong place, (c) the cement having been mixed for more than 1 minute before component insertion, (d) wrong cement being used, (e) vacuum mixing being used, or (f) taper drilling not being done.

The cancellous bone of the femoral head is opened up with pulse lavage (Fig. 22.37A). Brushing the femoral head is also used to open up the cancellous network (Fig. 22.37B).

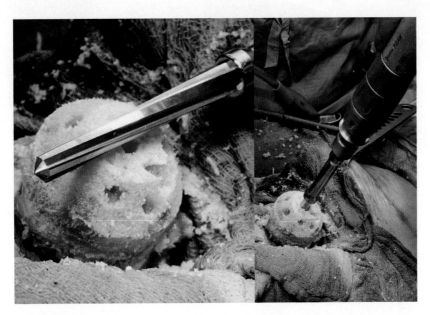

FIG. 22.36.

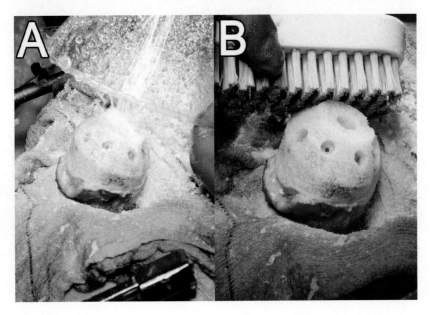

FIG. 22.37.

The guide bar is inserted and the head-neck template reapplied. A mark is made at the femoral head-neck junction so that the surgeon knows exactly where the femoral component must be advanced to (Fig. 22.38).

In former years, we had to insert a suction device down this central hole in the femoral head and neck to keep the femoral head free from blood at this stage, but the use of the suction vent through the lesser trochanter has greatly facilitated keeping the femoral head dry for cement fixation.

A sucker is in position down the femoral head and neck, the suction vent is sucking blood and keeping the femoral head dry, and final drying of the femoral head with a swab (sponge) is undertaken (Fig. 22.39).

The correct size of femoral component in its box is checked by the surgeon and then opened. The surgeon must check before the operating room staff open the box that the correct implant has been selected. In addition to the correct size of implant, which is marked on the box label, a color-coding

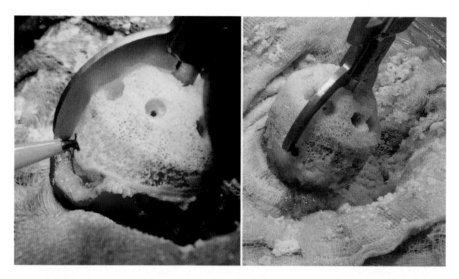

Fig. 22.38.

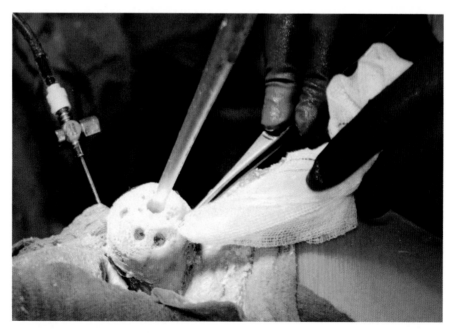

Fig. 22.39.

system is provided for those who are numerically challenged. The color surrounding the femoral component label on the box should be the same as the color surrounding the label on the box of the acetabular implant that has already been inserted (Fig. 22.40A).

When the femoral implant has been opened, the size of the component should be checked by the surgeon. This is laser marked on the femoral component stem (Fig. 22.40B).

History shows that packaging errors have occurred in orthopedics over many years, and this final check of implant size is sensible.

No vacuum mixing is used as this will remove monomer and increase viscosity in the cement early. Instead, traditional mixing in a bowl is used (Fig. 22.41).

The excellent work of Steve McMahon and Gabrielle Hawdon on cement technique for the BHR is presented in Chapter 7.

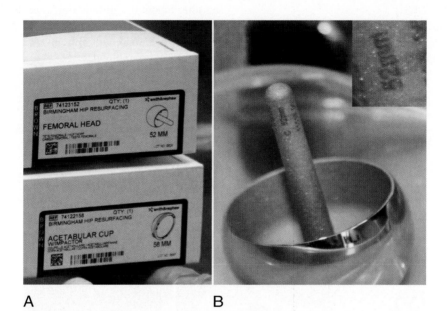

A   B

FIG. 22.40.

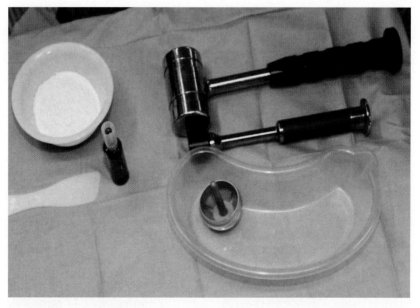

FIG. 22.41.

The antibiotic Simplex cement (Stryker Corporation, Kalamazoo, MI, USA) is mixed in a normal mixing bowl, and the scrub nurse is asked not to dither and waste time. When the liquid cement hits the powder, the second clock in the operating room is started. As soon as the cement goes fluid, the surgeon should draw up cement into a bladder syringe as this is the easiest, non-messy way of transferring liquid cement into the femoral component (Fig. 22.42A).

The femoral head is filled one-third full with antibiotic Simplex cement (Fig. 22.42B).

The femoral component is tipped so that the cement pours onto all the femoral fixation surfaces (Fig. 22.43). It is remarkable how well liquid cement adheres to the matt surfaces on the internal face of the femoral component. If the operating room protocol at your hospital calls for the use of vacuum mixing, it is wise to stand on the vacuum tube during mixing of the antibiotic Simplex cement for the BHR procedure. Surgeons usually find this easier than having to go through endless committees wasting their time getting permission not to use suction mixing for the cement. I first discovered the problem with vacuum mixing by accident when performing a demonstration operation at another hospital. I did not object to the use of their vacuum mixing because I didn't know better. The cement viscosity at 1 minute was high, and difficulty was encountered inserting the femoral component.

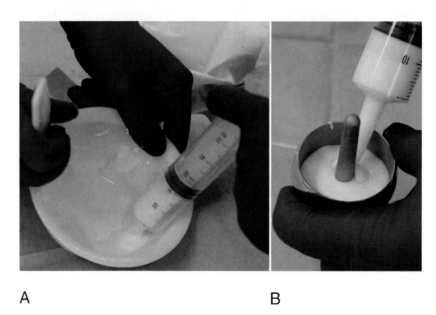

A   B

Fɪɢ. 22.42.

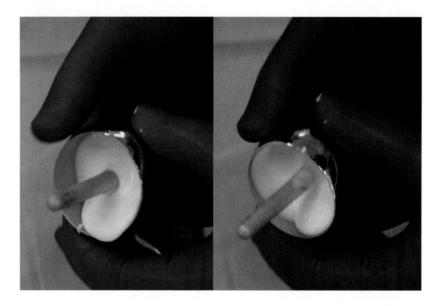

Fɪɢ. 22.43.

At precisely 1 minute from mixing, the femoral component is inserted onto the femur (Fig. 22.44).

The femoral head pusher is pushed hard on the femoral head, and this is tapped lightly with a hammer. This causes the femoral component to advance with each tap of the hammer. It is advisable not to fully insert the component at one go as this will overwhelm the suction vent and result in fat and marrow being driven through the femoral neck cortex from endosteal to outside. This is bound to cause embolization of small vessels in the femoral head and neck and may be one of the causes of femoral neck thinning and femoral neck fracture.

Instead after insertion of the femoral component about half way, I prefer to curette away cement from the periphery of the femoral component and establish by visualization how much further the femoral head has to be inserted (Fig. 22.45).

When the periphery of the femoral head reaches the mark at the femoral head-neck junction, then the femoral component is fully seated and no further hammering of the femoral component should be done. However, detail is very important. The surgeon should establish with the head-neck template, before the femoral component is inserted, exactly where on the mark the femoral component has to go to (e.g., does it need to go to the top of the mark, halfway point of the mark, or does it need to fully cover the mark). There is often a difference of 3 mm between the top and bottom of a mark made by an operating room sterile marker, and once the femoral component has bottomed out, no further advancement of the femoral component will occur. Attempts to advance the femoral component further will only lead to damage. One of the most potent reasons for the femoral component not reaching the mark is that the mark is in the wrong place!

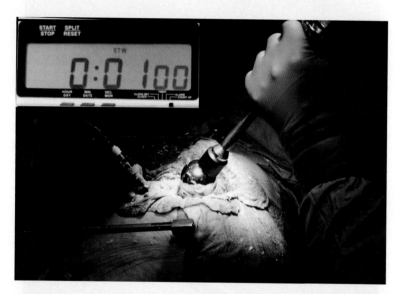

FIG. 22.44.

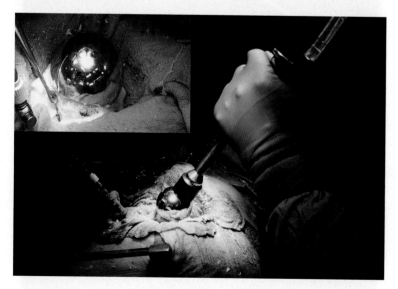

FIG. 22.45.

During the insertion of the femoral component, fat and marrow will continue to pour from the suction vent (Fig. 22.46).

Final curetting of cement at the component edge is undertaken (Fig. 22.47).

The protecting swabs around the femoral neck are carefully peeled away taking with them the bone and cement debris from the femoral head preparation and insertion part of the operation (Fig. 22.48). If protective swabs are

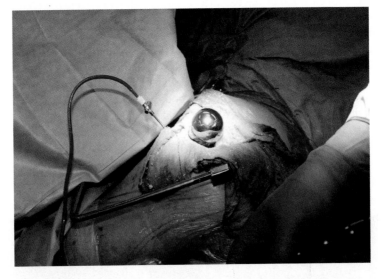

FIG. 22.46.

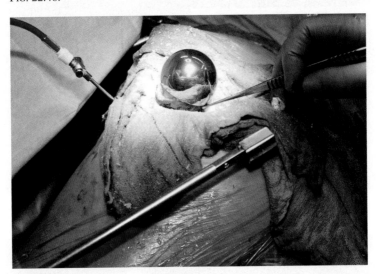

FIG. 22.47.

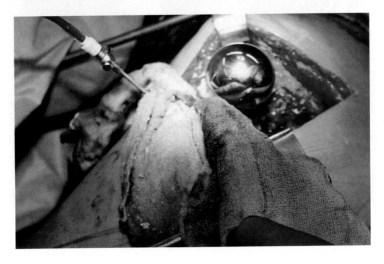

FIG. 22.48.

not used during the operation, then bone reamings are scattered into the soft tissues. It is very difficult to remove these bone reamings completely by lavage or any other technique. A better policy is to prevent such contamination of the soft tissues in the first place.

All cement debris is carefully curetted away from the periphery of the femoral component. A rongeur is used to remove any protruding osteophyte at the head-neck junction, but only protruding osteophyte that is likely to impinge should be removed. Care must be taken not to tear soft tissue off the femoral neck (Fig. 22.49).

A saline-soaked swab is placed over the femoral head and neck, and displaced fat and marrow in the femur is washed out through the suction vent (Fig. 22.50).

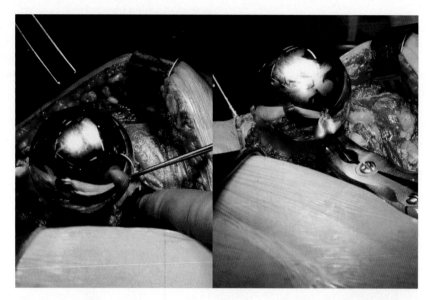

Fig. 22.49.

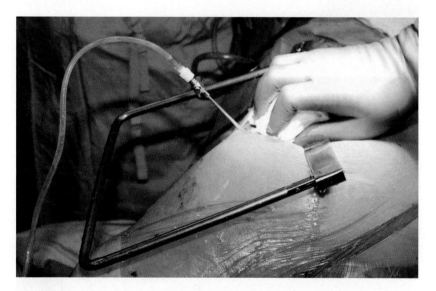

Fig. 22.50.

I started to use this suction vent about 9 years ago. The objectives were as follows: I wished to keep the intramedullary pressure down during femoral component insertion. The aims were first to reduce local embolization of blood vessels that supplied the femoral head and neck. Second, I wanted to reduce systemic fat embolization. A further objective was to flush the area with cool saline keeping the bone temperature down at the time of cement curing. A still further objective was to remove monomer from the curing bone cement, thus reducing monomer dissemination systemically.

At this stage, the wound is irrigated with pulsed lavage. The aim of this is to reduce any debris in the soft tissues to a minimum and to reduce the local bacteria count. It will be noticed when this procedure is performed that fluid at this stage also is sucked in through the femoral neck and irrigates out through the suction vent. At the completion of this stage, the cannula in the lesser trochanter is removed (Fig. 22.51). The cannula wall should be checked carefully because if significant side bending from the wound edge has occurred, then the cannula can become kinked and should not be reused. I have not had a cannula tip break off in the lesser trochanter, but I have had a cannula tip break off in the ilium when I used to vent the pelvis also. The bleeding from the pelvic vent was so severe that I stopped using this technique.

The soft tissue from the superior aspect of the acetabulum is retracted with a Langenbeck-type retractor, and the acetabular component is thoroughly cleaned with pulsed lavage. At the completion of this procedure, a thorough check is made to ensure that no bone, cement, or other debris lie within the acetabular component. The acetabular component is then filled with saline (Fig. 22.52).

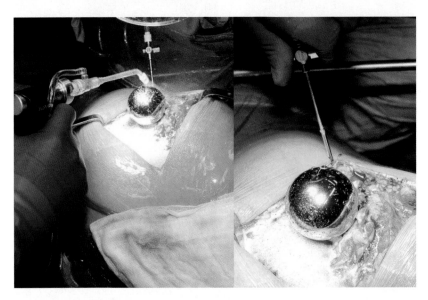

FIG. 22.51.

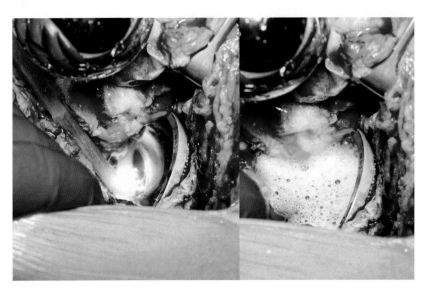

FIG. 22.52.

The first assistant places traction on the leg, and the femoral head component is reduced into the acetabulum, without scratching the femoral head on the edge of the acetabular component as reduction occurs (Fig. 22.53). Usually, the exit of fluid from the acetabular component upon femoral head reduction brings soft tissue out of the acetabulum and prevents entrapment of soft tissue between the head and cup. This is then checked visually and by palpation.

Tests of leg length, stability, range of movement, and impingement are carried out. Leg length assessments are important in DDH where the acetabular component is being brought down into a normal position and the leg lengthened at the acetabular part of the operation. Leg length is also important to assess in femoral conditions such as Perthes disease where the femoral head-neck complex is being

lengthened deliberately. However, in routine osteoarthritic cases, I do not carry out leg length assessment intraoperatively, as it is very difficult to inadvertently lengthen the leg with the resurfacing procedure. If lengthening of the leg after a resurfacing does occur, major errors have occurred on either the acetabular or femoral side of the procedure or both!

Impingement is important in DDH because with femoral neck anteversion, bony impingement can occur between the lesser trochanter region and the ischium in external rotation and extension. This is checked for by inserting a finger between the lesser trochanter and ischium and fully externally rotating the hip (Fig. 22.54).

Impingement can also occur in SUFE-type morphology where the anterior femoral head-neck offset has not

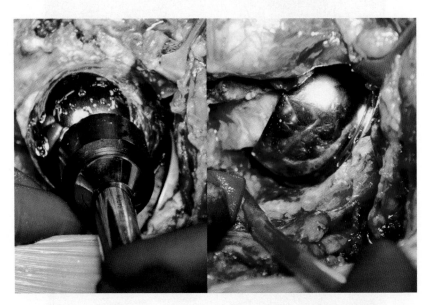

FIG. 22.53.

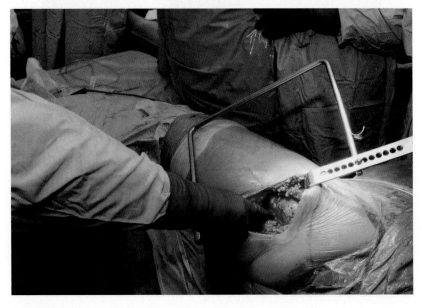

FIG. 22.54.

been correctly restored. This anterior impingement is being checked for in Fig. 22.55 and Fig. 22.56. The surgeon places a finger inside the capsule between the edge of the acetabular component and the anterior femoral neck, the hip is flexed, and then flexed and internally rotated to check for impingement. A squeal from the surgeon indicates impingement. It is claimed that navigation is a less painful way of detecting impingement.

Stability is not usually a problem with hip resurfacing. If instability with flexion and internal rotation occurs after hip resurfacing in the absence of impingement, the usual cause is impingement between the patient's thigh and the anterior pelvic support (Fig. 22.57).

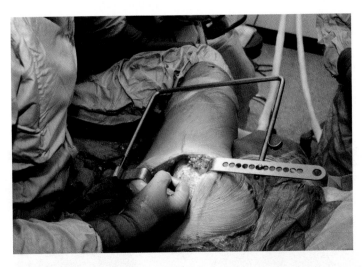

FIG. 22.55.

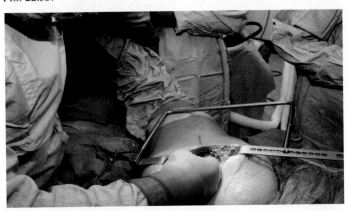

FIG. 22.56.

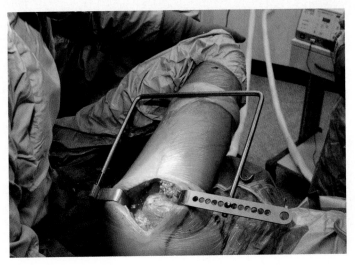

FIG. 22.57.

At the completion of reduction, the second dose of ropi-vacaine (Naropin), Adrenalin (epinephrine), and Toradol (ketorolac) (see Chapter 16) is injected into the posterior capsule, external rotators, and posterior soft tissue on the femur. An attempt is made not to allow local anesthetic fluid to flow around the sciatic nerve as this can lead to a sciatic nerve block and worry for the surgeon for the next 12 hours until the block wears off. The abductors and gluteus maximus muscle fibers are also infiltrated through their exposed surfaces (Fig. 22.58).

Closure

The first two or three stitches are easy, with a good bite being obtained into the junctional area between the abductors and the greater trochanter, and the external rotators and capsule can easily be picked up (Fig. 22.59).

At the tip of the greater trochanter, the needle is inserted from superficial to deep through the posterior corner of the tendon of gluteus medius. The piriformis tendon and the

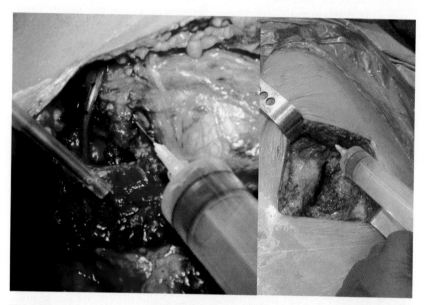

Fig. 22.58.

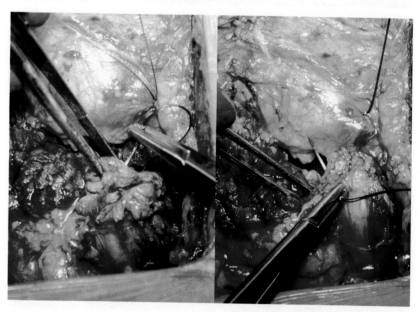

Fig. 22.59.

postero-superior capsule are then picked up, and the needle is inserted from deep to superficial through the posterior corner of the gluteus medius and the suture locked.

I do hear surgeons saying on occasions that they have stopped bothering to repair the external rotators and capsule after a posterior approach, but I cannot support this stance. As will be seen in Chapter 28, I have two patients who sustained trauma and dislocation of their resurfaced hips; both went on to recurrent dislocation. When these patients were treated with a soft tissue repair/reconstruction, their dislocation episodes ceased. I therefore repair the external rotators and the capsule, but for many years I have done this all as one mass closure using continuous 0 looped PDS (Ethicon, Livingston, UK) (Fig. 22.60).

When one reaches the back of the greater trochanter, two circumstances can make life difficult. If one has not left a good soft tissue cuff on the posterior aspect of the greater trochanter, closure is difficult, and drill holes need to be made in the posterior aspect of the trochanter. The other situation that can occur in elderly people is that the quadratus femoris muscle is very atrophic, and a satisfactory cuff is just not available. In those patients also, drilling of the posterior trochanter should occur to get a satisfactory closure. After about 3 to 4 cm of the closure, the capsule can no longer be picked up with the external rotators as this turns the corner toward the inferior femoral neck, and the closure from here on is of quadratus femoris only (Fig. 22.61).

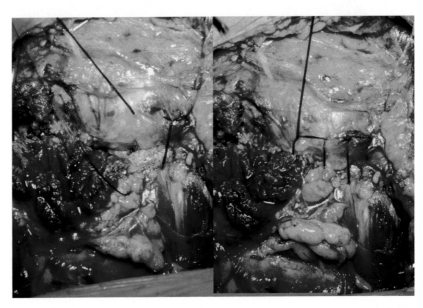

FIG. 22.60.

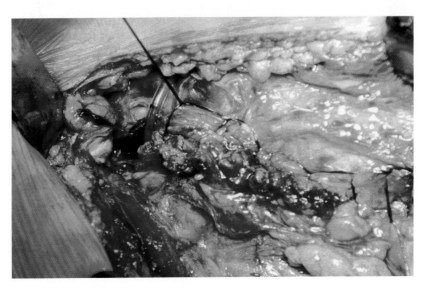

FIG. 22.61.

As the closure moves inferiorly, the risk of inadvertently picking up the sciatic nerve increases as this structure comes closer to the posterior aspect of the femur. It is advisable to expose or at least feel where the sciatic nerve is in the inferior aspect of this closure. The other catch is that the suction drain can be incorporated in the suture line.

In the inferior aspect of the closure, I aim to pick up the edges of the divided tendon of gluteus maximus and approximate these also (Fig. 22.62).

All the sutures so far have been of the mattress type with locking of each stitch. I regard it as very important not to pull too hard on this suture line. When surgeons really want something fixed firmly together, they tend to apply too much force. Experienced surgeons will know that if they explore a hip after a few days, all the tissues are markedly swollen. A tight suture line would inevitably cause necrosis of the muscle edge and breakdown of the suture line, so I aim for a loose approximation of soft tissue rather than strangulation of soft tissues. The suture line is then carried from distal to proximal, and the greater trochanter bursa is approximated with a running suture (Fig. 22.63).

My impression is that I have much less trouble with greater trochanter bursitis in recent years since I started closing the

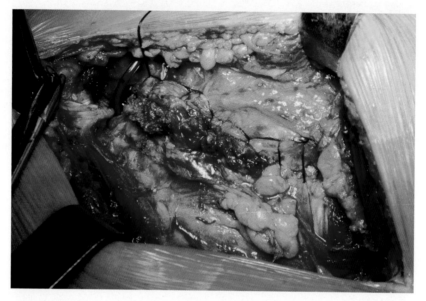

Fig. 22.62.

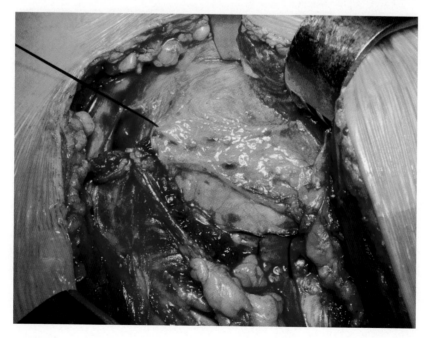

Fig. 22.63.

incised greater trochanter bursa compared with former years where I did not. However, I do not have hard data on this. I would never be prepared to do a trial of nonclosure versus closure of the greater trochanter bursa, so the reader will just have to take my word that it is a good thing to close this structure to where it was found (Fig. 22.64).

A final check for bleeding vessels in the divided gluteus maximus muscle is undertaken and electrocautery performed as required.

The length of the skin incision is recorded for the notes. As explained earlier, I do not regard this as a very important issue and far more important is whether an accurate placement of components has been achieved with the minimum disruption of soft tissue. A short skin incision does not necessarily imply a lack of trauma deep to that incision in the same way as a small bullet-hole entry point does not imply a small amount of trouble deeper in the body (Fig. 22.65).

A second suction drain is inserted. I insert one drain deep to the capsule and one drain between the external rotators and the undersurface of gluteus maximus. I was considering giving up drains, but I have been influenced not to by visiting surgeons. I learn a lot from visiting surgeons, and three different groups of

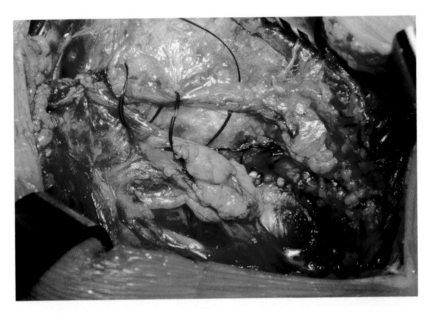

FIG. 22.64.

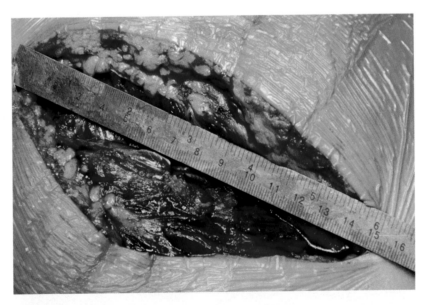

FIG. 22.65.

them now have told me the same story. Having given up drains several years previously, they reviewed their deep infection rate at the 5-year period and found that they had a much higher infection rate than previously. This, of course, is anecdote, but I have no good reason to give up drains at present. Until the evidence in favor of abandoning drains is overwhelming, I will continue to use these. In the past, we had regular complaints from patients that removing their drains on the first postoperative day was the most painful aspect of the hip arthroplasty operation, but we have now solved this problem. At the time

of the third administration of ropivacaine (Naropin), Adrenalin (epinephrine), and Toradol (ketorolac) into the superficial soft tissues, we also infiltrate this mixture into the region of the exit wounds of the drains through the skin of the thigh (Fig. 22.66). We know from experience that this local anesthetic cocktail gives anesthesia for 12 hours. We now routinely have the nursing staff remove our drains at 10 hours postoperatively, and the patients no longer complain of pain.

The inferior 2 or 3 cm of divided fascia lata are approximated using loop 0 nylon running sutures (Fig. 22.67). The separated

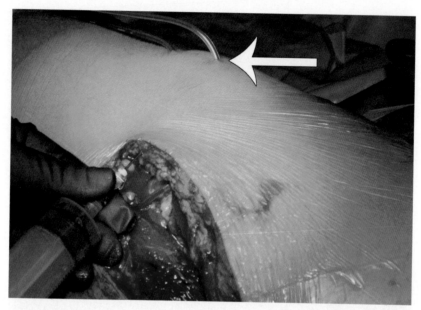

FIG. 22.66.

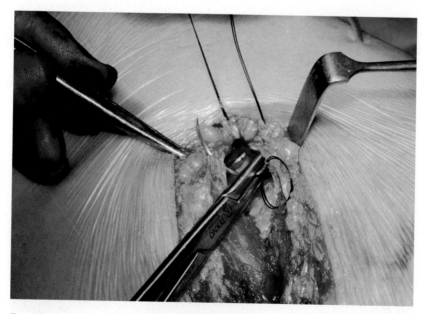

FIG. 22.67.

fibers of gluteus maximus are approximated, taking care not to strangle them. I still use nylon when repairing an incision in the fascia lata as in my revision practice it is common to find a hernia in the fascia lata when an absorbable suture has been used at the previous surgery.

Charnley understood this issue 40 years ago. He recognized that healing of the fascia lata was slow, and he advised the use of a nonabsorbable suture to repair it. The problem with using a nylon suture is the knot, and if one leaves spikes protruding toward the skin, then the patient can start to feel this when they sit on that area of the incision. When using a nylon suture, therefore, it is very important to use a Miller's hitch and bury the knot (Fig. 22.68).

The subcutaneous tissues are closed with Vicryl (Ethicon, Livingston, UK). Again, it is important not to pull the sutures too tight as this causes fat necrosis. In addition to picking up the subcutaneous tissue, it is a good idea to also pick up the fascia covering the gluteus maximus muscle. The object of this is to not leave a space under the fat where a hematoma can collect. We also bury the knot of the Vicryl suture, but this is not so important as with the nylon suture knot (Fig. 22.69). We use skin clips as these cause less cross-hatching

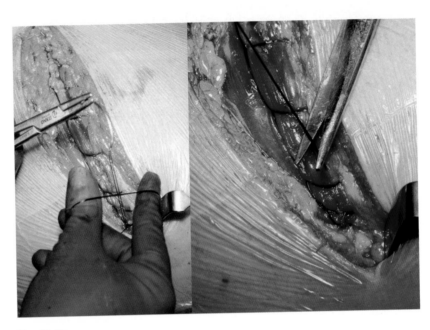

FIG. 22.68.

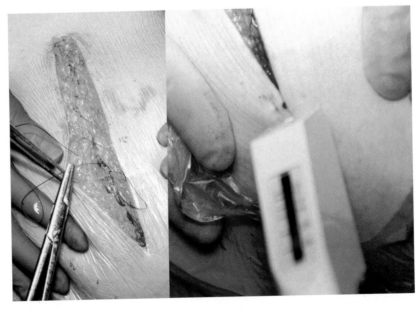

FIG. 22.69.

in our experience than do interrupted sutures. I do not like the reddening and thickening of the skin edge caused by an absorbable subcuticular suture.

A long compression stocking that goes over the hip region and is secured with a waist band is applied (Credenhill Surgical Hosiery Ltd., Ilkeston, UK) (Fig. 22.70). These long stockings have markedly reduced the amount of hip and thigh swelling we get after hip surgery. Unfortunately, the company that manufactures these stockings only supplies them in three sizes but my patients tend to come in more than three sizes. The patient is now transferred to his or her bed and moved to the recovery room. An x-ray is taken in the recovery room when the patient is wide awake to ensure that dislocation has not occurred in moving from the operating room table.

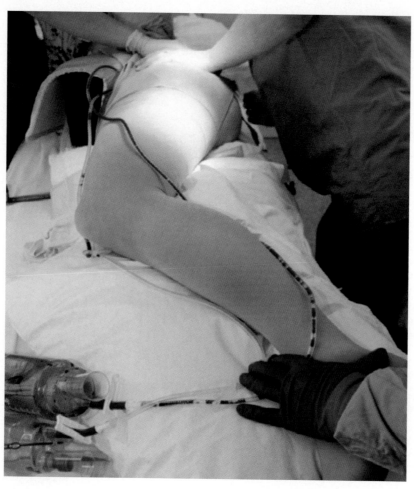

FIG. 22.70.

23

Birmingham Mid-Head Resection Prosthesis and Its Implantation

Derek J.W. McMinn

It is always a difficult consultation with young patients who come specifically wanting a hip resurfacing to have to tell them that their femoral head bone is of suspect quality. This poor-quality bone classically occurs in avascular necrosis (AVN) but can also be seen in osteopenia or osteoporosis or when large femoral head cysts are present (usually provoked by long-term anti-inflammatory medication). Other conditions such as severe slipped femoral capital epiphysis or Perthes disease can render the bony anatomy unsuitable for hip resurfacing. When I see poor-quality bone, I warn the patient that a hip resurfacing may not be a wise procedure. If they still insist on having the highest chance of a resurfacing, then we leave the decision on which procedure to perform to intraoperative findings. In these patients, I obtain consent for either a Birmingham Hip Resurfacing (BHR), a Birmingham Mid-Head Resection

(BMHR) prosthesis, or a stemmed total hip replacement. The BMHR prosthesis was developed because moving from a hip resurfacing to a stemmed total hip replacement is a major leap in aggressiveness with respect to (a) femoral shaft invasion, (b) proximal femoral stress shielding, and (c) the ease of subsequent revision surgery if it should be required. We started developing our BMHR prosthesis some years ago with first implantation approximately 4.5 years ago. The incentive to develop this implant came from our observation that the BHR did not perform as well in patients with avascular necrosis as in patients with osteoarthritis (see Chapter 27). I do not intend to show any successes with hip resurfacing in avascular necrosis, although there have been many, and instead I want to focus on the failure pattern. Figure 23.1 shows the x-ray and magnetic resonance imaging (MRI) scan of a man

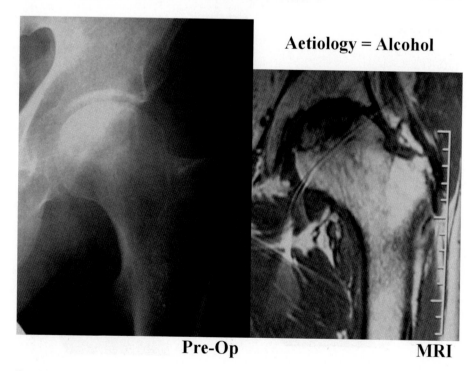

Aetiology = Alcohol

Pre-Op   **MRI**

Fig. 23.1.

whom we thought would be suitable for a BHR. His disease process seemed relatively localized on MRI scan, but it was believed that the etiology of his problem was alcohol abuse. I carried out a BHR and as can be seen in Fig. 23.2, the 2-month postoperative x-ray is fine but the x-ray at 2 years 10 months shows collapse of the femoral head. Further collapse of the femoral head is the most common cause of failure in my patients with a pre-existing diagnosis of AVN having been treated with the BHR.

In Fig. 23.3, we can see the different levels of head and neck resection used in modern hip arthroplasty surgery.

Level A is the resection level for a conventional total hip replacement. Level B is the resection level for neck retaining prostheses such as the Freeman implant or the Pipino device. These types of implants, however, require fixation in the shaft of the femur. The mechanical situation for short-stem total hip replacements is difficult because from level B down, the femoral canal widens. To obtain secure fixation of the implant, therefore, designers have extended their implant to take purchase on the inner aspect of the cortex of the upper femur. The downside of this is that as soon as the implant fixes into the cortex of the femur, proximal stress shielding

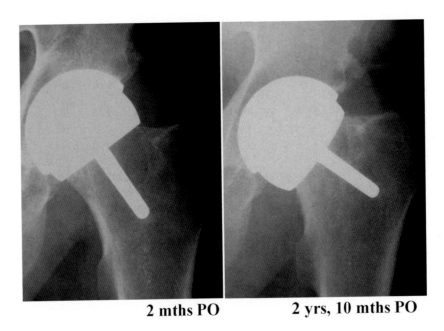

2 mths PO   **2 yrs, 10 mths PO**

FIG. 23.2.

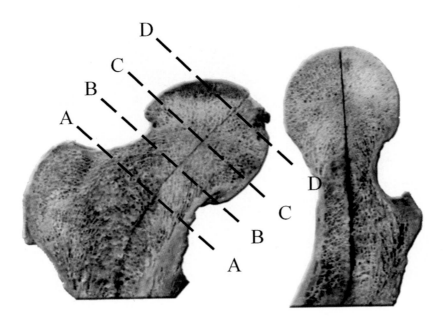

FIG. 23.3.

will occur. Level D is the traditional level of resection for a resurfacing prosthesis. Level C is the resection level for the BMHR implant. I chose this level of resection because it gets rid of the vast majority of bad bone in the femoral head that is encountered, for example, in avascular necrosis. It has, however, the massive advantage that the head-neck transition area is retained, and particularly on the lateral view of Fig. 23.3, one can see that this area is conical in shape. Conical shapes offer good fixation for orthopedic implants. As can be seen in Fig. 23.4, a stopper in a decanter is quite stable without

the need for a distal extension. I chose to have a short curved stem on our prototype implant of this design so that rotational stability would be obtained.

To understand the template overlays shown in Fig. 23.5, it needs to be appreciated that the tip of the curved stem in no way aims to take purchase on the inner aspect of the cortex of the femur as this would defeat the object and cause proximal stress shielding. The curved stem of this implant lies totally within cancellous bone and was designed purely to resist early torsional movement. The principal load transfer area in this

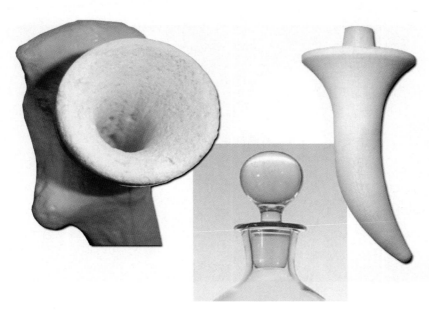

Fig. 23.4.

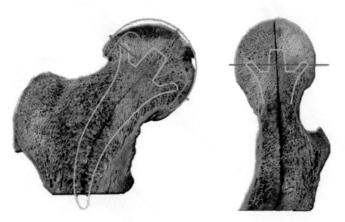

Fig. 23.5.

implant is seen in the lateral view where the cone of the implant engages in the conical head-neck transition zone. This conical head-neck transition zone is, of course, resected in all of the short-stem total hip replacement designs used hitherto. In Fig. 23.6, the x-rays of a patient with severe avascular necrosis are shown. At surgery when machining of the head-neck transition area was performed, good-quality viable bone was left, allowing satisfactory fixation and purchase of the prototype BMHR implant. At 1 year and 2 years, no stress shielding of the femoral neck seems to have occurred. We take this as a positive indication that the bone is being proximally rather than distally loaded. Our series of this prototype implant have all had RSA migration measurements (see Chapter 8). At 2 years, no detectable migration of these femoral components was seen.

There were, however, some technical problems at implantation surgery (Fig. 23.7).

It is possible to machine the head-neck transition by rotating a suitable cutter instrument on a guide bar. However, the curved stem meant that the bone for the stem had to be rasped

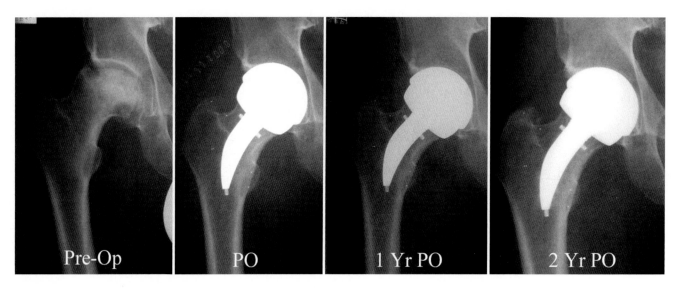

FIG. 23.6.

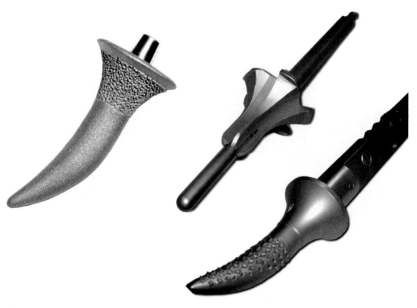

FIG. 23.7.

freehand. This led to slight inaccuracy where the bone cut for the proximal and distal aspects of the stem did not match. The inaccuracies were minor, but it seemed to us that freehand rasping was not an ideal bone preparation method. Because the only purpose of this stem was to resist torsional movement, then we reasoned that this could be easily accomplished by a straight-stem device having longitudinal flutes. Such a device is shown in Fig. 23.8.

There are two considerable advantages with this straight-stemmed BMHR device. The first is that bone preparation can all be done on the same intramedullary guide bar, thus removing potentially inaccurate bone preparation from free-hand rasping. The second advantage is that the BMHR can be designed into the same family of implants as the BHR so a surgeon can start the operation with the same bone cuts and then carry out either a BHR or a BMHR depending on the quality of bone discovered at surgery.

The BMHR prosthesis allows the surgeon to prepare the femoral head for resurfacing, determine if the bone is satisfactory for a resurfacing, and if it is not then to move seamlessly to the BMHR implant. The initial stages of the BMHR operation therefore are identical to the steps involved in performing a BHR. After insertion of the acetabular prosthesis, the femur is exposed as in the standard BHR (see Chapter 22) (Fig. 23.9).

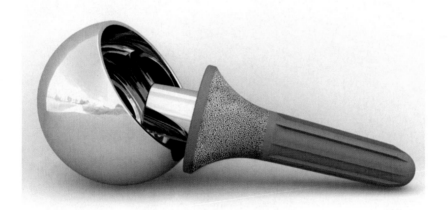

FIG. 23.8.

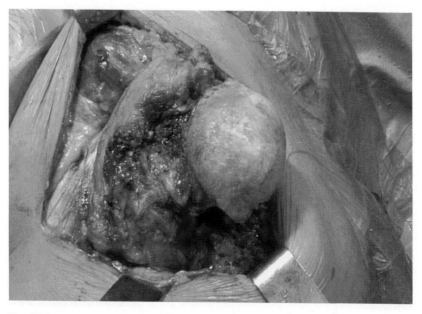

FIG. 23.9.

The templated entry point for the guide pin is measured up from the lesser trochanter tip and the guide pin inserted through the aperture in the short-arm jig (Fig. 23.10). The x-ray templating to determine this entry point is exactly the same for the BHR and the BMHR.

Correct lateral plane alignment is achieved and the jig adjusted and fixed accordingly (Fig. 23.11). The lateral plane alignment for the BMHR implant is more critical than for the BHR. The stem of the BHR implant is, of course, thin, and there is scope for lateral plane alignment error without perforating the cortex of the anterior or posterior femoral neck. The stem of the BMHR implant is much broader, and a determined effort should be made to obtain the midlateral axis using the jig.

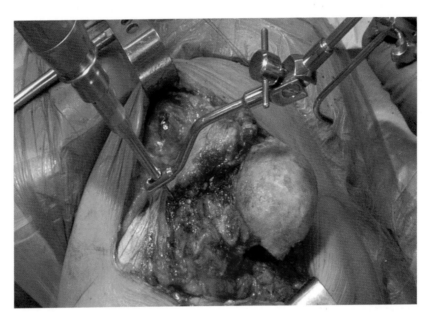

FIG. 23.10.

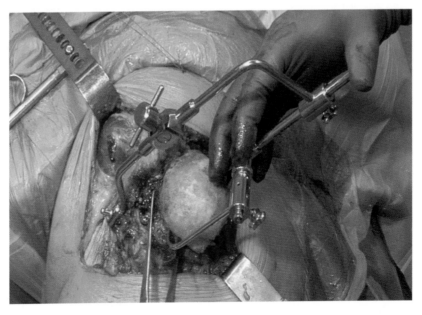

FIG. 23.11.

The correct entry point into the femoral head for the guide wire is determined by stylus rotation around the femoral neck, and the guide wire is inserted (Fig. 23.12). This is exactly the same as for the BHR except that, when performing the BHR in difficult pathology like slipped upper femoral epiphysis, one is tempted to make compromises to achieve peripheral femoral head support for the implant. This compromise in effect reduces the anterosuperior head-neck offset. With the BMHR, no such compromise should be made, and the aim is to restore the anatomy, with respect to offset, to normality. Taking fixation at the head-neck transition area gives the surgeon total freedom to put the BMHR prosthesis in the ideal position.

The correct placement of the guide wire is checked by rotating the stylus around the femoral neck, and any adjustment for malposition of this guide wire is corrected at this stage (Fig. 23.13). Except in slipped upper femoral epiphysis, as already discussed, this step is exactly the same for both the BHR and the BMHR.

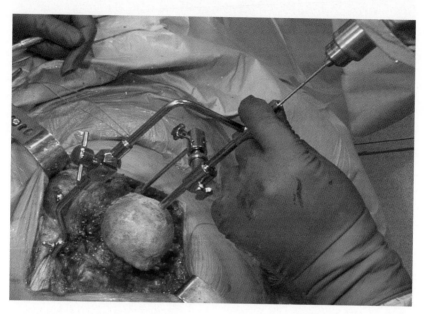

FIG. 23.12.

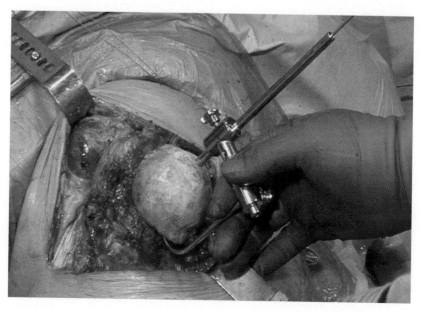

FIG. 23.13.

The venting hole through the lesser trochanter is made exactly as the standard BHR procedure with drilling into the canal of the femur, but the vent is only inserted into the lesser trochanter and not into the canal of the femur as the vent can be damaged by stem preparation for the BMHR prosthesis (Fig. 23.14).

If there is a possibility that the BMHR implant may be used, then the BMHR overdrill is used at this stage. This is thinner than the standard BHR drill (Fig. 23.15A).

The BMHR guide bar is then inserted. This has the same diameter as the BHR guide bar proximally but the intraosseous portion is thinner (Fig. 23.15B). This allows the same cutter instruments to be used for both the BHR and the BMHR. This makes the BMHR system surgeon-friendly as a decision does not have to be taken on whether to use it or not until a late stage.

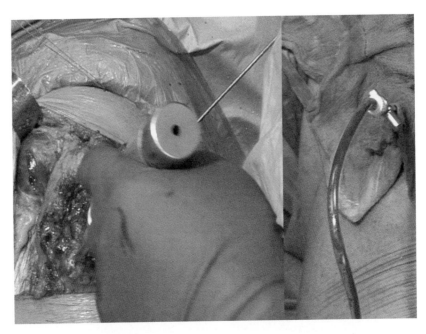

Fig. 23.14.

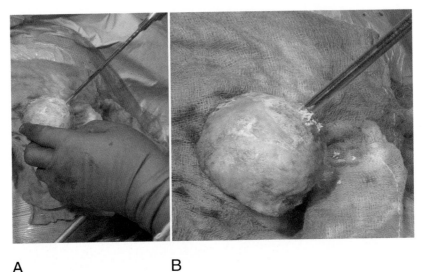

A   B

Fig. 23.15.

Correct placement of the guide bar is then checked with the stylus (Fig. 23.16A).

The anti-notch device stylus is advanced to a safe position on the superior femoral neck (Fig. 23.16B).

An appropriate thickness of anti-notch plastic spacer is applied over the guide bar to prevent shoot-through of the peripheral femoral head reamers.

Peripheral reaming of the femoral head proceeds in the usual way again using a head-neck template to hold the swabs away from the teeth of the cutter instrument (Fig. 23.17).

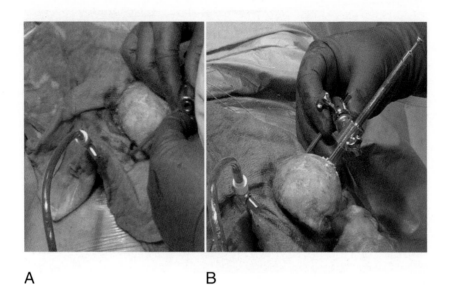

A   B

FIG. 23.16.

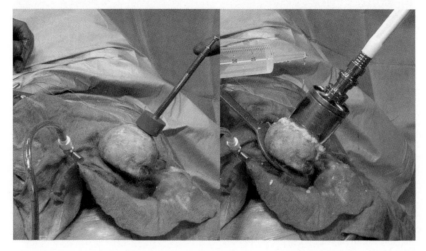

FIG. 23.17.

When peripheral reaming of the femoral head is complete, the inferior peripheral head is cracked off using a periosteal elevator. The inferior peripheral femoral head bone is detached from the soft tissue connection on the femoral neck by sharp dissection (Fig 23.18).

Osteophyte around the periphery of the head-neck junction is excised using a rongeur and taking care not to tear soft tissue off the surface of the femoral neck (Fig. 23.19).

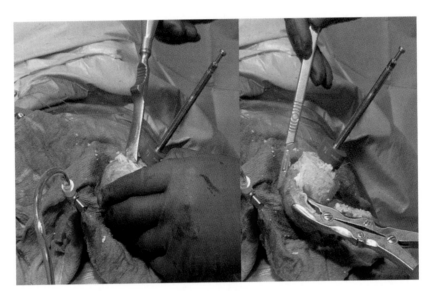

Fig. 23.18.

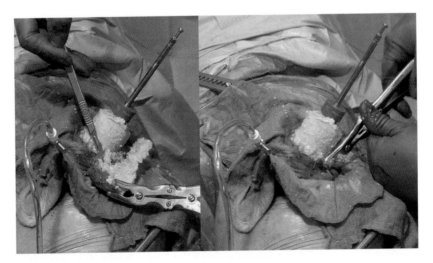

Fig. 23.19.

We now discover that this patient's anatomy is just as bad as it looked on preoperative x-ray, and there is a large cyst present in the superior femoral head extending down close to the femoral head-neck junction. Dissecting forceps have been inserted into the depth of the cyst, and one can see that this is a large cyst (Fig. 23.20).

Cysts are also present in the medial femoral head, and the presence of a large cyst plus multiple small cysts makes this femoral head unsuitable, in my view, for hip resurfacing (Fig. 23.21).

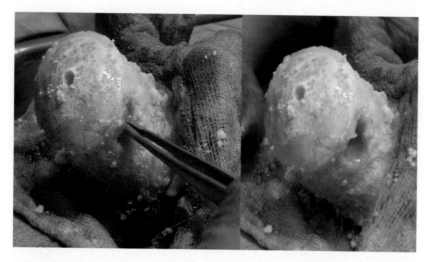

FIG. 23.20.

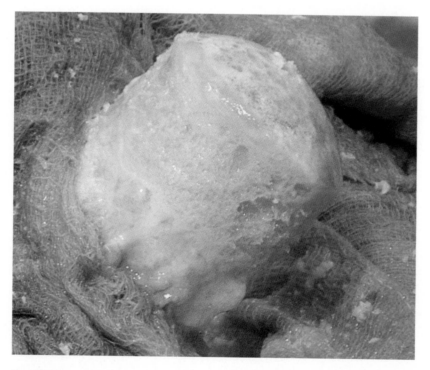

FIG. 23.21.

This picture shows the difference in depth of the two napkin rings. The BMHR napkin ring is inferiorly placed on the femoral head. The BHR napkin ring is more proximally placed on the femoral head.

The proximal femoral head bone is being resected with a reciprocating saw. One is, of course, resecting more bone from the femoral head in the BMHR procedure than is performed in the BHR procedure (Fig. 23.22).

Now that the bone is resected, it can be seen that the resection line goes through three cysts in the superior part of the femoral head (Fig. 23.23). If this patient's femoral head had been resurfaced, then these cysts would have been left within the substance of the bone supporting the resurfacing implant. It is not hard to see why femoral head collapse in the face of such cystic destruction could easily occur after hip resurfacing.

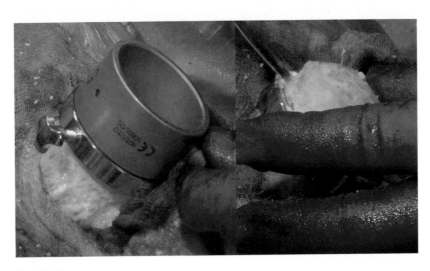

FIG. 23.22.

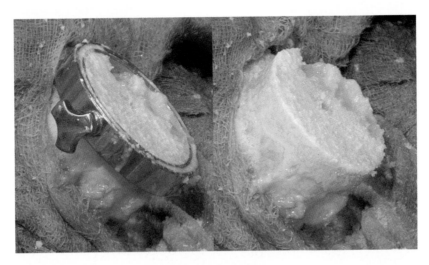

FIG. 23.23.

It can be seen by using the BMHR head-neck template that too much bone has been left in the base of the femoral head, but with this procedure, I prefer to leave excess bone and then trim the bone down to the desired position using a face cutter. The face cutter is used to plane the resected surface down to the correct level (Fig. 23.24).

The head-neck template is reapplied, and it is confirmed that the head has been planed down to the correct level. Now that the head planing has occurred down to the correct level, only the base of one cyst persists superiorly. The dual-thickness guide bar is replaced with the single-thickness short guide bar and this is tapped in until the tip of the guide bar hits the lateral inner cortex of the femoral shaft (Fig. 23.25).

An inverse ruler is now used to measure the maximum length of BMHR stem that can be inserted into this particular patient. There is no need to insert the longest stem possible, but it must be ensured that too long a stem is not attempted, because it might abut on or penetrate through the lateral femoral cortex.

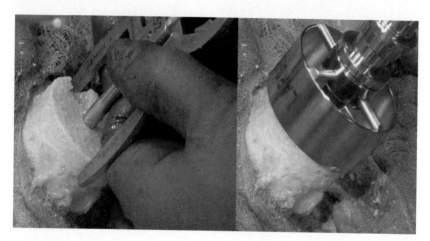

Fig. 23.24.

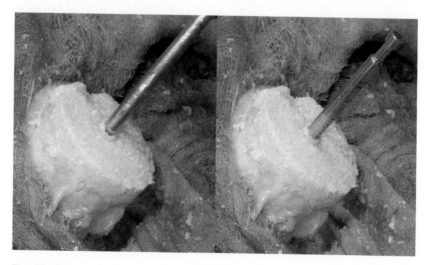

Fig. 23.25.

The proximal cone reamer is mounted on the appropriate sleeve. The sleeve size must be the same as the peripheral femoral head cutter used (Fig. 23.26).

On the ream setting on the power unit, the proximal conical cutter is inserted until the stop makes contact with the planed cut surface of the femoral head.

When proximal conical reaming has been completed, the proximal reamer is removed from the guide bar (Fig. 23.27).

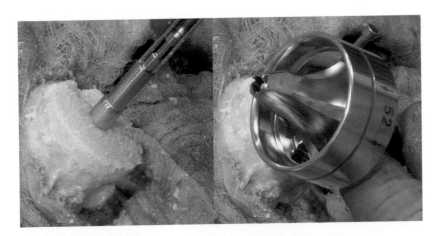

FIG. 23.26.

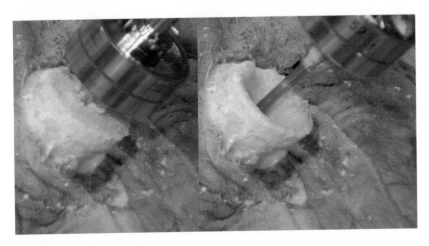

FIG. 23.27.

The stem drill is then substituted for the proximal reamer, and this is attached to the appropriate sleeve. Reaming for the stem then occurs, and initially guidance is provided by the guide bar (Fig. 23.28A).

As the instrument is advanced, guidance is additionally obtained from the fit of the sleeve over the peripheral femoral head base (Fig. 23.28B).

The guide bar is then removed.

Now one can see the extensive cone that has been made in the head-neck transition area. Cones, of course, are very efficient at transferring load. The cyst is curetted of all remaining soft tissue (Fig. 23.29).

The cyst is autografted, and the BMHR implant on its introducer is ready for impaction (Fig. 23.30).

Distally, the longitudinal splines on the BMHR implant give a tight press fit and rotational control of the implant.

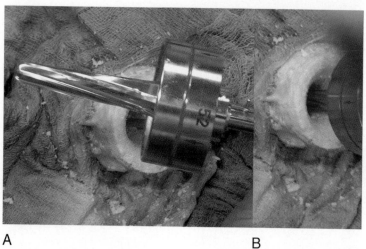

A   B

Fig. 23.28.

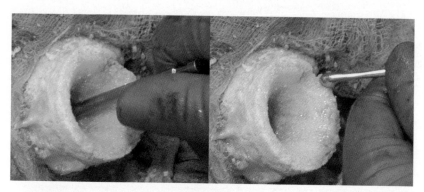

Fig. 23.29.

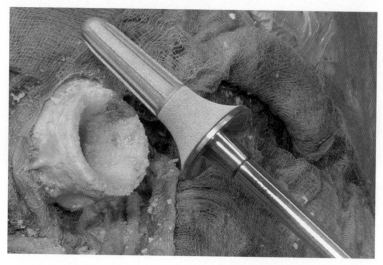

Fig. 23.30.

Proximally, the fit of the implant in the bone is line to line (Fig. 23.31). When the BMHR implant is fully seated, there is no point in attempting to hit the implant in any further, otherwise the implant acts like a log splitter.

The introducer is removed, and a guide bar with distal threads is screwed into the top of the BMHR implant. The peripheral femoral head cutter is passed one last time just to ensure that no spicules of bone protrude from the head-neck junction region, which could cause hang up of the prosthetic femoral head (Fig. 23.32).

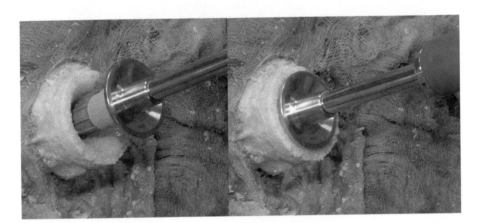

Fig. 23.31.

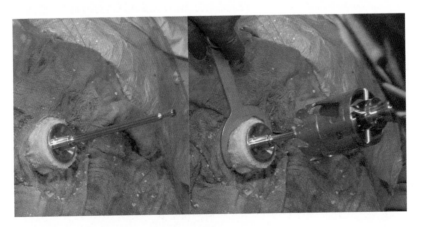

Fig. 23.32.

The BMHR modular head is offered up to the cone on the proximal implant. The cone is locked by impaction with an introducer (Fig. 23.33).

A final check is made for any protruding osteophytes at the femoral head-neck junction, and the prosthetic head is reduced into the acetabular component (Fig. 23.34).

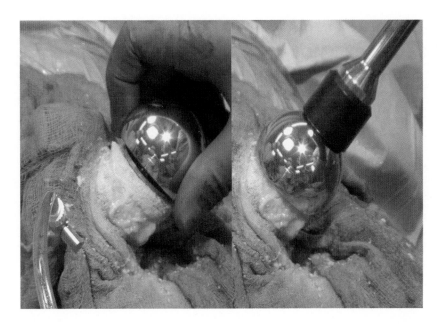

Fig. 23.33.

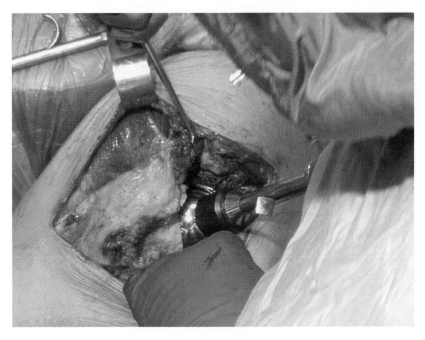

Fig. 23.34.

24
Guides, Jigs, and Navigation-Assisted Birmingham Hip Resurfacing

Derek J.W. McMinn

Total hip replacement has been successfully performed since 1960. It could be argued that as surgeons have managed to perform successful total hip replacements all these years without the aid of navigation, navigation is not required now. However, surgeons who assess their results accurately understand that the problem is not the average; it is the outliers. If one considers the issue of acetabular cup inclination angle, then there is good evidence that high inclination angles are associated with edge loading of the implant and excess wear, which can lead to premature failure. This has been seen with the Birmingham Hip Resurfacing (BHR) and other hip resurfacing devices. (See Chapter 6 to observe the effects of edge loading on the wear of these metal on metal devices.) No doubt, with experience, surgeons improve their implantation technique. There is also the problem of realizing that acetabular inclination angle is important. I know that I was tricked into thinking that because we had virtually no instances of dislocation of these large-headed metal on metal articulations in the early years, our inclination angles must have been perfectly satisfactory.

With a realization that inclination angles were important, my performance in this respect did improve over the years. If we consider a cohort of Birmingham Hip Resurfacings that I performed in 1997 when my experience of metal on metal hip resurfacing was circa 400, and compare this with a cohort of Birmingham Hip Resurfacings that I performed in 2004 when my experience was circa 2500 metal on metal hip resurfacings, then improvements can be seen. The mean inclination angle has reduced from 43 degrees to 40 degrees. The number of outliers at or above 50 degrees of inclination has also decreased, but outliers are still present (Fig. 24.1). Accuracy is also desirable in acetabular component anteversion.

Figure 24.2 shows radiographs of a 50-year-old man with osteoarthritis of his right hip. I carried out a Birmingham Hip Resurfacing, and he made an excellent recovery. He returned to sport and 3 years later had his contralateral hip resurfaced also. The initial BHR had perfect function and no discomfort, but the x-ray showed a "bite" in the superior femoral neck. I undertook screening of this man's hip under Image Intensification.

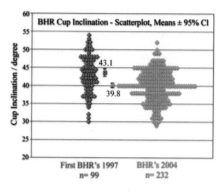

FIG. 24.1. BHR inclination angles from 1997 and 2004.

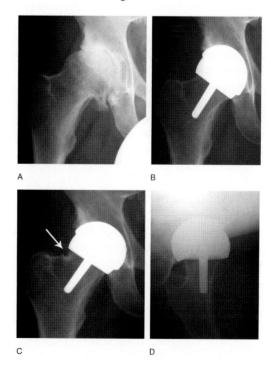

FIG. 24.2. (A) Preoperative x-ray showing osteoarthritis. (B) Satisfactory postoperative x-ray. (C) Three-year postoperative x-ray showing large "bite" in the superior femoral neck (arrow). (D) Three-year postoperative lateral x-ray giving impression of excessive cup anteversion.

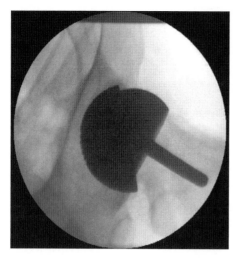

FIG. 24.3. Same patient as in Fig. 24.2; image intensifier screening without anaesthetic 3 years postoperatively. With 90 degrees of hip flexion and full abduction, the "bite" area of the superior femoral neck comes close to the posterior cup edge.

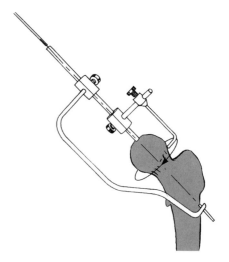

FIG. 24.4. Original McMinn femoral jig.

With the hip extended and with abduction of the hip, the superior femoral neck would not approach the lateral border of the acetabulum. However, in flexion with abduction, the "bite" in the superior femoral neck did come close to the posterior acetabular component edge. I consider that this is an area that previously was impinging, where bone has resorbed and the impingement resolved without any clinical mishap (Fig. 24.3). Even for experienced surgeons, therefore, technological improvements to assist with accurate acetabular component placement would be useful. It has been recognized since the 1970s that avoidance of severe varus placement of the femoral component of a resurfacing and avoidance of neck notching are important in reducing the incidence of femoral neck fracture. Technological advances, to assist with avoidance of severe varus component placement and avoidance of femoral neck notching, would also be helpful.

Femoral Alignment Jigs

We have used various alignment jigs. My first jig was very satisfactory at obtaining correct varus-valgus alignment and at preventing femoral neck notching (Fig. 24.4).

The downside of that jig was that it was poor at getting the correct lateral plane alignment of the femoral guide wire and therefore the femoral component. There were three requirements for that jig: (1) The surgeon needed conventional x-rays with a believable magnification factor. This was no problem back in the early 1990s because all of us were working on conventional x-rays. The problem now is that with digital x-rays in many hospitals, one cannot be so assured of the magnification factor and hence templating is a real problem. (2) It required the use of a large incision to insert the guide pin through the lateral femoral cortex, but as it was normal to use large incisions at that time, this also was no problem. (3) Although many surgeons have become accustomed to this jig in a number of different countries, there are some surgeons who still cannot use it correctly. These surgeons sought other solutions like simpler, pin-less jigs. At the beginning of the Midland Medical Technologies (MMT) era, we decided to try and simplify the femoral alignment jig to make life easier for surgeons.

I used this jig (Fig. 24.5) during 1997. It was also good at obtaining the correct varus-valgus alignment, but it was poor at gaining correct lateral plane alignment and poor also at siting exactly the correct entry point for the guide wire. I therefore abandoned it and returned to the McMinn jig, with a modification to allow correct lateral plane alignment to be achieved (Fig. 24.6).

Figures 24.7 to 24.31 demonstrate the correct use of the long arm jig with lateral plane correction.

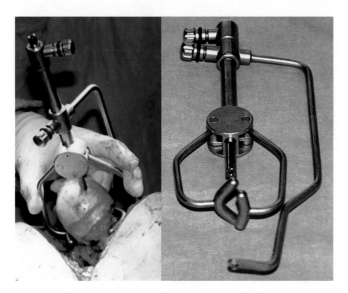

FIG. 24.5. Simplified jig used in 1997. The jaws clamp the femoral neck and "self-center" the cannulated guide bar and hence the guide wire within the femoral neck.

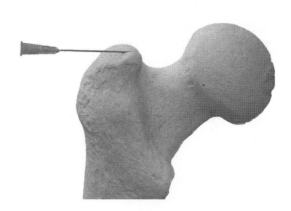

FIG. 24.7. The greater trochanter tip is marked with a needle.

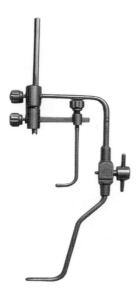

FIG. 24.6. McMinn long-arm jig with lateral plane alignment adjustment in the long arm.

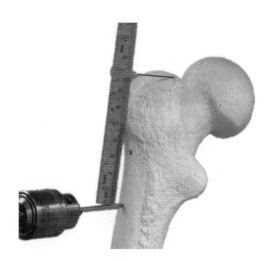

FIG. 24.8. The guide pin is inserted at the measured, templated distance from the greater trochanter tip (see Chapter 17).

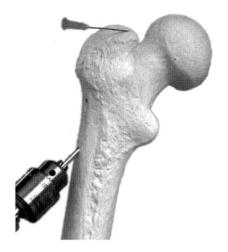

FIG. 24.9. When the guide pin enters bone, the handle of the power unit is directed towards the femoral head.

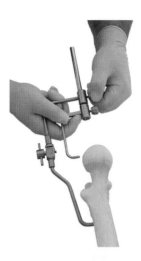

FIG. 24.12. The locking nuts for the long arm and the stylus are released. It is important for the surgeon to hold onto the stylus when this is done.

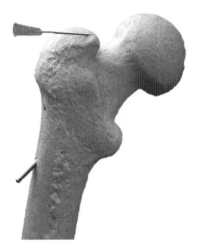

FIG. 24.10. The guide pin will therefore give the correct alignment, irrespective of the bulk of vastus lateralis.

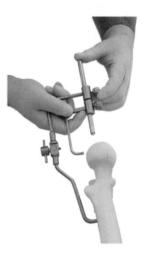

FIG. 24.13. The surgeon then advances the cannulated bar toward the femoral head, and the stylus tip is passed around the femoral head.

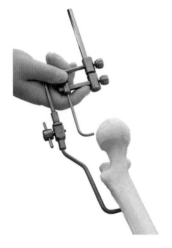

FIG. 24.11. The scrub nurse has set the stylus to the correct femoral size. The surgeon hooks the long arm of the jig onto the guide pin. Assistant delivers head into the wound.

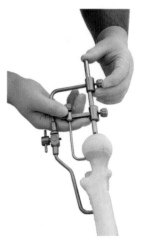

FIG. 24.14. The cannulated bar now rests on the summit of the femoral head, and the stylus tip has cleared the femoral head and now rests near the femoral neck.

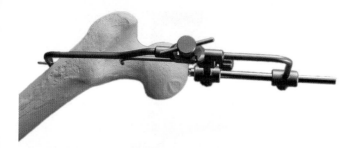

FIG. 24.15. When viewed posteriorly, the varus-valgus alignment has now been set. The long arm must remain at right angles to the back of the femur, and it is the second assistant's job to not allow it to rotate by holding it with finger and thumb. If angulation of the long arm is used to achieve correct lateral plane alignment, then rotation either clockwise or anti-clockwise can introduce unwanted varus or valgus guide-wire positioning.

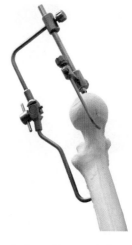

FIG. 24.18. The lateral plane alignment is incorrect. The guide wire would exit from the front of the femoral neck.

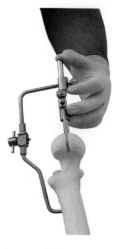

FIG. 24.16. The stylus is rotated 90 degrees in preparation for lateral plane alignment adjustment.

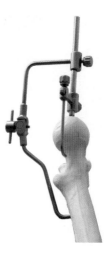

FIG. 24.19. The lateral plane alignment here is also incorrect. The guide wire would exit from the back of the femoral neck.

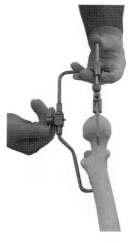

FIG. 24.17. If desired, the locking nut for the stylus can be tightened at this stage. The adjustment hinge in the long arm of the jig is released by undoing its locking nut.

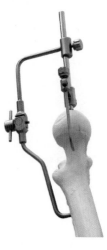

FIG. 24.20. This lateral plane alignment is correct. The guide wire will pass down the center of the femoral neck.

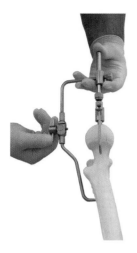

Fig. 24.21. The hinge in the long arm is locked by tightening the locking nut.

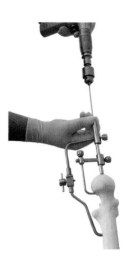

Fig. 24.24. The teeth on the end of the cannulated bar are tapped into the femoral head. The guide wire is now inserted.

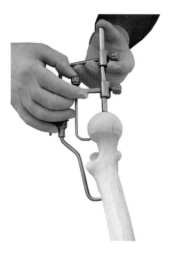

Fig. 24.22. The entry point position is now determined by translating the cannulated bar on the femoral head and observing the position of the stylus tip as it is rotated around the femoral neck.

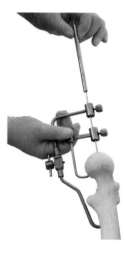

Fig. 24.25. The cannulated bar is now removed, and the long arm jig unhooked from the lateral pin in the femur.

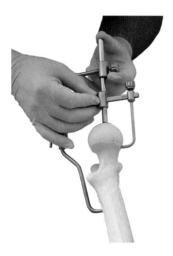

Fig. 24.23. The object is to recreate the normal anterosuperior prosthetic head-femoral neck offset. In addition, clearance of the stylus tip all around the neck should be achieved.

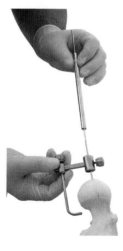

Fig. 24.26. The cannulated bar is replaced on the guide wire and in the body of the stylus.

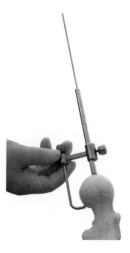

Fig. 24.27. A thorough checking now follows of the guide-wire position. The first requirement is clearance of the stylus tip all around the femoral neck.

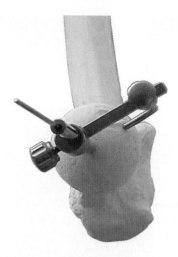

Fig. 24.30. It is common that more bone will be resected from the periphery of the femoral head posteroinferiorly compared with anterosuperiorly.

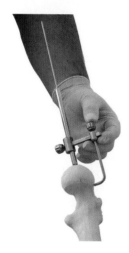

Fig. 24.28. The second requirement is that the anterosuperior head-neck offset after resurfacing will be equal to the normal head-neck offset.

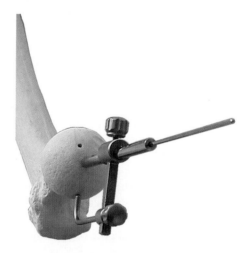

Fig. 24.31. This becomes a difficult task in severe slipped capital femoral epiphysis. It may be impossible to have stylus clearance on the femoral neck yet achieve contact on the periphery of the anterosuperior femoral head (see Chapter 25).

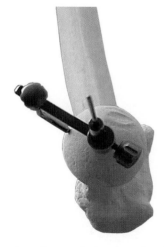

Fig. 24.29. The next requirement is that the stylus should touch the femoral head through 360 degrees.

The long-arm jig, just demonstrated, also required the use of a large incision. I moved to smaller-incision surgery so was not able to use the jig that had shown itself to be extremely reliable. Instead, I had to use various designs of pin-less jigs, and although I could show examples of perfectly good alignment with these, unfortunately they did not prove reliable on a bad day.

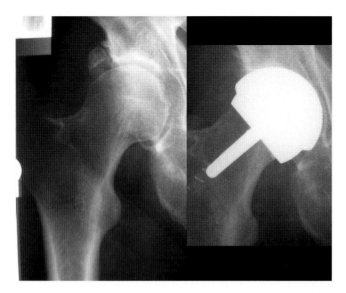

FIG. 24.32. Preoperative and immediate postoperative x-rays of BHR inserted with pinless jig. Note varus placement of femoral component and barely noticeable notching of superior femoral neck.

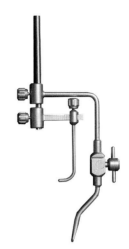

FIG. 24.34. Short-arm jig developed for reduced incision length surgery.

Figure 24.32 shows the preoperative and postoperative radiographs of a patient whose BHR I carried out using a pin-less jig in the early stages of my MIS learning curve. The postoperative x-ray shows that the femoral component is in varus alignment and there is also notching of the superior femoral neck. The radiograph 8 weeks later (Fig. 24.33) shows a fracture of the femoral neck and the adjacent radiograph shows the revision to a cemented, stemmed total hip replacement with a modular head articulating on the original acetabular component. I eventually decided that I could not live with the inaccuracy of these pin-less jigs and the unnecessary complications that poor component positioning

was causing. A modification of the original McMinn jig was made to allow this to be used with small-incision surgery (Fig. 24.34).

With a reduced incision length in a posterior approach, it is not possible to get comfortable access to the lateral aspect of the femur. Instead of measuring down from the tip of the greater trochanter, the lesser trochanter can just as easily be used as the fixed bony point (Fig. 24.35).

During x-ray templating, the position for the guide pin in the intertrochanteric crest is determined that will give the desired varus-valgus alignment (see Chapter 17). On this dry bones demonstration, I am using a ruler to measure up from the lesser

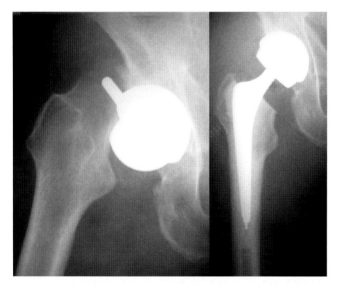

FIG. 24.33. Eight-week postoperative x-ray showing fracture of the femoral neck. Postrevision x-ray showing cemented polished taper stem with modular head matching original cup.

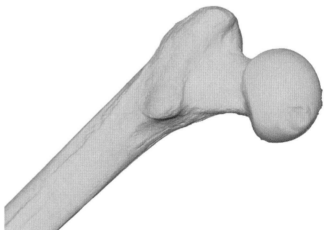

FIG. 24.35.

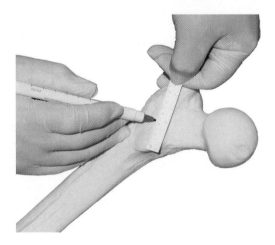

Fig. 24.36.

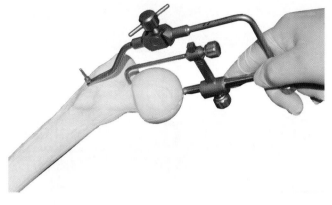

Fig. 24.38.

trochanter tip to the templated point on the intertrochanteric crest, and the point is being marked with a pen (Fig. 24.36).

At surgery, it is much easier to use the dedicated ruler instrument for this purpose (Fig. 24.37).

In addition, the mark on the intertrochanteric crest is marked using electrocautery (see Chapter 22). The short-arm jig is now attached by the guide pin into the intertrochanteric crest, piercing this at the marked, templated point. This particular variety of short-arm jig is shown deliberately as this was a prototype that was very quickly changed. Just like the long-arm jig, this particular variant of short-arm jig could rotate clockwise or anti-clockwise and if the arm was angulated to achieve desired lateral plane alignment, the clockwise or anti-clockwise rotation would alter the desired varus-valgus alignment (Fig. 24.38). It was rapidly appreciated that a simple redesign would prevent rotation once the guide pin had been inserted into the intertrochanteric crest. However, the jig shown in Fig. 24.39 does depend on the surgeon fixing the short arm to the femur in the desired alignment. The guide pin must be at right angles to the back of the intertrochanteric region (see Chapter 22). The use of the short-arm jig from hereon is exactly the same as that of the long-arm jig. The only difference is that with the *current*

design of short-arm jig, the second assistant no longer has to control the rotational position.

This is the current version of the short-arm jig. This device has a slot at the distal end of the short arm that prevents unintended rotation during surgery thus guaranteeing the varus-valgus alignment. The stylus adjustment for different head sizes is also much better than that of previous versions. In Fig. 24.39, the instrument has been handed to the surgeon by the scrub nurse in a useable fashion. The worst thing that can happen is as the scrub nurse hands the instrument to the surgeon, part of the instrument falls on the floor. The next worst thing that can happen is that the jig has been put together in an unusable configuration. In the next six figures (Figs. 24.40–24.45), I will show some of the common scrub nurse mistakes. So that my life is easier, I should point out that these mistakes never occur at Birmingham Nuffield Hospital.

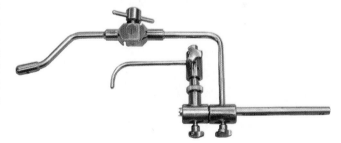

Fig. 24.39.

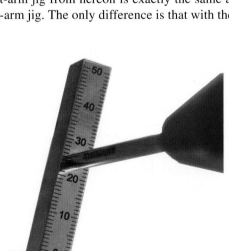

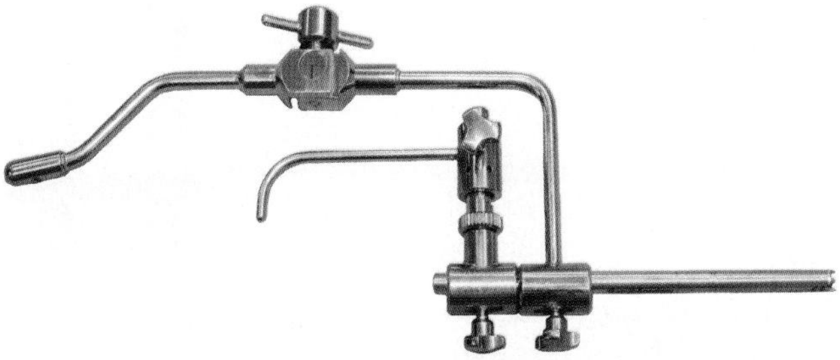

Fig. 24.37.

Fig. 24.40. The cannulated bar has been inserted the wrong way round with the teeth pointing at the surgeon end. When the surgeon presses on the guide bar to hold the instrument against the femoral head, the teeth will tear his gloves. In addition, when the surgeon wishes to fix the entry point position, no teeth will be present to fix into the femoral head.

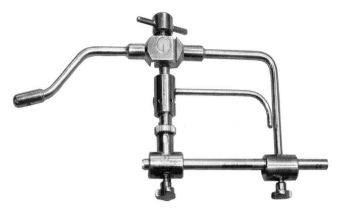

Fig. 24.41. The scrub nurse is cross-eyed.

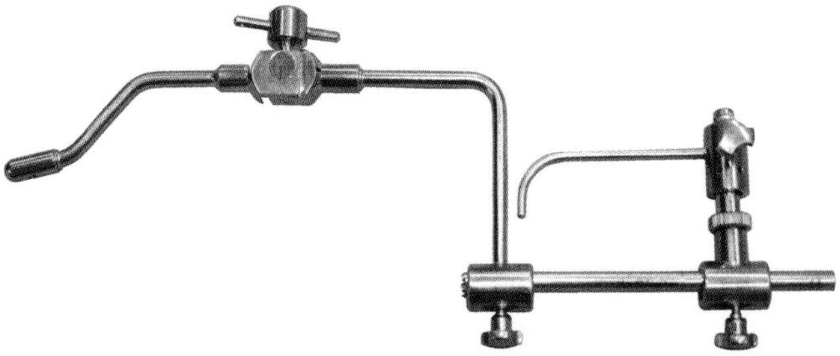

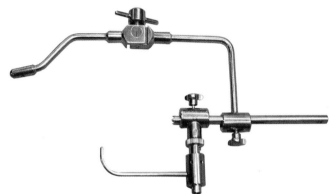

Fig. 24.44. The scrub nurse ought to pursue an alternative career.

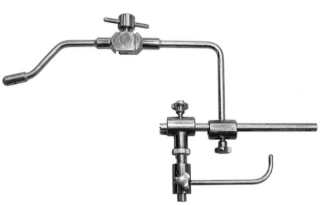

Fig. 24.42. Only just better than dropping it on the floor.

Fig. 24.45. It is a Monday morning!

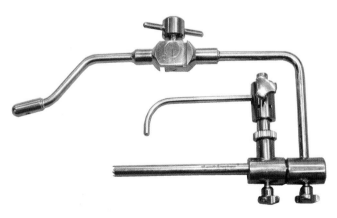

Fig. 24.43. The surgeon has annoyed the scrub nurse during the previous operation.

Experience with BrainLab Navigation for the Femoral Component of the BHR

Several years ago I was trained, both in the BrainLab factory and in a cadaver lab, in the use of their navigation system for the BHR. I was very happy with the navigation system both in BrainLab's laboratory facility and in the cadaver lab. Back home at surgery, however, on the femoral side, I found the system very consuming of time (Fig. 24.46). In addition, I checked the guide wires manually with my alignment jig after they had been inserted using navigation. Unfortunately,

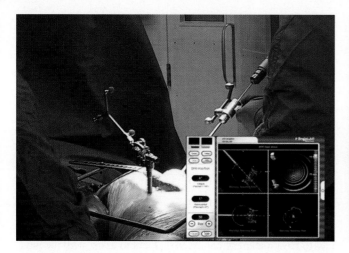

FIG. 24.46. The author inserting a femoral guide wire using BrainLab navigation.

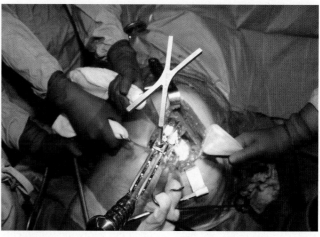

FIG. 24.47. Acetabular alignment guide used to estimate acetabular component anteversion.

whereas the varus-valgus and lateral plane alignment were quite accurate, the entry point determined by navigation was not accurate enough in my judgment. All guide wires were reinserted using a short-arm jig.

Even with a point accuracy of +1 to −1 mm, this on occasion is not accurate enough for the guide-wire insertion point. A difference of 2 mm in the insertion point can make the difference between notching and not notching the femoral neck. I decided very early on in my navigation experience that the femoral side of the navigation operation was not for me as I was much quicker and more accurate with a manual jig.

Jigs and Alignment Devices to Assist with Acetabular Component Placement of the BHR

A discussion of patient positioning has occurred in Chapter 19. The uncomfortable fact for surgeons, however, is that no matter how good the positioning system is, and no matter how careful the surgeon is in setting up the patient pre-operatively, a certain amount of movement of the patient occurs during surgery. This is made worse if the patient is grossly obese, has a very stiff hip that requires heavy retraction by the assistants, which can tilt the pelvis, or is very flexible, such as a hypermobile young woman with DDH. I do use alignment rods attached to the acetabular component introducer, but one has to understand the limitation of these devices (Fig. 24.47).

Provided the acetabular anatomy is reasonably normal, an experienced surgeon can better appreciate acetabular component alignment by referring to the normal acetabular anatomy. It needs to be understood that the acetabular wall inclination is around 55 degrees in the normal patient, yet the desired inclination angle for a metal on metal resurfacing acetabular component is 40 degrees. There is some leeway, however, and 45 degrees of inclination for a BHR acetabular component is perfectly satisfactory, 50 degrees is tolerable but undesirable, and 55 degrees is unacceptable. Today, if a patient of mine had 55 degrees of acetabular inclination on the recovery room x-ray, I would bring the patient back into the operating room and revise the acetabular component. When one starts to discuss degrees of acetabular component anteversion, then one needs to know whether one is talking about operative anteversion, radiographic anteversion, or anatomic anteversion. The reader is referred to the paper of Murray to acquire an understanding of the differences [1]. Without the aid of navigation devices, I find it almost impossible to give an answer to the question, "How much anteversion did you put on that acetabular component?" Inserting the acetabular component with respect to anteversion measurement is a question of educated guesswork, and one has to use as much of the normal acetabular anatomy as possible for clues as to correct component orientation. For example, the anterior edge of the acetabular component should not protrude beyond the bony margin of the anterior acetabulum, but determining exactly what is osteophyte on the anterior acetabular wall and what is normal acetabular wall is very difficult.

If ever there was a place for navigation-assisted component placement, then it is with the insertion of the acetabular component.

I used the BrainLab navigation system as an observational tool while inserting the Birmingham Hip Resurfacing cups. I would decide using traditional methods what the acetabular orientation should be, and the navigation was used merely to record the position of the acetabular component chosen (Fig. 24.48).

Table 24.1 shows rather disappointing differences between the measured inclination angle from the anteroposterior (AP) radiograph of the pelvis postoperatively and what the navigation apparatus recorded as the inclination angle during surgery. As can be seen, there was up to 12 degrees difference between the actual inclination angle measured from x-ray and what the navigation apparatus recorded as the inclination angle. I have heard it said that the measurement of cup inclination angles from plain x-ray is inaccurate. We have checked our x-ray measurements against those derived from CAD overlays. There is near perfect agreement. I had very simple requirements from this navigation apparatus. I was not interested in navigating the acetabular reamer, I could see this perfectly well. I was not interested in knowing about the center of rotation of the acetabulum, nor was I interested in knowing when the acetabular component was bottomed-out, as it is rare in my practice not to bottom-out the BHR cup. I was only interested in knowing exactly what the inclination and anteversion angles were of the component being inserted at surgery. It must be confessed that I am not very good

with computers, and each time that this apparatus was used, I had to have a team of engineers/helpers to assist with the navigation part of the operation. Given the extra time that navigation added to my surgery, my operating room staff were not sad to see me give this procedure up, when I discovered that the inclination angles recorded on the computer were incorrect.

It always did seem to me excessive that such a cumbersome, expensive, and time-consuming computerized apparatus was being used for such a simple task. The whole of the acetabular positioning with this computer depends on obtaining registration from the two anterior superior iliac spines and the symphysis pubis (Fig. 24.49).

TABLE. 24.1. BHR Acetabular Cup Inclination Angle

Name	Navigation Inclination Angle	Measured Actual Inclination Angle
Mr I.K.	44	45
Mr E.S.	36	46
Mr P.N.	49	38
Mr A.P.	39	37
Mr D.G.	27	39
Mr D.S.	42	43
Mr B.K.	40	37
Mr L.H.	27	34

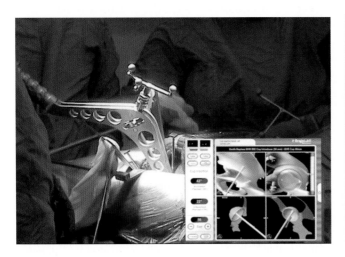

FIG. 24.48. Acetabular navigation being used to "measure" the author's cup position.

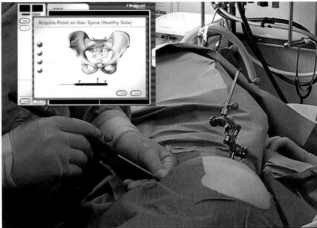

FIG. 24.49. Registration of pelvis.

When I gave up computerized navigation, I set about attempting to transfer the information from these three points into a positioning gadget for the acetabular component without the aid of a computer. The acetabular cup positioning system that we have devised, Lasernav™, is at an early stage of clinical development but is presented to show the principle involved with this means of assisting acetabular cup placement. The device consists of four subassemblies.

In the anesthesia room, the surgeon attaches the datum subassembly to the anterior-superior iliac spine using a self-tapping screw. A second screw is inserted for rotational stability. (Fig. 24.50). This is shown diagrammatically in Fig. 24.51.

The framework subassembly is then placed on the pelvis referencing the opposite anterior superior iliac spine and the symphysis pubis (Fig. 24.52). The datum subassembly is then locked in this adopted position capturing all necessary registration information.

The patient is moved into the lateral position for skin preparation and draping. In the operating room, the acetabulum is exposed and reamed, and at the trial cup stage Lasernav is used. The desired radiographic anteversion angle and the desired acetabular inclination angle are dialled into the reflector subassembly part of the instrument (Fig. 24.53).

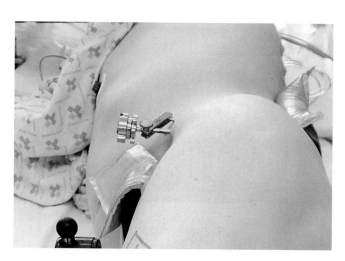

FIG. 24.50.

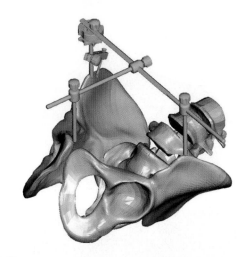

FIG. 24.52.

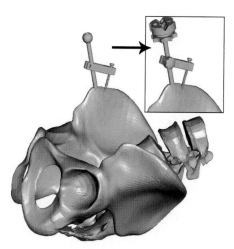

FIG. 24.51.

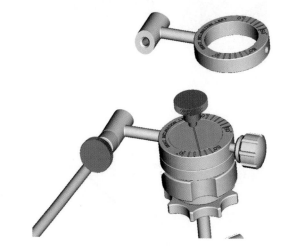

FIG. 24.53.

The reflector arm and the reflector itself are connected with magnetic couplings (Fig. 24.54).

The reflector, attached by a magnetic coupling to the reflector arm, is shown during surgery (Fig. 24.55). The reflector arm also has a magnetic coupling to the datum subassembly.

The laser light pen is inserted by an unsterile assistant into the sterile slot in the light source subassembly and locked with a sterile cover in position (Fig. 24.56).

The light source subassembly is then positioned on the acetabular cup introducer, and the orientation of the acetabular

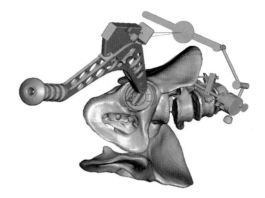

Fig. 24.57.

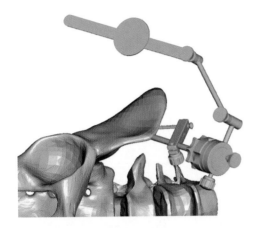

Fig. 24.54.

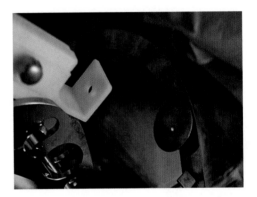

Fig. 24.58.

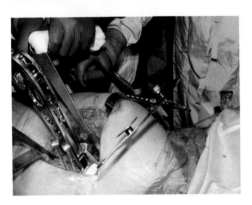

Fig. 24.55.

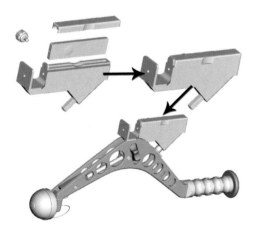

Fig. 24.56.

cup is altered until the laser light reflected beam is coincident with the exit beam (Fig. 24.57).

The reflector is shown with a red dot of laser light. The reflector is parallel to the desired cup face inclination and anteversion angles. The goal of the surgeon is to get the acetabular component positioned with the acetabular cup face parallel to the reflector. To do this, the reflected laser light has to be coincident with the exit beam of laser light. In Fig. 24.58, the dot of the reflected laser light is seen just to the side of the laser beam exit hole. This means that the cup is not quite in the perfect position and needs minor alteration.

My experience with this device is still very early, but it seems to have some advantages over computerized navigation. It uses the same reference points as computerized navigation but there is much less electronic wizardry to go wrong in the surgery. The only electronic failure possible with this device is that the disposable laser light pen fails to work. In these circumstances, one further dollar will have to be spent using a second laser pen.

References

1. Murray DW. The definition and measurement of acetabular orientation. J Bone Joint Surg Br 1993;75:228–32.

25
Management of Complex Anatomy

Joseph Daniel, Chandra Pradhan, Hena Ziaee, and Derek J.W. McMinn

Hip Dysplasia

Traditionally, there have been attempts to classify hip instability into two distinct entities (i.e., congenital and developmental). This distinction is rather poorly defined, and instability of the hip due to acetabular insufficiency presents as a broad spectrum of conditions with varying severity. Crowe et al. [1] classify dysplastic hips into four grades on the basis of proximal displacement of the femoral head. In grade I, the femoral head is displaced by a distance that is equivalent to 50% of its diameter. In grades II, III, and IV, the displacement is 50% to 75%, 75% to 100%, and greater than 100% of the femoral head, respectively. Hartofilakidis et al. [2] classify dysplasia into three types: (a) dysplasia, in which the socket is shallow but the femoral head is contained within the original true acetabulum, (b) low dislocation, in which the femoral head articulates with a false acetabulum, which is distinct from the true acetabulum but overlaps it, and (c) high dislocation, in which there is no contact between the true and the false acetabulum.

Sir John Charnley initially warned against the use of arthroplasty in severe hip dysplasia and stated that the policy in Wrightington in 1973 was "not to attempt the operational reconstruction of late cases of … congenital dislocation of the hip" [3]. However, with the advances made in bearing materials and device fixation today, hip arthroplasty is being successfully used to manage hip arthritis secondary to severe dysplasia.

Dysplasia Before the Development of Severe Hip Arthritis

Hip-preserving options such as realignment osteotomies of the acetabulum and/or femur (Figs. 25.1 and 25.2) are an option in symptomatic dysplastic hips in young patients before the development of arthritic change. By redistributing the load on the hip over a wider area, it is possible to delay or prevent the development of arthritic change or the need to replace the hip. Furthermore, if a resurfacing or replacement should become necessary at a later stage, a well-aligned socket and proximal femur, and well-distributed load-bearing

through the hip over the years, retain better anatomy and bone quality. This augurs well for a successful outcome with a resurfacing or a replacement.

However, it is important that these osteotomies are performed after accurate preoperative imaging and assessment to determine the optimum reconstruction that will restore anatomy around the hip. We have encountered a number of patients with dysplasia who had undergone "shelf procedures" of different varieties in the past, performed in the hope of providing better weight-bearing containment of the femoral head. We find that invariably the "shelf" is always located a distance above and anterior to the true acetabulum, and when the time for hip arthroplasty comes, the shelf does not support the acetabular component. In fact, we have on several occasions had to resect a shelf at hip arthroplasty to solve the problem of extraarticular impingement.

Dysplasia with Arthritis (Preoperative Considerations)

Total dislocations (Crowe grade IV and Hartofilakidis' high dislocation type) are not suitable for a resurfacing because the true acetabulum is too small. Either the acetabulum would need to be overreamed or a very small femoral component would be needed, and both options are unacceptable. A total hip replacement (THR) with a head diameter that is best suited for the individual hip is a more acceptable solution (Fig. 25.3). Furthermore, Crowe IV hips are known to be asymptomatic until later in life, as the articulating hip surfaces are not subjected to the weight-bearing stresses in the same manner as in a regular or a subluxing hip.

At the other extreme, mild to moderate insufficiencies of the acetabulum (Crowe I and less severe forms of Crowe II) can be managed with a small shift in the placement of a regular resurfacing cup either medially or proximally. In comparison, the dislocating/subluxing hips seen in the more severe forms of Crowe grade II and all Crowe III dysplasias provide too little socket coverage for primary fixation stability with a regular acetabular component (Fig. 25.4). They are better developed

333

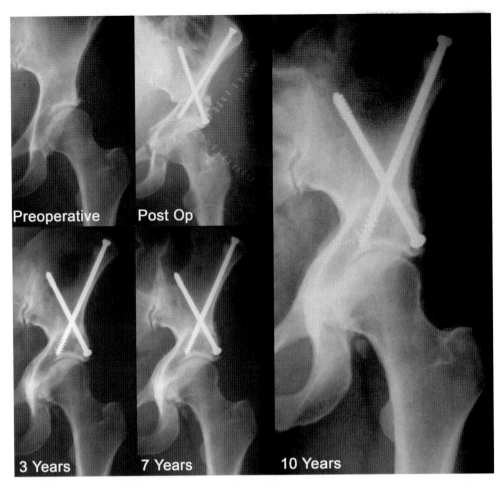

FIG. 25.1. A painful dysplastic hip in a 47-year-old woman. Her radiographic series at 3, 7, and 10 years shows the improved coverage of the hip after the osteotomy and internal fixation. She has been able to return to all her regular activities and no recurrence of symptoms. Ten years after her initial symptoms had started, there is no evidence of an arthritic change. If the hip turns arthritic subsequently, the improved anatomy is better suited for cup fixation.

than the dislocated Crowe IV hips and have bony anatomy that lends itself to a resurfacing procedure. If the surgeon attempts to use a regular cup in such severe acetabular insufficiency, he is often tempted to overream the socket. Furthermore, in order to obtain sufficient bony coverage, the regular cup may have to be left relatively open leading to instability, impingement, and edge wear. This is made worse by a valgus femoral neck, which often accompanies developmental dysplasia and necessitates cup placement in a more closed position than is required with a regular neck-shaft angle. It is for such hips that the Dysplasia Birmingham Hip Resurfacing (BHR) component was developed (Fig. 25.5).

A subluxing hip poses several other technical problems too. The stiletto-type loading of the subluxing femoral head on the edge of the socket leads to stress-shielding of the lateral half of the femoral head and the medial portion of the socket, which then turns osteopenic (Figs. 25.6 and 25.7). If this osteopenic change is severe, the risk of femoral head collapse is increased. Although preoperative imaging is useful in this

assessment, it is not always conclusive. A careful reevaluation at operation may be needed, and the patient must be warned preoperatively of the possibility of an intraoperative conversion to a Birmingham Mid Head Resection (BMHR) device or a THR if the situation demands.

Dysplastic hips are often associated with severe leg length discrepancies, excess femoral neck valgus, and/or anteversion (Fig. 25.8). These are not always easy to correct with a resurfacing. In relation to equalizing leg length, restoring the hip center of rotation to its original position adds true length. Correction of preoperative fixed deformities and improved range of motion after the procedure reduce apparent length discrepancy.

It is important that femoral anteversion is assessed carefully preoperatively. If there is a suspicion that this is excessive, a computed tomography (CT) scan assessment is useful. Minor abnormalities of femoral version can be compensated for by implanting the socket in a less anteverted position. If femoral anteversion is in excess of 45 degrees, a femoral derotation

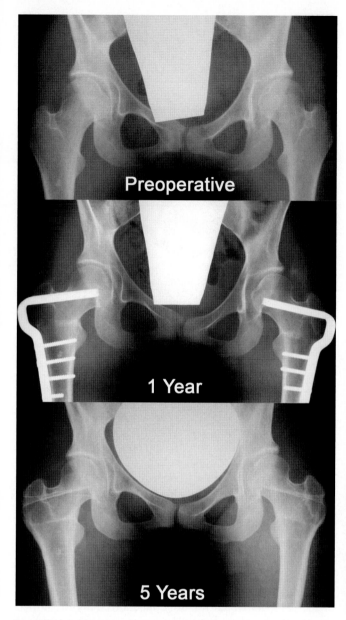

FIG. 25.2. A 20-year-old woman presented with a 3-year history of progressively worsening pain in her hips especially on weight-bearing activities. Her radiographs show coxa valga with poor superior femoral head cover, resulting in abnormal load concentration. She underwent bilateral femoral realignment (varus and derotation) osteotomies followed by removal of implants after osteotomy union. Sixteen years after the first operation, she has had no recurrence of symptoms, thereby delaying and possibly averting the need for an arthroplasty procedure.

osteotomy is required along with hip resurfacing (Fig. 25.8). However, rehabilitation after a combined osteotomy plus resurfacing procedure is very slow and arduous and is only a reasonable procedure in young, fit patients. In older patients, a total hip replacement with correction of excess femoral neck anteversion is a better procedure. If excess anteversion is suspected, we always perform a CT scan assessment preoperatively and discuss carefully the risks and benefits of

resurfacing versus THR with the patient before proceeding with further planning.

Some of these patients have been through one or more childhood hip operations (Fig. 25.9) altering the bony anatomy around the hip (and sometimes damaging the soft tissues as well). Appropriate imaging studies will be necessary in order to plan the reconstruction and restore the anatomy to nearly normal.

Finally, patients with dysplasia are often young and of childbearing age. Blood metal ion levels are elevated in patients with metal on metal (MM) devices and in those with conventional devices as seen in Chapter 13. Cobalt and chromium are essential to the mother and to the developing fetus and these ions pass through from the mother to the fetal circulation in everyone. Current knowledge indicates that in those with elevated metal ion levels, the placenta exerts a modulatory effect on metal transfer and withholds a significant portion of the excess from being passed on to the fetus. However, it is not known for certain whether the raised metal ion levels have

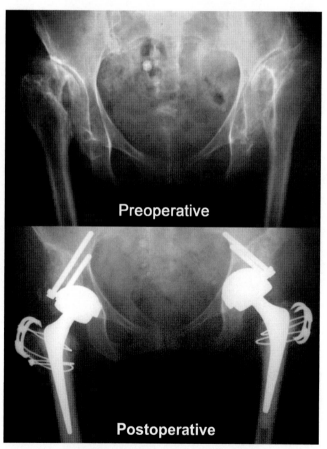

FIG. 25.3. This 63-year-old woman with bilateral congenital dislocation of hips (CDH) had operations on both hips at the age of 18 months. She walked with a limp and suffered from backache but remained pain-free in the hips until a few years ago as is typical in patients with Crowe IV dysplasia. The acetabulum in such patients is too poorly developed to accommodate a resurfacing femoral head. She underwent primary total hip arthroplasties with dysplasia cups, supplementary screws, and bone grafting.

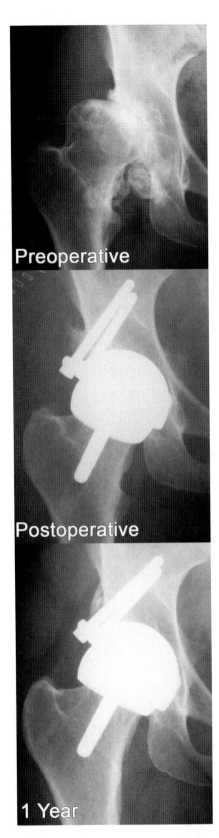

Fig. 25.4. Preoperative, postoperative, and follow-up radiographs of a 38-year-old woman with developmental dysplasia and severe arthritis treated with a dysplasia BHR and bone grafting.

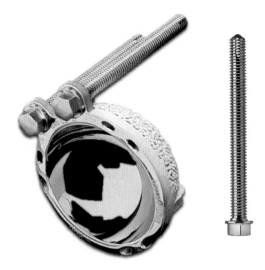

Fig. 25.5. The Dysplasia BHR socket and screws

an effect on the unborn child. We always inform women in child-bearing age about elevated metal levels and discuss options as outlined in Chapter 13.

BHR in Mild to Moderate Dysplasia (Manageable with a Regular BHR Cup)

Mild to moderate insufficiencies of the acetabulum can be managed with a regular resurfacing cup. A small medial or proximal shift in its placement often provides sufficient cover for stable primary fixation. The medial wall of the dysplastic acetabulum is often hypertrophied. The socket can be safely and effectively deepened and shifted proximally in order to get adequate coverage.

The technique to implant a regular BHR cup in the treatment of mild to moderate insufficiency is similar to that described in Chapter 20. Preoperative templating is used to determine the desired position of cup implantation in terms of the depth to which it can be medialized and/or shifted proximally (see Fig. 25.8). We clear the medial osteophyte in the socket adequately to clearly visualize the tear drop and the true acetabular floor, and use that as a guide to control medialization of the cup. Deepening is performed starting with a small-diameter reamer and progressively advancing, without widening, to the predetermined level. Repeated checking of the reamed depth is essential to avoid overshooting the true floor of the socket. Once the necessary depth is reached, gradual widening of the socket is undertaken. The size of component that can be inserted into a dysplastic acetabulum is limited by the front to back dimension of the bony acetabulum. The surgeon must judge carefully the largest safe size of reamer that can be used, and if that does not allow a cup with a corresponding femoral size to clear the femoral neck, then a THR must be performed. Care must be taken not to ream away the anterior acetabular wall, which is often deficient and poorly developed.

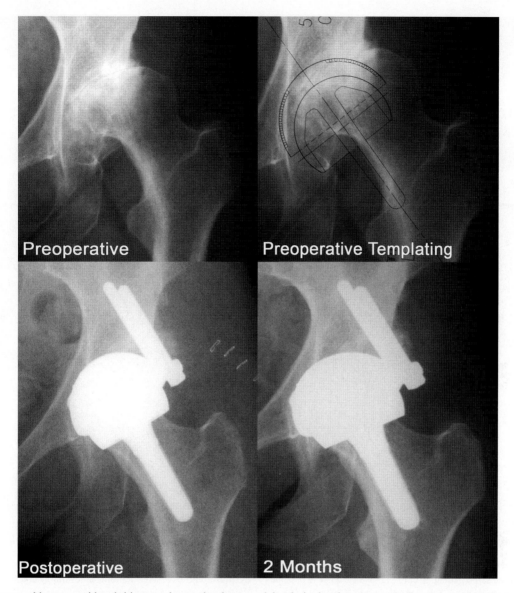

FIG. 25.6. A 52-year-old woman with arthritis secondary to developmental dysplasia showing osteopenia due to stress-shielding in the lateral part of the femoral head. She agreed to proceed with an exploration of the hip and, depending on bone quality found at operation, receive a BHR, a BMHR prosthesis, or a stemmed THR. At operation there was cystic change in the femoral head, and the bone quality in the osteopenic area of the bone was too poor to be suitable for a BHR. A BMHR was performed on her with a matching Dysplasia cup.

Reamers need to be biased posteriorly so that the thickened posterior acetabular wall is reamed and the thin anterior wall is preserved.

It is also important that femoral neck anteversion is assessed before embarking on acetabular component positioning. Minor abnormalities of femoral anteversion can be compensated for by implanting the socket in a less anteverted position. If the sum total of femoral neck anteversion and acetabular component anteversion is more than 45 degrees, a femoral derotation osteotomy is required along with the hip resurfacing.

After reaming to the desired diameter, the trial cup is inserted before making the final decision whether to use a regular or a Dysplasia cup. The stability of the trial component is assessed using the introducer handle. The extent of the unsupported cup is measured with a depth gauge from the edge of the component to the margin of the available bony coverage at the deepest point. Trial cup stability and the depth of unsupported cup are the factors on which the decision to use a regular or a Dysplasia cup has to be based. As a rough guideline, if the uncovering is more than 10 mm, one should consider carefully if stable primary fixation is possible with a regular cup. The senior author has, on some occasions, used a regular cup with more than 15 mm of lateral uncovering, but those were specific cases where excellent fixation was possible with the regular cup in patients with very good bone quality.

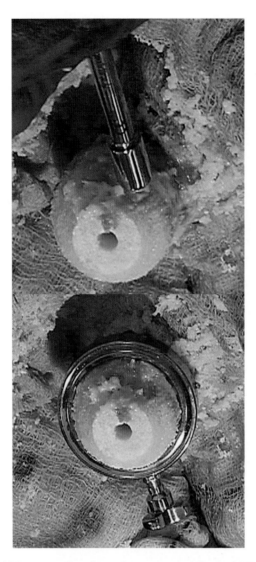

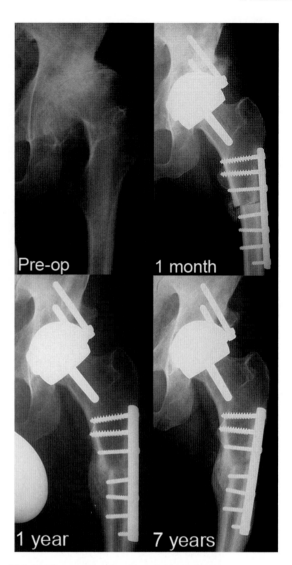

FIG. 25.7 Intraoperative views after preparation for the BHR of the femoral head of the same patient as in Fig. 25.6 showing the osteopenic bone in the femoral head. The BMHR napkin ring is in position, and the osteopenic superolateral femoral head bone is then resected.

FIG. 25.8. A 50-year-old man with arthritis secondary to developmental dysplasia and excessive femoral anteversion underwent a dysplasia BHR along with a femoral derotation osteotomy with autograft from the socket reamings placed at the osteotomy site. The osteotomy restored Shenton's line and improved the offset. His osteotomy progressed to union, and he has returned to an active lifestyle. Seven years on, he has had no problem with his hip.

BHR in Severe Acetabular Insufficiency (Managed with a Dysplasia Cup)

Several strategies for cup stabilization have been described in total hip arthroplasty for severe acetabular insufficiency. Good results have been reported with controlled medialization. In this technique the medial wall of the pelvis is fractured with a gouge [4] or deepened [5], and the cup is implanted with its medial aspect lying medial to the ilioischial Kohler's line. Encouraging early results have also been reported with supplementary block allograft fixed with bolts and nuts [6]. However, the 12-year results with this technique were not encouraging [7]. Morcellized graft with a metal mesh, reinforcement rings, or different combinations of the above have all been advocated in the past with varying degrees of clinical success. Kobayashi et al. [8] showed excellent results with a compromise combination of block bone graft

and proximal cup placement in order to obtain coverage of the most proximal point (apex) of the socket by the ilium. However, they advice this procedure only in patients over the age of 48 years, socket coverage of at least 50%, and restricted physical activity later on.

With a regular THR cementless acetabular component, screw fixation is used in the metal cup where bony support is available. Because socket floor screws are not an option with a resurfacing cup, the dysplasia resurfacing component was devised with offset screws. The Dysplasia cup is an adjunct to the BHR system and consists of a BHR cup fitted with two threaded lugs for screw fixation as already shown in fig. 25.5. The socket deficiency is filled with morcellized bone graft, which is held in place with Surgicel (Ethicon, Livingston, UK) and suture. The screws obtain purchase into sclerotic bone in

FIG 25.9 (A) This 21-year-old woman presented with a history of having had hip problems from bilateral CDH. She underwent open reduction at the age of 18 months followed later by pelvic osteotomy/shelf operations. A repeat left femoral osteotomy was performed at around 9 years of age. (B) Templating shows the cup being restored closer to the true hip center than the current position of the false acetabulum and the extent to which deepening of the socket can be performed to reach the true floor. This adds stability to the cup and helps leg length equalization. The wide and curved femoral canal from the previous osteotomy makes it very awkward for the implantation of a THR stem. (C) A dysplasia BHR implanted at the site of the true hip center led to equalization of leg lengths. Abductor tightness as seen from the severe pelvic tilt leads to transient apparent lengthening. The residual old shelf can be seen riding high and not adding any bony support to the cup. (D) A 2-year radiograph showing leg length equalization, good incorporation of the autograft above the socket, and gradual remodeling of the old shelf.

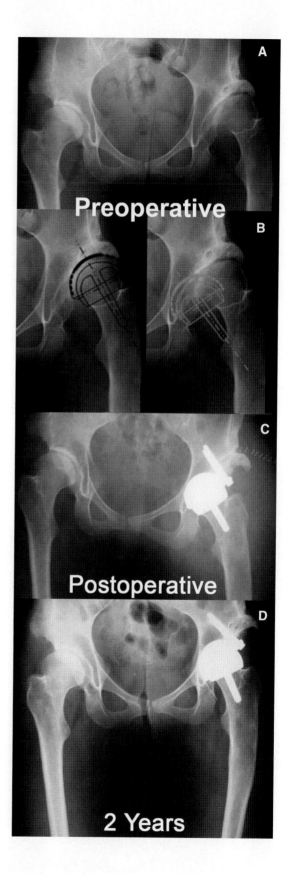

the false acetabulum rather than in the osteopenic acetabular roof. The cup articulates with a regular BHR femoral head component or the modular head of a stemmed THR or a BMHR device.

The need to use a Dysplasia cup (as opposed to a regular cup) is initially established on the basis of preoperative templating. If a significant portion of the cup is likely to remain uncovered by the bony socket, a dysplasia component may be needed.

The technique to implant a Dysplasia cup has been described in detail in Chapter 21. Once the decision to use a Dysplasia cup has been made, the false acetabulum is inspected to choose a good position for screw fixation. The lugs in the Dysplasia cup are rotated anteriorly toward it.

The two supplementary screws are self-tapping neutralization screws (see Fig. 25.5). The posterior screw is fixed first as described earlier (Chapter 21). When the screw reaches the surface of the prepared drill hole in the bone, further advancement is done slowly and with firm forward pressure applied on the screwdriver in order to allow the screw to tap its own threads and obtain purchase in the bone. The neutralization principle dictates that the screw will flip the cup out if it fails to engage the bone but continues to advance in the component. If this happens, the cup has to be removed and reloaded on to the introducer and impacted back into the socket before starting all over again. Only after both screws are securely fixed should the introducer wires be cut.

The femoral component is implanted as described in Chapter 22. After implantation, the wound is washed out thoroughly with pulsed lavage before proceeding to bone grafting the defect in the socket. The bony defect is denuded of soft tissue, freshened with appropriate curettes, and filled in with morcellized autograft as described in Chapter 21.

The hip is then reduced and tested for intraarticular and extraarticular impingement and stability by moving it through the full range of movement, including rotations. Equal ranges of internal and external rotations must be possible. Excess femoral anteversion severely restricts external rotation while allowing abnormally high internal rotation, in which case a subtrochanteric derotation osteotomy is necessary. The difference between the range of internal and external rotations is an approximate guide to the degree of derotation required.

340

J. Daniel et al.

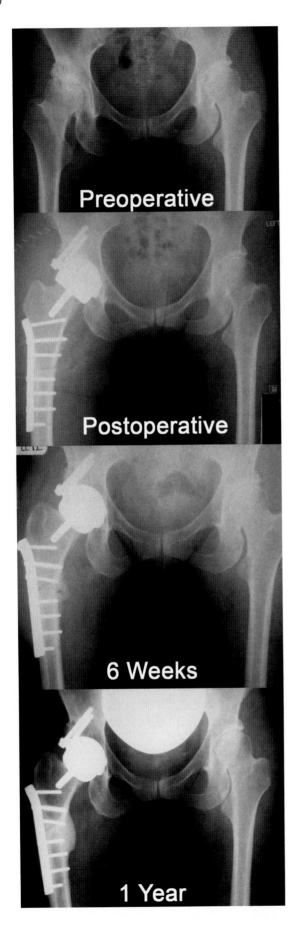

Preoperative

Postoperative

6 Weeks

1 Year

Fig. 25.10. A 39-year-old woman with developmental dysplasia and femoral anteversion underwent a dysplasia BHR with a femoral derotation osteotomy, which restored femoral offset and Shenton's line. She ignored the advice to mobilize non–weight bearing and returned to weight bearing too soon. At 6 weeks, she started experiencing pain, and radiographs showed angulation at the osteotomy site. She then started complying with the mobilization regimen. Her osteotomy united at 10 months albeit with an angulation.

Femoral Derotation Osteotomy

The incision is extended distally to access the lateral surface of the femur. For adequate fixation, we use a broad AO Dynamic compression plate (DCP) with a minimum of 7 holes. The plate is first contoured and held against the femur with appropriate clamps. The proximal part of the plate is then fixed with a provisional screw in the second-from-top screw hole. A longitudinal mark is made with a saw blade superficially on the surface of the femoral shaft across the site of the intended osteotomy below the level of the lesser trochanter. A transverse osteotomy is then performed at the predetermined level, and the fragments are rotated to the needed extent as read by the angle between the two halves of the mark. The distal fragment is fixed with screws applying compression at the osteotomy site. Fixation of the rest of the screws in the proximal fragment is then completed. The hip is retested for stability, impingement, and range of motion. Autograft from the reamings is applied around the osteotomy site before closure.

Patients who undergo an osteotomy are advised non–weight-bearing toe touch mobilization until osteotomy union. In our overall series of more than 197 Dysplasia BHRs, nine patients needed a combined resurfacing and femoral osteotomy. Of these, eight have progressed uneventfully to osteotomy union. One patient started weight-bearing mobilization before the recommended period and developed pain at the osteotomy site at 6 weeks follow-up (Fig. 25.10). X-rays showed that her femur had begun to angulate at the osteotomy site with the screws partially pulling out. Only after that did she start paying heed to our advice regarding strict adherence to the non–weight-bearing mobilization regimen. The osteotomy eventually united at 10 months albeit with a small medial angulation. She uses a small shoe raise but has since returned to her profession and to an active lifestyle, which includes regular workouts in the gym and cycling.

The Dysplasia cup along with its neutralization screws together transform the Dysplasia acetabular component into one solid composite three-dimensional construct, whose stability in any plane is a function of the area circumscribed by the cup and the screws as a whole. This allows the morcellized autograft filling the bony deficiency superolaterally to incorporate and consolidate without the fear of displacement during weight-bearing mobilization. The good primary stability of the dysplasia component construct allows patients to weight-bear from the first postoperative day.

An arthritic dysplastic hip remains a therapeutic challenge. In Chapter 27, we describe the results of a consecutive series of regular BHRs in mild to moderate dysplasia, from the Royal Orthopaedic Hospital and our experience with a Dysplasia

BHR, in a series of young, active patients with severe acetabular insufficiency. The absence of socket loosening in the series with the Dysplasia BHRs is very reassuring in terms of the reliability of the system. Furthermore, the excellent graft incorporation in the reconstructed socket will stand the patient in good stead should a subsequent revision become necessary later.

Summary

- Mild to moderate acetabular insufficiencies can be managed with a regular socket with a small medial and/or proximal shift of the hip center.
- Severe acetabular insufficiencies (Crowe grades II and III) often need the use of a Dysplasia BHR with supplementary screws for secure primary fixation stability.
- High dislocations (Crowe grade IV hips) are not suitable for a hip resurfacing because the acetabulum is too underdeveloped to accommodate a femoral head of a reasonable diameter without overreaming the socket.
- Beware of unnoticed excess femoral neck anteversion. This should be assessed preoperatively with computed tomography (CT) scanning if necessary as it may necessitate a concomitant femoral osteotomy. Osteotomy slows down recovery and rehabilitation considerably and should be discussed with the patients preoperatively.
- In the presence of osteopenic change in the stress-shielded lateral femoral head, counsel patients preoperatively about the possibility of an intraoperative conversion to a BMHR or a THR.

Perthes Disease

The active phase of Legg-Calvé-Perthes disease (LCPD), or idiopathic osteonecrosis of the capital femoral epiphysis, typically affects children before skeletal maturity and leads to femoral head deformation of varying severity. If the deformation is minimal and has occurred at an early age (before the age of 8 years), remodeling results in a near-spherical congruity between the opposing surfaces of the femur and acetabulum, thereby delaying or preventing secondary change in later life [9]. However, if the deformity is severe or has occurred closer to skeletal maturity, remodeling is ineffective and results in a flattened, mushroom-shaped femoral head, a short wide neck, and a secondary dysplastic acetabulum, all of which contribute to premature degenerative change.

Femoral osteotomies and acetabuloplasties have been described to improve hip function and containment of the femoral head before the development of severe arthritic changes. Once arthritic change develops, the only treatment that reliably improves function and quality of life is an arthroplasty.

Preoperative Considerations

In addition to providing pain-free movement and hip function, the goal in the management of post-Perthes secondary arthritis (as in any other pathology) is to restore the biomechanical parameters of the hip (such as neck shaft angle, femoral offset, and head-neck offset) to as near normal as possible, with the least possible intervention. We have seen good clinical results with the BHR in post-Perthes hip arthritis even though the radiographs do not look as good as those with regular osteoarthritis (Fig. 25.11). If necessary, the neck can be lengthened but to a limited extent with the BHR (Fig. 25.12). In order to achieve this, it is necessary to sculpt additional neck length out of the femoral head. The femoral component is then placed proud of the original medial head neck junction. We have performed this reconstruction with the BHR in the past, see Fig. 25.12, but it can be better achieved with a

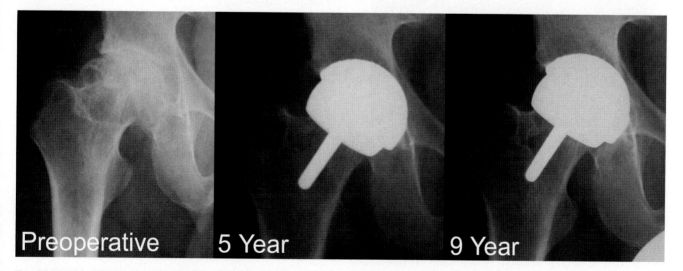

FIG. 25.11. This 53-year-old man had been treated for Perthes disease as a child aged 8 years, with 18 months in bed and traction, and a further 18 months in calipers. His preoperative radiograph shows signs of post-Perthes sequelae including a "sagging rope" sign. In addition, he has had regular anti-inflammatory medication for his pain. He was treated with a regular BHR and is pleased with his results 9 years on, but the femoral offset and neck length have remained undercorrected.

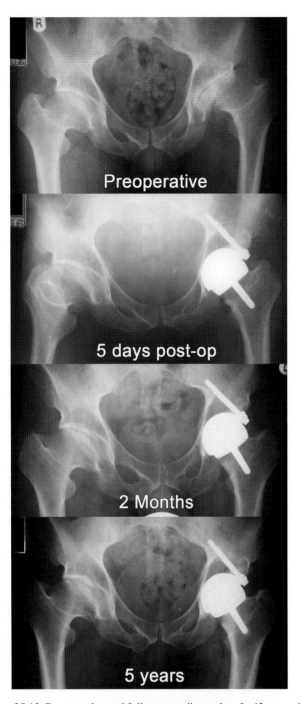

FIG. 25.12. Preoperative and follow-up radiographs of a 42-year-old man showing all the classic signs of severe post-Perthes sequelae bilaterally with symptomatic severe arthritis in his left hip and experiencing occasional twinges in his right hip. In addition to a distorted femoral head and neck, he had secondary acetabular dysplasia, which required the use of a Dysplasia cup. It was possible to add length to his femoral neck through femoral head sculpturing. He is pleased with his results 5 years on, and the re-created femoral neck shows evidence of corticalization. His right hip symptoms have eased off as well. He is a keen cyclist and on occasion cycles 100 miles at a stretch without any problem from either hip. He wishes to start jogging now.

BMHR device now (Figs. 25.13–25.15). The magnitude of anatomic correction possible with the BMHR is much greater than the correction achieved with a BHR.

It is easier to correct the proximal femoral anatomy with a stemmed THR, and this should be the option of choice in an older patient. However, the sequelae of a previous corrective osteotomy of the femur such as an angled or curved femoral shaft can make stem placement a problem. Furthermore, most post-Perthes patients are young and are likely to outlive their prosthetic device, hence the need to go conservative.

Sculpting the femoral head to provide this additional neck length exposes cancellous bone at the re-created medial head-neck junction, which eventually remodels and becomes cortical. The patient is therefore advised to restrict weight bearing in the early weeks. Loading is cautiously and progressively increased to allow time for the remodeling to occur. The slower rehabilitation and the possible need to intraoperatively convert to a BMHR or even a THR if required should be discussed with the patient at the consultation.

Operative Technique

The large mushroom-shaped femoral head and the dysplastic socket require the use of a generously large incision and approach. The femoral neck should be carefully defined by trimming all the osteophytes as templating and guide-wire placement will need to be centered on the true femoral neck rather than neck plus osteophyte. It is sometimes necessary to first debulk the mushroom-shaped femoral head using the jig, stylus, guide wire and bar, and cylindrical cutter in order to gain access to the acetabulum. It may also be necessary to trim the edges of the head to allow the stylus to move freely in the first instance.

After the cup is implanted, the final preparation and implantation of the femoral component are undertaken. The shape of the femoral head has the potential to disorientate the surgeon while determining the point of entry of the guide wire. Guide-wire placement should be based solely in relation to the femoral neck as determined by the jig and not based on the shape of the femoral head.

If there is no need to add length to the femoral neck, the reference point for the transverse cut of the femoral head is the medial head-neck junction (HNJ) as always. The lower end of the napkin ring is advanced until the medial HNJ and the rest of the procedure continues as described in Chapter 22. If the neck is foreshortened, then the lower end of the napkin ring is allowed to stay proud of the medial HNJ. The extent to which this is done depends on the required increase of neck length as determined by preoperative measurements and templating. In most cases, nothing but the bare minimum skimming of the femoral head summit is allowed. When the neck needs substantial lengthening, as seen in Figs. 25.14 and 25.15, we

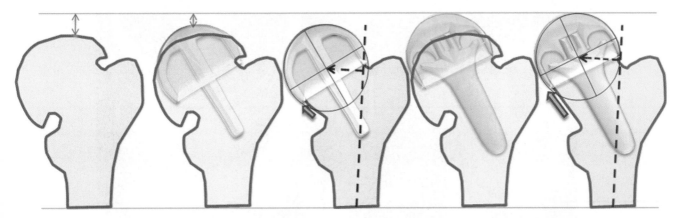

FIG. 25.13. It is possible to gain some neck length (blue arrows) and leg length (red arrows) with the BHR. However, in such severe cases we now routinely use a BMHR device in order to provide a greater advantage in both these parameters and a beneficial effect with femoral offset (interrupted lines).

FIG. 25.14. This 40-year-old man with post-Perthes secondary arthritis had 2-cm shortening of his left leg. His postoperative and 2-month follow-up radiographs show good neck reconstruction and leg length equalization made possible with the BMHR prosthesis. The BMHR offers much more scope to restore proximal femoral anatomy than what is possible with a resurfacing.

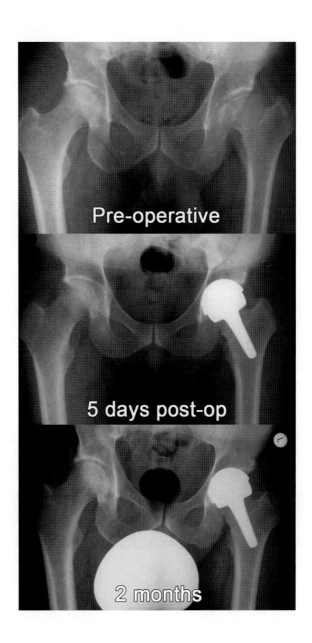

use the BMHR device for better reconstruction of the proximal femoral anatomy and improved hip function and range of motion. We have used the BMHR in four cases of post-Perthes secondary arthritis with excellent reconstruction of the femoral head and neck. The patients have been perfectly satisfied with the results. It must be stated that our experience with the BMHR in complex anatomy is still early. However, it is very appealing to be able to achieve a good anatomic restoration and stay conservative in these young patients. With full informed consent of the patient, we believe this approach is reasonable.

Summary

- The wide foreshortened femoral neck, wide flattened femoral head, reduced offset and neck length, and the dysplastic socket present special difficulties in restoring anatomy in post-Perthes patients who need a resurfacing.
- Careful measurements and preoperative templating are essential to plan the procedure.
- It is preferable to convert to a BMHR or a THR and restore the anatomy rather than settle for a compromised outcome with a BHR. This need for an intraoperative conversion and the possibility of delayed weight bearing should be discussed with the patient at the consultation.

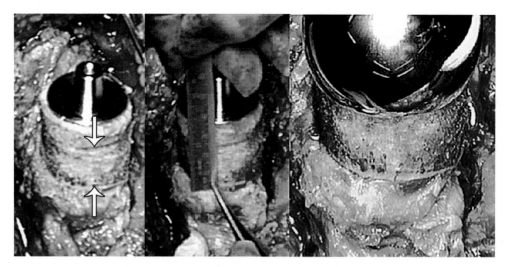

FIG. 25.15. Intraoperative view showing the additional neck sculptured out of the erstwhile femoral head. The arrows indicate the original head-neck junction and the marked position of the new head-neck junction to give a 2-cm neck lengthening in this patient.

Slipped Capital Femoral Epiphysis

The prevalence of slipped capital femoral epiphysis (SCFE) as a primary pathology leading on to degenerative arthritis has been variously estimated as between 5% and 40% of those presenting with early primary osteoarthritis. Some of these cases are minor slips and pose no difficulty in doing a resurfacing procedure. Slightly more severe slips can be effectively treated using a regular BHR with careful minor adjustments (Fig. 25.16). However, severe cases of SCFE present a really awkward situation for a good outcome with a resurfacing (Fig. 25.17).

The anterosuperior deficiency in the femoral head can give insufficient peripheral support for the femoral component preventing its correct placement and alignment. In order to obtain support, the component will have to be shifted to an eccentric position posteroinferiorly or tilted posteriorly and into varus. Both these situations result in compromised anterior head-neck offset leading to impingement in flexion and are unacceptable. Sometimes, the deficiency will have to be built up with excess cement, which is also undesirable. Furthermore, there is significant femoral neck retroversion, which adds to the problem of anterior impingement necessitating excess acetabular

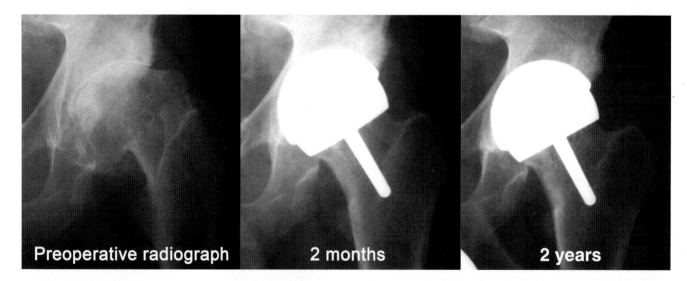

Preoperative radiograph   2 months   2 years

FIG. 25.16. The preoperative, 2-month, and 2-year radiographs of a 50-year-old man who suffered from SCFE during adolescence for which he underwent *in situ* pinning at the age of 16 years, followed by pin removal a year later. Although the femoral head was inadequate anterosuperiorly, there was just enough peripheral support for the femoral component to be placed in an ideal position. When the femoral head can be safely implanted in the optimal position, then a BHR provides a good conservative alternative to total hip replacement.

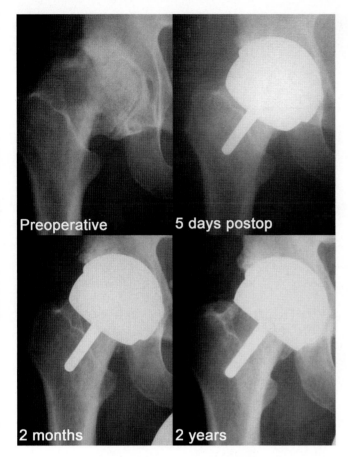

FIG. 25.17. Radiographic series of a 50-year-old man who suffered from SCFE during adolescence. The anterosuperior inadequacy in his femoral head was compounded by the presence of cysts in the substance of the femoral head. At surgery, a varus position with poor restoration of anterosuperior head-neck offset had to be accepted in order to obtain peripheral support for the BHR femoral component. This situation can lead to reduced head-neck offset and result in anterior impingement. At follow-up, the patient reported that he has been doing fine. Nowadays, however, we prefer to use the BMHR prosthesis to get a better anatomic restoration.

anteversion in order to compensate. The femoral neck is often foreshortened leading to compromised abductor offset and unequal leg lengths. In severe cases, especially where reduction procedures have been attempted during adolescence, femoral head avascular necrosis (AVN) may be an associated feature but lies unrecognized in view of the other overbearing features.

In such cases, it is better to convert to a device such as a BMHR prosthesis or even a total hip replacement and correct these inadequacies better, rather than persist in performing

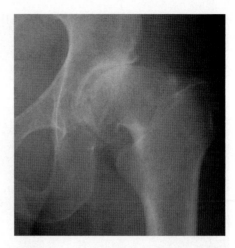

FIG. 25.18. Preoperative radiographs of a 38-year-old man who suffered from SCFE during adolescence for which he underwent autograft epiphysiodesis at the age of 14 years. He went on to develop severe arthritic change. On CT scan, the femoral neck and head showed a relative retroversion of 10 degrees.

a resurfacing in a suboptimal position. We have found that a BMHR (Figs. 25.18–25.20) is extremely useful, allowing better reconstruction of proximal femoral anatomy, which is critical for a successful long-term outcome. The BMHR does not rely on the deficient femoral head. It obtains its support from the interior of the head-neck junction, which is unaffected however severe the slip. It can be used safely in the presence of AVN because the resection line runs distal to the avascular zone. The BMHR does not need to be placed eccentrically or in varus in order to obtain support. Neck length can also be added as described in the section on Perthes disease.

Summary

- Less severe forms of SCFE can be managed effectively with a BHR.
- Severe forms of SCFE presents particular difficulties. The anterosuperior deficiency in the femoral head often falls short of providing the essential 360-degree peripheral support leading the surgeon to misplace or misalign the femoral component and result in poor head-neck offset.
- Accurate preoperative assessment of these factors and the possible need to use a BMHR should be discussed with the patient.
- It is better to convert to a BMHR or even a THR rather than compromise with a poor anatomic restoration using the BHR.

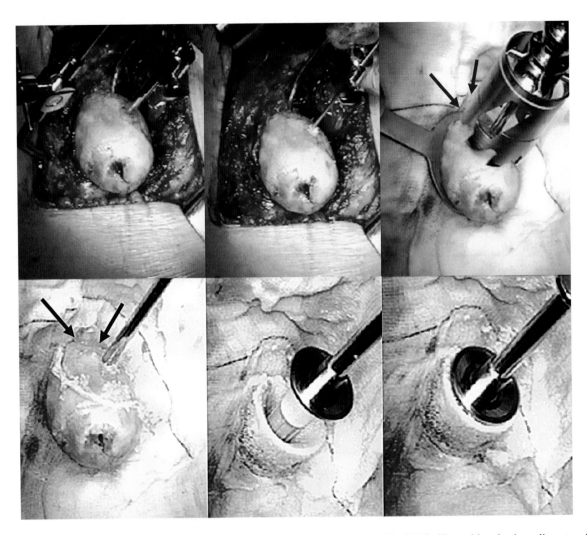

FIG. 25.19. Intra-operative views of femoral head preparation in the same patient as in Fig 25.18. The guide wire is well-centered on the femoral neck but gives the appearance of being very eccentrically placed on the femoral head. The pathology (SCFE) creates a femoral head deficiency anterosuperiorly (arrows). A resurfacing femoral component would therefore not receive adequate anterosuperior peripheral support in a case like this. Shifting the femoral component into an eccentric position or tilting it into varus is an unacceptable compromise. The BMHR stem can be effectively used in such a situation, since it receives support from the interior of the femoral head and head-neck junction rather than the periphery of the femoral head.

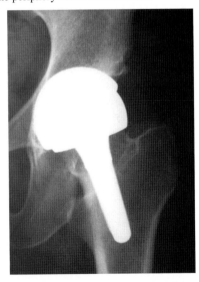

FIG. 25.20. Follow-up radiograph of the same patient as in Figs. 25.18 and 25.19 showing the neck lengthening achieved.

References

1. Crowe JF, Mani VJ, Ranawat CS. Total hip replacement in congenital dislocation and dysplasia of the hip. J Bone Joint Surg Am 1979;61:15–23.
2. Hartofilakidis G, Stamos K, Karachalios T, Ioannidis TT, Zacharakis N. Congenital hip disease in adults. Classification of acetabular deficiencies and operative treatment with acetabuloplasty combined with total hip arthroplasty. J Bone Joint Surg Am 1996;78:683–92.
3. Charnley J, Feagin JA. Low-friction arthroplasty in congenital subluxation of the hip. Clin Orthop 1973; 91:98–113.
4. Hess WE, Umber JS. Total hip arthroplasty in chronically dislocated hips. Follow-up study on the protrusio socket technique. J Bone Joint Surg Am 1978;60:948–54.
5. Dorr LD, Tawakkol S, Moorthy M, Long W, Wan Z. Medial protrusio technique for placement of a porous-coated, hemispherical acetabular component without cement in a total hip arthroplasty in patients who have acetabular dysplasia. J Bone Joint Surg Am 1999;81:83–92.

6. Harris WH, Crothers O, Oh I. Total hip replacement and femoral-head bone-grafting for severe acetabular deficiency in adults. J Bone Joint Surg Am 1977;59:752–9.

7. Jasty M, Anderson MJ, Harris WH. Total hip replacement for developmental dysplasia of the hip. Clin Orthop Relat Res 1995;311:40–5.

8. Kobayashi S, Saito N, Nawata M, Horiuchi H, Iorio R, Takaoka K. Total hip arthroplasty with bulk femoral head autograft for acetabular reconstruction in developmental dysplasia of the hip. J Bone Joint Surg Am 2003;85:615–21.

9. Herring JA, Kim HT, Browne R. Legg-Calve-Perthes disease. Part II: prospective multicenter study of the effect of treatment on outcome. J Bone Joint Surg Am 2004;86:2121–34.

26
Outcomes and Standards for Hip Resurfacing

Callum W. McBryde and Paul B. Pynsent

Introduction

Only in the past decade has the routine use of outcome instruments been introduced into orthopedic practice. Early arthroplasty literature was dominated by actuarial survival analysis and the outcome instruments of Harris [1] and Charnley [2] hip scores. These latter two traditional approaches to outcome required both signs and symptoms to be measured, thus when regular follow-up was required, these instruments imposed a large burden on clinical and hence financial resources. The emphasis has now moved to the design of patient self-reporting questionnaires, which are much more practical to implement. This is a reasonable approach as a patient presents with symptoms and the "healing physician" is expected to relieve these symptoms.

Results given in this chapter are extracted from the Royal Orthopaedic Hospital's audit database. This comprises a MySQL database running on an Apple file server connected to the hospital's intranet. In addition to outcomes, the database stores related information such as patient demographics and operative details. The system also incorporates software for automatically uploading the required subset of the information to the National Joint Registry [3]. Results have been extracted from the database and analyzed using the R statistical package [4]. Interquartile ranges (iqr) are expressed as ranges between limits rather than the absolute differences to emphasize asymmetry about the median. Where 95% confidence intervals have been quoted, the abbreviation c.i. is used.

Outcomes from hip arthroplasty can be broadly divided into five groups:

1. Signs and investigations (e.g., range of movement, radiographs).
2. Complications: These can be divided into systemic, such as DVT, and local, for example wound infection (Chapter 28).
3. Component survival: Examples of these outcomes are also considered in Chapter 27 of this book.
4. Various other nonanatomic measurements such as health status and satisfaction.
5. Symptoms.

Only the last three groups will be considered in this chapter.

Component Survival

The primary question in both the surgeon's and the patient's mind is, how long will my resurfacing last? Thus survival analysis dominates the arthroplasty outcome literature including the early metal on metal total hip arthroplasties [5] to the current resurfacing devices [6]. Figure 26.1 shows the results of a survival analysis of resurfacing procedures from our database over a 9-year period. Notice the importance of providing confidence intervals. There are several methods of calculating these, and it is always useful to indicate the method to the reader as the different methods do return very different values. The hazard rate is not generally constant for arthroplastic hip surgery so that nonparametric methods, usually the Kaplan-Meier, are used to estimate the survival function. The log-rank test is a nonparametric method that can be used to test if survival curves are identical. However, the Cox proportional hazards method may be preferred, as this allows several variables to be modeled; these variables can be continuous or discrete and even time-dependent themselves, thus giving greater flexibility in modeling an analysis. This method is actually equivalent to a regression analysis with the assumption that the log-hazard is linear, thus diagnostics and checks on the residuals for the Cox model should be made. Details of survival methods can be found in most medical statistics books (e.g., [7]), although one may have to dig a bit deeper to find help on diagnostics for the Cox model (e.g., [8]).

Health Status

Health status together with comorbidities may have an important influence on outcome. Health status instruments are sometimes termed *quality of life measures*. Although, in our minds, there may be a distinction between these terms, the distinction does not exist in the literature. It is worth reminding the reader that the WHO definition of health is "health is a state of complete physical, mental and social well-being and not merely the absence of disease or infirmity" [9]. There

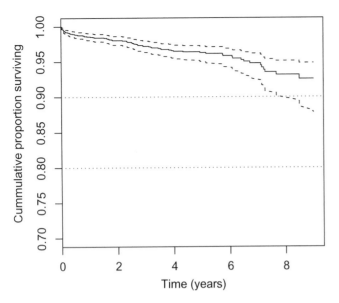

FIG. 26.1. A Kaplan-Meier survival plot of resurfacing arthroplasty at our institution. The confidence limits (dashed lines) have been calculated using the Peto method.

TABLE 26.1. The question stems for the COOP health status questionnaire.

Q1. During the past 4 weeks, what was the most strenuous level of physical activity you could do for at least 2 minutes?

Q2. During the past 4 weeks, how much have you been bothered by emotional problems, such as feeling unhappy, anxious, depressed, or irritable?

Q3. During the past 4 weeks, how much difficulty did you have doing your daily work, both inside and outside the house, because of your physical health or emotional problems.

Q4. During the past 4 weeks, to what extent has your physical health or emotional problems interfered with your normal social activities with family, friends, neighbors, or groups?

Q5. During the past 4 weeks, how much bodily pain have you generally had?

Q6. How much would you rate your physical health and emotional condition now compared with 4 weeks ago?

Q7. During the past 4 weeks, how would you rate your overall physical health and emotional condition?

Q8. During the past 4 weeks, was someone available to help you if you needed and wanted help?

Q9. How has the quality of your life been during the last 4 weeks? (that is, how have things been going for you?)

are many instruments available to assess health status. Some of these, such as the Short Form-36 (SF-36) [10], are inappropriate for standard auditing of elective orthopedic treatments, as the depth of questioning puts an unnecessary burden on the patient. There should be a specified need for such a precision assessment of health to justify concomitant imposition on the patient.

For many years, our hospital has been using the COOP health status instrument [11] and more recently the COOP/WONCA scale [12]. (Reproduced with kind permission of the Trustees of Dartmouth College/Dartmouth COOP Project.) The COOP chart comprises nine questions (Table 26.1) with a time span of 4 weeks. The dimensions of health status measured are physical, emotional, daily activities, social activities, social support, pain, and overall health. The COOP/WONCA score reduced the number of questions to six, omitting questions 5, 8, and 9 and reduced the "capture" time period to 2 weeks together with some slight modifications to the question wording. Both scores comprise a 5-point response scale with 1 representing the best and 5 the worst level. In clinical use, the instruments do not have an index but each question taps a health dimension and is scored individually. The results of this instrument applied to patients with hip resurfacing and total hip arthroplasty are shown in Fig. 26.2 for the six COOP questions that are equivalent to the COOP/WONCA charts. However, although this method is useful in a clinical setting where the physician can quickly scan the individual responses and be concerned for any score above three, this is not a particularly manageable method in the research setting. Indeed, finding published data with each question scored individually has proved very difficult. Van Weel [13] suggested that the scores could be summed

for research purposes. This approach allows us to compare the preoperative health status of patients within our institution for total hip and resurfaced hip arthroplasties against the status for the population and other diseases (Table 26.2). The instrument suggests that, preoperatively, our hip groups have the worst health status of those compared, even those on palliative chemotherapy.

Disability Outcomes

The WHO has defined disability as "the functional limitation caused by an impairment, which interferes with something a patient wishes to or must achieve" [14], and this is the concept we use here. In particular, we produce results using the Oxford Hip Score (OHS) [15], which is freely available and meets the psychometric requirements for such an instrument [16]. The higher the Oxford Hip Questionnaire scores, the greater the disability. Each question has a stem and five graded alternatives that are scored from 1 to5 in the original paper. Throughout, we have adopted the scoring system proposed by Pynsent et al. [17] for the OHS, where the scores are presented as a percentage of the questions answered and scored from nought to 4. This removes the anomalies in the score that were present in the original paper when data were missing, it also provides a score ranging from nought to a 100%. The layout of paper questionnaire is also as given in the latter publication. In the case of the results given in this chapter, if more than two questions were missing, the data were discarded. A box-and-whisker plot showing the distribution of the scores for resurfacing

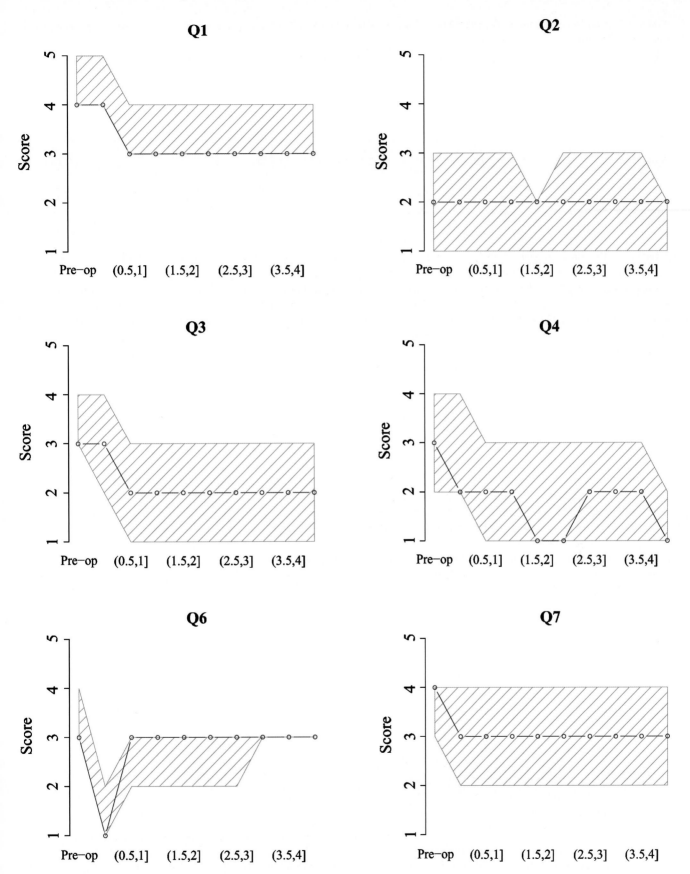

Fig. 26.2. Six plots showing the COOP health status outcome. The headers (Q1, Q2, etc.) refer to the question numbers given in Table 26.1. The points are the median values at the time intervals. The shaded part represents the area between the 25th and 75th quantiles (iqr).

TABLE 26.2. Published results for mean COOP/WONCA scores and our own data (ROH) for preoperative BHR (mean age 54.5 years) and THR (mean age 67.2 years).

Dimension	Resurfacing	Total hip replacement	Palliative chemotherapy	Migraine	Population (age 20 y)	Population (age 70 y)
				Essink-Bot et al., 1997 [23]	Bruusgaard et al., 1993 [24]	Bruusgaard et al., 1993 [24]
	ROH	ROH	Detmar et al., 2002 [22]			
Physical fitness	4.01	4.60	3.2	1.72	1.42	2.61
Feelings	2.25	2.45	2.3	1.88	2.03	1.85
Daily activities	2.92	3.37	2.8	1.74	1.42	2.09
Social activities	2.71	3.09	2.2	1.54	1.41	1.63
Change health	3.14	3.12	–	2.62	2.87	2.12
Overall health	2.84	2.92	3.4	2.65	2.92	2.52
Average	2.98	3.26	2.78	2.03	1.88	2.27

relative to the date of operation is given in Fig. 26.3); this is based on 5164 questionnaires and 2186 hips. The scores have been grouped into 6-month intervals with the x-axis showing the range of each interval. The superimposed means on this plot demonstrate how skewed these scores tend to be and why we usually refer to the median result rather than the average. The results show that the scores quickly fall from their preoperative value of 62% (iqr = 48.1 to 75.2) to approximately 10% (iqr = 0.0 to 23.7). This is lower than the results for total hip arthroplasty 70.8% (iqr = 58.3 to 81.2) to 20.8% (iqr = 10.4 to 35.4) given in Pynsent et al. [17] where 4086 scores were used on 1554 hips. Figure 26.4 shows the contribution each question makes to the scores of Fig. 26.3 preoperatively and over the 2- to 2.5-year period. For these groups, the mean age was 50.6 years with a preoperative median score of 52.0% and a 2-year score of 8.3%. It is encouraging to see that the median value of all the questions is 1 (i.e., symptomless) except for pain, which is at the second point (i.e., very mild). The greatest changes are for questions 8 and 12 where both medians have dropped

from 4 to 1. Question 8 concerns standing from sitting on a chair, with an improvement from "very painful" to "not at all painful." Question 12 concerns night pain, which has diminished from "most nights" to "no nights."

In order to establish lines that could be used for measuring outcome against some standard, smooth lines have been fitted through the data using an equation of the form

$$y = b_1 + b_o e^{kt} \tag{26.1}$$

where y is the modeled OHS, b_0, k is the rate constant (i.e., the rate of change for the score to go from $b_0 + b_1$ to b_0 and t is the time from operation. As this change with time is exponential, it may be easier for the reader to think in terms of the time taken for the score to change by half, as in the half-life of a radioactive element. This is calculated by

$$t1/2 = \ln(2)/k \tag{26.2}$$

Figure 26.5 shows the result of a best fit for resurfacing. These are compared with the results for total hip joint arthroplasty. In this figure, the resurfacing and total hip data have a median starting value of $b_0 + b_1 = 62.5$ and 72.8, respectively, and fall

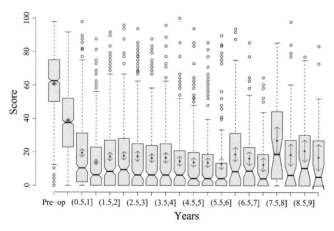

FIG. 26.3. A box-and-whisker plot of the OHS for hip resurfacing. The scores are accumulated into six monthly intervals over 9 years. The mean and 95% confidence intervals of the means are superimposed onto the plot.

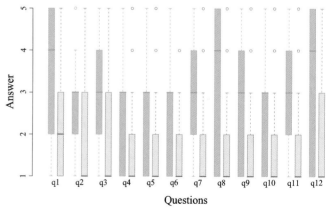

FIG. 26.4. Box-and-whisker plots showing the distribution of 12 questions scores preoperatively (pink) and at the 2.0- to 2.5-year time interval (blue) to show the change in individual questions. The numbers on the left represent the response to an item on the questionnaire, so 1 is the first alternative.

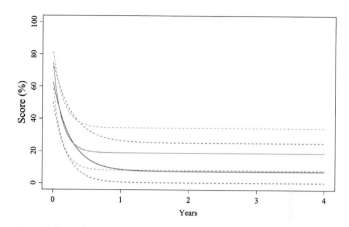

FIG. 26.5. A plot comparing the OHS for resurfacing (blue) and total (red) hip joint arthroplasty using fitted lines through the median (solid) and interquartile ranges (dashed lines).

to half their final values (*b0*) in 2.2 and 1.1 months. Having standard set by these lines enables these results to be used as a tool for auditing resurfacing procedures [17].

Up to now, the discussion of the OHS has only been in terms of a measurement made at a given point in time. Also of interest is how individual patients' scores change with time. The sensitivity to change (responsiveness) of the Oxford scores were established at the time of publication and subsequently by the original authors [18]. One approach to this problem is to use so called growth curves. Thus, rather than using an average change in scores, the change of each individual is measured and then these results used for a statistical analysis. We have already seen that on average the change in scores with time is an exponential drop, so it would seem reasonable once again to use equation (26.1) to fit the data for each individual patient; two examples of this fit are shown in Fig. 26.6. The result of the fits to all the resurfacing data is summarized in Fig. 26.7, giving an average fall in score of *b1* = 47.2% to an asymptotic value of *b0* = 15.0% at a rate of k = 13.1 years^{-1}. That is, it takes a patient 23 weeks to drop to 50% (i.e., the half-life) of the preoperative value. These analytical data can now be used for further analysis; for example, do these parameters vary between sexes? Figure 26.8 shows the result of such an analysis, the plots suggest there is only a difference in parameter *b0*, this significance is confirmed with a Wilcoxon test. This means that the drop (*b1*) and rate of drop (*k*) in OHSs are not different between sexes, but the final level reached (*b0*) is significantly lower for males (median = 4.2) than females (median = 10.0). Further analysis would now be required to explain this difference; this is beyond the remit of this chapter.

The main point is that these so-called hierarchical methods [19] have an important role to play in the analysis of outcomes.

Since the disability results of modern metal on metal resurfacing have been published, there has been concern that the OHS is not sensitive enough to find changes in activities. That

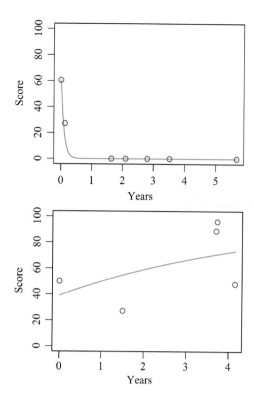

FIG. 26.6. Two examples of fitting growth curves to individual patients using equation (26.1). Left: An ideal result (*b0* = 0, *b1* = 60.4, and k = −10.7). Right: A poor fit, this patient went on to be revised 3 months after the last score (*b0* = 100, *b1* = −60.9, and k = −0.20).

is, the patients do so well that there is a "flooring effect" where many patients attain a very low score. This has prompted researchers to apply methods that delve into physical activities to a greater extent than the OHS. In particular, instruments that look at hip-loading activity rather than just patient energy consumption are required. Daniel et al. [20] has published results using the UCLA Activity Level Assessment [21].

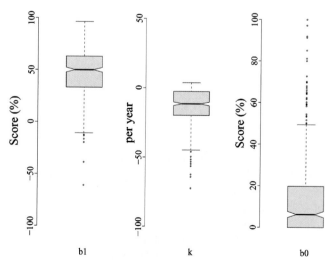

FIG. 26.7. A box-and-whisker plot showing the results of fitting growth curves to each resurfacing using equation (26.1).

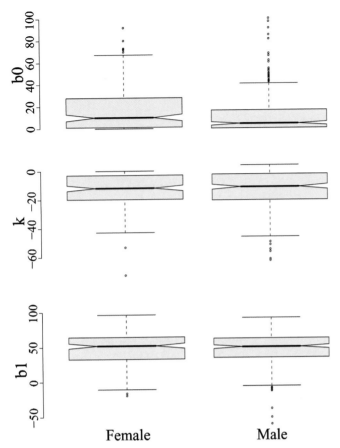

FIG. 26.8. An example of using the model to look for differences. Here the final level (*b*0) is shown to be significantly different.

Conclusion

The measurement of outcome is essential to both the orthopedic surgeon and the patient. Production of standards using validated instruments allows comparison between an array of different factors such as new prostheses, different diagnoses, and even different surgeons. Traditionally, the success or otherwise of an arthroplasty device has been determined by the measurement of survival. The BHR survival (not revised) is above 95% at 10 years for this young and active group in which traditional hip replacement has not demonstrated such success. As has been detailed in this chapter, using revision as an outcome measure is only one of many measurements that can be employed. With such low rates of revision and with patients' expectations of a return to "normality" after surgery, the use of measurements such as the OHS, COOP/WONCA, and UCLA Activity Level Assessment are necessary. These provide a greater insight into the impact of any procedure on the patient's symptoms and functional limitations. In comparing the OHS results of resurfacing with total joint arthroplasty, it can be seen that the latter start with a higher score and end with a higher score than do the former, with a similar mean drop seen in both groups. Does this mean that both operations are equally successful?

In summary, there are a large number of potential confounders causing differences in outcome. Use of the statistical methods described in this chapter allows comparison of outcomes for all the variables that have been recorded during data collection. From this, variables that have a large influence on outcome can be identified and corrected for. These influential variables can also be investigated as to the reason for the effect seen, both positive or negative. It is apparent, from the results presented here, that in the population treated by metal on metal hip resurfacing, there is an excellent improvement in a variety of outcome measurements. Further analysis and research is required to acquire a true understanding of the role of hip resurfacing in the management of patients with painful conditions of the hip joint.

References

1. W H Harris. Traumatic arthritis of the hip after dislocation in acetabular fractures: treatment by mould arthroplasty. J Bone Joint Surg Am, 51:737–755, 1969.
2. J Charnley. Long term results of low friction arthroplasty of the hip performed as a primary intervention. J Bone Joint Surg Br, 54:61–76, 1972.
3. National Joint Registry Centre. 2nd Annual Report — September 2005. Annual report, National Joint Registry for England and Wales, 2006. Available at www.njrcentre.org.uk.
4. R Development Core Team. R: A Language and Environment for Statistical Computing. R Foundation for Statistical Computing, Vienna, Austria, 2007. Available at http://www.R-project.org.
5. A C August, C H Aldam, and P B Pynsent. The McKee-Farrar hip arthroplasty. A long-term study. J Bone Joint Surg Br, 68:520–527, 1986.
6. J Daniel, P B Pynsent, and D McMinn. Survival analysis of metal-on-metal hip resurfacing in young patients with osteoarthritis. J Bone Joint Surg Br, 86:177–184, 2004.
7. J M Bland. An Introduction to Medical Statistics. Oxford University Press, 3rd edition, 2000.
8. T M Therneau and P M Grambsch. Modeling Survival Data: Extending the Cox Model. Statistics for Biology and Health. Springer, 2000.
9. World Health Organization. Constitution of the World Health Organization. Available at http://www.searo.who.int/en/section898/section1441.htm.
10. J E Ware. SF-36 Health Survey. Manual and Interpretation Guide. Nimrod Press, The Health Institute, New England Medical Centre, 2nd edition, 1997.
11. E C Nelson, J H Wasson, D J Johnson, and R D Hays. Dartmouth COOP functional health assessment charts: Brief measures for clinical practice. Available at http://www.dartmouth.edu/ coop-proj/index.html.
12. J M Landgraf and E C Nelson. Summary of the WONCA/COOP International Health Assessment Field Trial. the Dartmouth COOP Primary Care Network. Aust Fam Physician, 21:255–7, 260–2, 266–9, 1992.
13. C van Weel. Functional status in primary care: COOP/WONCA charts. Disabil Rehabil, 15:96–101, 1993.
14. World Health Organization. International classification of impairments, disabilities and handicaps. World Health Organization, Geneva, 1986.

15. J Dawson, R Fitzpatrick, A Carr, and D Murray. Questionnaire on the perceptions of patients about total hip replacement. J Bone Joint Surg Br, 78:185–90, 1996.

16. P B Pynsent. Choosing an outcome measure. J Bone Joint Surg Br, 83:792–794, 2001.

17. P B Pynsent, D J Adams, and S P Disney. The Oxford hip and knee outcome questionnaires for arthroplasty. J Bone Joint Surg Br, 87:241–248, 2005.

18. J Dawson, R Fitzpatrick, D Murray, and A Carr. The problem of 'noise' in monitoring patient-based outcomes: generic, disease-specific and site-specific instruments for total hip replacement. Journal of Health Services & Research Policy, 1:224–31, 1996.

19. A S Bryk and S W Raudenbush. Hierarchical Linear Models: Applications and Data Analysis Methods. Sage, Newbury Park, CA, 1992.

20. J Daniel, H Ziaee, C Pradhan, P B Pynsent, and D J W McMinn. Blood and urine metal ion levels in young and active patients after Birmingham Hip Resurfacing arthroplasty: Four-year results of a prospective longitudinal study. J Bone Joint Surg Br, 89:169–73.

21. H C Amstutz, B J Thomas, R Jinnah, W Kim, T Grogan, and C Yale. Treatment of primary osteoarthritis of the hip. a comparison of total joint and surface replacement arthroplasty. J Bone Joint Surg Am, 66:228–41, 1984.

22. S B Detmar, M J Muller, J H Schornagel, L D V Wever, and N K Aaronson. Health-related quality-of-life assessments and patient-physician communication: a randomized controlled trial. JAMA, 288:3027–3034, 2002.

23. M L Essink-Bot, P F Krabbe, G J Bonsel, and N K Aaronson. An empirical comparison of four generic health status measures. the Nottingham Health Profile, the Medical Outcomes Study 36-item Short-Form Health Survey, the COOP/WONCA charts, and the EuroQol instrument. Med Care, 35:522–537, 1997.

24. D Bruusgaard, I Nessiy, O Rutle, K Furuseth, and B Natvig. Measuring functional status in a population survey. The Dartmouth COOP functional health assessment charts/WONCA used in an epidemiological study. Fam Pract, 10:212–218, 1993.

27
Results of Birmingham Hip Resurfacing in Different Diagnoses

Joseph Daniel, Callum McBryde, Chandra Pradhan, and Hena Ziaee

The results of total hip arthroplasty in young patients have been uniformly worse than those in older patients. In a recent series [1], the Swedish Hip Arthroplasty Register reports 10-year survival rates of 65.8%, 66.6%, and 64.0% with cemented, uncemented, and hybrid implants, respectively, in male patients under the age of 55 years with osteoarthritis (OA). This led them to the conclusion that this young cohort is epidemiologically and demographically different from older patients with OA and that there is an obvious need to increase the usage of alternative and conservative methods in the treatment of these patients. It is this high incidence of early failures of conventional total hip arthroplasties that drove the search for a more conservative solution and led to the resurgence of modern resurfacing.

When it was first introduced, the goal of resurfacing was to provide an interim solution that would buy time until the patient reached an age at which he would be suitable for conventional arthroplasty, without jeopardizing the chances of a future conversion to a total hip replacement (THR). The expectation therefore had been that if the resurfacing offered 10 symptom-free years, it had achieved its goal.

More than 16 years after the introduction of modern metal on metal (MM) resurfacings and 10 years after the release of the Birmingham Hip Resurfacing (BHR), we review the results of the BHR in our patients with hip arthritis from different etiologies. The results of the earlier series of resurfacings are presented in Chapter 1.

We included all patients operated on by Mr. McMinn between 30 July 1997 (when the first BHR was performed) and 31 July 2005. Nearly 50% of the failures that have occurred so far occurred in the first 2 years. In order to allow the capture of every short-term event for each patient, we have used our BHR cohort with a minimum 2-year follow-up. The cohort includes 2600 consecutive BHRs with a mean age of 53 years (range, 13.5–86.6 years) (Fig. 27.1) and a male:female ratio of 7:3. The median and the 10th and 90th percentiles of age are 54, 40, and 64.4 years, respectively. For the avoidance of doubt, there have been no revisions or reoperations in our resurfacings performed in the 2 years since 1 August 2005.

Nearly 75% of patients in the above-mentioned cohort had a primary diagnosis of either osteoarthritis (1875) or an early destructive form of osteoarthritis (81). Other diagnoses include avascular necrosis, inflammatory arthritis, sequelae of childhood hip disorders, post-septic arthritis, and so forth (Fig. 27.2).

Forty of these patients (51 hips) died during the follow-up period at an average duration of 7.4 years after the operation, due to unrelated causes. There were 43 revisions in all, giving an overall failure rate of 1.65%. Kaplan-Meier survival analysis gives survival probabilities of 98.6%, 97.5%, and 96.1% at 5, 9, and 10 years, respectively (Fig. 27.3).

Currently, there is one published source that gives comparative failure rates with different types of resurfacings; that is, the Australian Joint Replacement Register 2006 [2]. The results of several different types of resurfacings with a combined total of 15,181 component years are shown in the register (Fig. 27.4). In addition to the BHR, three other resurfacings have logged more than 100 component years in their series. The failure rate of BHRs (0.9% per component year) is significantly lower than that of the other three devices (2.2% to 4%). The overall failure rate in our series is 0.27% per component year. The total number of component years in our series, 15,838, compares well with the combined series of all types of resurfacings put together in the Australian Joint Replacement Register. Compared with our series, which is a single-surgeon series, the Australian Register includes 89 surgeons from all over Australia, and therefore it is understandable that our series has an advantage.

Osteoarthritis, Destructive Arthritis, Traumatic Arthritis, and Avascular Necrosis

The warning of Sir John Charnley that in the absence of other physical restraining factors, young patients with osteoarthritis would experience early failures has proved correct over the years. However, the biggest group of patients presenting with a need for hip resurfacing in any series has been those with primary osteoarthritis, in particular, those with no other physical restraining factors.

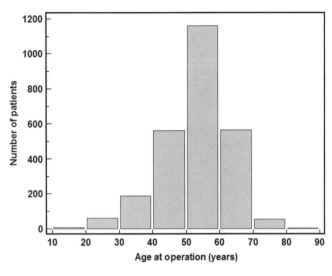

Fig. 27.1.

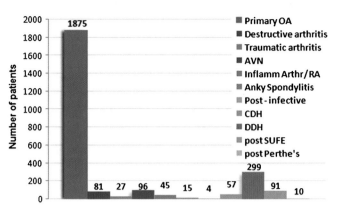

Fig. 27.2.

Osteoarthritis

Our 10-year results show that the survival probability of BHRs in patients with primary osteoarthritis (96.7%) is as good as those in the overall series (Figs. 27.5 and 27.6). We analyzed the first 100 patients with osteoarthritis treated with BHRs at their 8- to 9-year follow-up with a clinicoradiologic assessment. Out of the first 100 BHRs performed for primary OA, there were four revisions. Four patients (six hips) died, of an unrelated cause, at an average of 5.9 years after the operation. The rest were evaluated at their 8- to 9-year follow-up. The mean Oxford score of the patients with surviving hips was 14.7 and the median 13. None of the unrevised patients is awaiting a revision. Five patients have not been

radiographed at their final evaluation because of unavoidable reasons (e.g., the patient being or possibly being pregnant). A summary of the radiographic findings in the rest is given in Table 27.1.

Radiologic Evaluation

Anteroposterior and Johnson shoot-through lateral views were used to evaluate the radiographic results. Femoral neck narrowing of more than 10% was considered significant. Radiolucent lines of more than 1 mm in thickness around the femoral stem were recorded in the zones described by Beaule et al. [3] and around the cup according to the zones described by DeLee and Charnley [4]. The inter-teardrop line was used

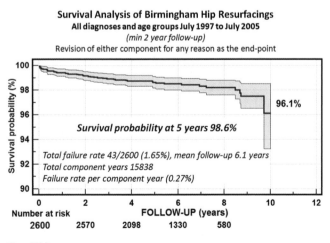

Fig. 27.3.

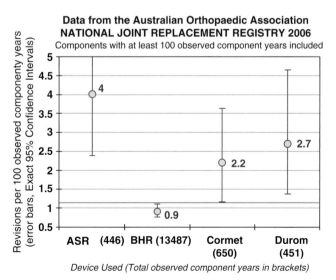

Fig. 27.4.

Survival Analysis of BHRs in patients with primary OA
Revision for any reason as the end-point

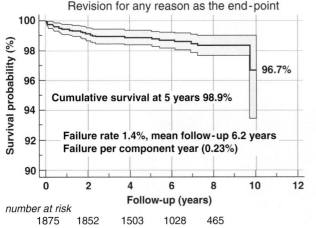

Cumulative survival at 5 years 98.9%

Failure rate 1.4%, mean follow-up 6.2 years
Failure per component year (0.23%)

96.7%

number at risk
1875   1852   1503   1028   465

FIG. 27.5.

TABLE 27.1. 8- to 9-year radiological evaluation of the first 100 BHRs.

Radiologic findings	Incidence
Femoral	n=100
Osteolysis	1
Loosening/change in orientation/migration	0
Lucent lines	
1 zone	1
2 zones	1
3 zones	1
Neck thinning (greater than 10% loss of neck width)	4
Punched-out impingement lesion at head-neck junction	6
Acetabular	
Osteolysis	4
Loosening/change in cup orientation/migration	0
Lucent lines	
1 zone	0
2 zones	1
3 zones	0
None of the above adverse features	82.1%
Heterotopic ossification (HO)	
Brooker I or II HO	15
Brooker III or IV HO	3

as the reference for acetabular inclination. Femoral component diameter was used for correction of radiographic magnification in the measurement of neck thinning.

Where there were adverse features of unknown significance such as atypical osteolytic lesions, these were further investigated with computed tomography (CT) scanning. In cases with localized punched-out lesions in the femoral neck, we used pulsed image intensifier radiography to see if it was possible that these were caused as a result of mechanical impingement.

None of the radiographs showed evidence of loosening, change in orientation, or migration of either the femoral or acetabular components. A male patient who underwent a BHR at the age of 54 years developed an area of osteolysis in the femoral neck, which appeared to extend from the region of the base of the greater trochanter to around the midcervical area. This first appeared as faint fuzziness in his 5-year radiographs and has become better delineated in his 9-year radiographs (Fig. 27.7). Multislice CT scanning was performed to see if there were more extensive changes in his femoral head or neck.

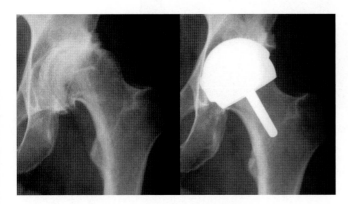

FIG. 27.6. Preoperative and follow-up radiographs of a 48-year-old man with severe osteoarthritis treated with a Birmingham Hip Resurfacing.

The CT scanner we used had metal artifact correction software, which allows clear visualization of the rest of the femoral neck and the femoral head contained within the femoral component. The CT revealed the presence of a localized well-demarcated lesion with a sclerotic margin leading to a diagnosis of bone cyst. No other periprosthetic adverse reaction was found in him adjacent to either component.

There was one patient with a radiolucent line in two zones (Fig. 27.8) on the acetabular side. He is a very active man who underwent a BHR at the age of 52 years. He continues to be active and pleased with his result, but his radiograph reveals a lucent line around zones 1 and 2 of his acetabular component. Three patients had radiolucent lines around the femoral stem, of which only one has these in all three zones. All of them are pleased with their result and have no symptoms in their operated hips, including the one with lucent lines in all 3 zones (Fig. 27.9).

It was pleasing to note that the incidence of radiolucent lines around the BHR femoral stem is very low. The BHR stem is designed to prevent osseo-integration and stress-shielding. It is made of smooth cobalt-chrome and has a distal gap. It is tapered from top to bottom, and the tube created in the bone to receive it is a parallel tube. The distal part of the stem is therefore a deliberate loose-fit (Fig. 27.10). The stem press-fits proximally as the bone in that area becomes compressed to allow its seating. Now we use a taper drill proximally in order to make even the proximal stem-bone interface line-to-line rather than press-fit. At revision of well-fixed femoral components, when a neck osteotomy is made, the stem lifts out without any difficulty, and we have always observed a thin fibrous membrane around the stem. Given that the BHR stem remains loose-fitting from day one, we are puzzled why all BHRs do not show a radiolucent line around the stem. This

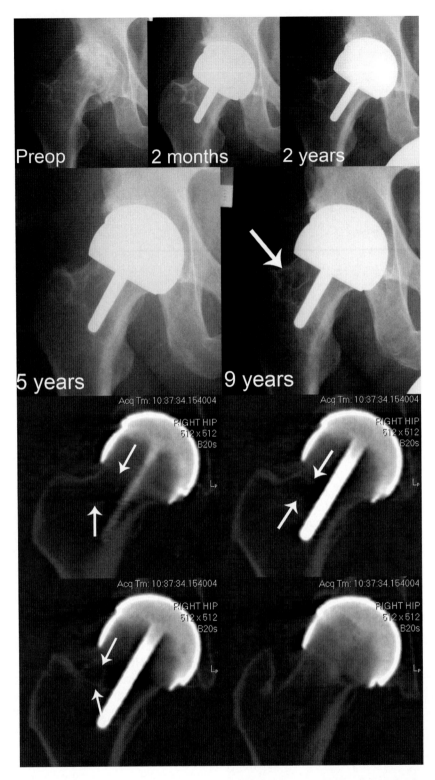

FIG. 27.7. Radiographic series of a man who underwent a BHR at the age of 54, showing the development of an area of osteolysis in the femoral neck that first appeared faintly in his 5-year radiographs and has persisted and become well-delineated in his 9-year radiographs. Multislice CT scanning however revealed the presence of a localized well-demarcated lesion with a sclerotic margin leading to a diagnosis of bone cyst (arrows). No other periprosthetic adverse feature was found adjacent to either component, including the portion of the femoral head contained within the femoral component.

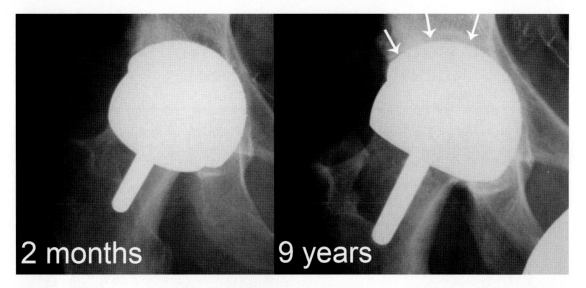

FIG. 27.8. The radiographs of a man who underwent a BHR at the age of 52 years showing a lucent line around zones 1 and 2 (arrows) of his acetabular component at 9-year follow-up.

shows clearly that you need a substantial gap in order to see a radiolucent line on an x-ray.

On the acetabular side, there were four patients who showed osteolysis. Three of these were in zone 3 of the acetabulum and another in zone 2. Two of them have been CT scanned and two are awaiting a scan. The one who has apparent osteolysis in zone 2 was diagnosed as having a degenerative cyst on his CT scan. Figure 27.11 shows the CT results of one of the patients who showed osteolysis in zone 3. She underwent a BHR at the age of 58 years. At the 5-year follow-up, she showed evidence of neck thinning. At 9 years, her

radiographs showed a localized area of osteolysis in zone 3 of the acetabulum. She is perfectly pleased with her 9-year results and has no symptoms at all in spite of a physically demanding job. Multislice CT scanning revealed that there is a large iliopsoas bursa 6.2 × 8.5 × 8 cm which was creating pressure effects on the medial femoral neck and the posterior column. In the view of the radiologist, this external pressure erosion is responsible for the medial neck thinning and for the appearance of the erosion in the ischium. No debris was detected in the fluid filling the bursa. We have observed this phenomenon before, in which an iliopsoas bursa has caused

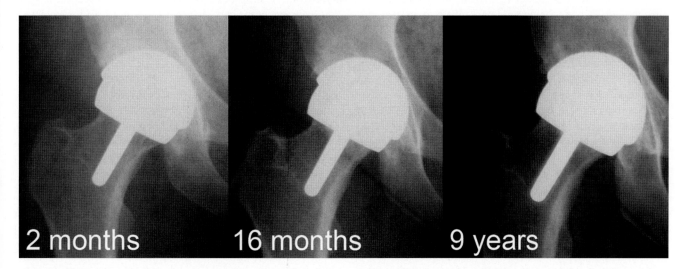

FIG. 27.9. Radiographic series showing radiolucent lines in all three zones of the femoral stem in the 9-year radiographs of a woman operated at the age of 55 years.

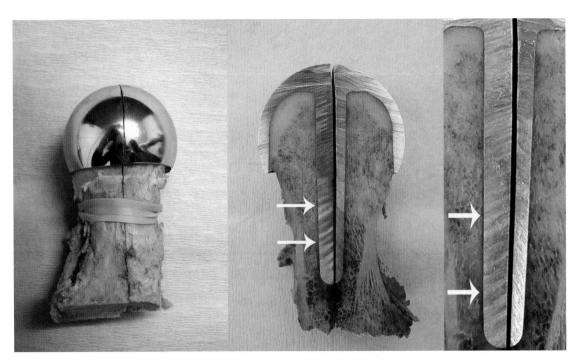

Fig. 27.10. A BHR implanted on to a cadaver femur and divided longitudinally to show the tapered stem in relation to the parallel walls of the tube drilled in the bone. The stem is designed to press-fit proximally and retain a gap along the stem-bone interface distally (arrows). Now we achieve a noninterference fit throughout the length of the stem by expanding the proximal part of the drill hole with a taper drill.

medial neck thinning, as explained later in Chapter 28 and Fig. 28.14. Three other patients in the present cohort had neck thinning greater than 10%.

It must be noted that although CT scanning has revealed that the etiology and the true nature of the lesions seen in Figs. 27.7 and 27.11 are different from the osteolysis seen due to wear-induced debris, we have still included them as osteolysis in our list of radiologic findings.

We investigated the series of patients who manifested a punched-out lesion in the femoral neck. We present the radiographs of a man who underwent a BHR at the age of 57 years. His 2-year radiographs showed the presence of a lesion at the medial head neck junction. This has persisted in his recent radiographs as well. On manipulation of the hip under image intensifier fluoroscopy, we found that this lesion was caused by an impingement of the femoral neck on the edge of the cup in a position of flexion, adduction, and external rotation (Fig. 27.12). The fact that it has not worsened in the past 8 years suggests that it is an adaptive process rather than a progressive pathologic lesion. We have observed such localized defects in five other patients. Image intensifier–guided manipulation of the hip showed that all of them were a result of such an impingement. We have also observed in another patient with a BHR, although he is not from this cohort, the development of a similar punched-out lesion on the superior neck due to impingement in a position of flexion, abduction, and external

rotation (see Figs. 24.2 and 24.3). He was a pilot, and sitting in the cockpit, he had to keep his leg in that position of flexion, abduction, and external rotation for long hours.

From this radiographic analysis, we have made two new observations that have helped us to understand the reason for some of the radiologic findings in patients with hip resurfacings. The first observation is that it is possible that some cases of medial neck thinning are due to external pressure erosion from an iliopsoas cyst. The second observation is that impingement of the cup on the neck is responsible for localized punched-out lesions on the femoral neck.

Young Patients with Osteoarthritis

Failure rate in young patients under the age of 55 years with osteoarthritis (n = 887) in this cohort (1997 to 2005) is 1.35% (12/887) and Implant survival at 5, 9 and 10 years are 98.9%, 98.6% and 95.1% respectively. The drop in the survival rate between 9 to 10 years is due to late failure from infection in one of the early patients. They compare well with the published rates of THRs from the Swedish Register mentioned earlier (64 to 67% at ten years). Six of these failures were due to a collapse of the femoral head and occurred at a mean follow-up of 2 years (0.63 to 6.93). In all but one case the cup was left in situ and the femoral head was replaced with a modular head THR that matched the existing cup.

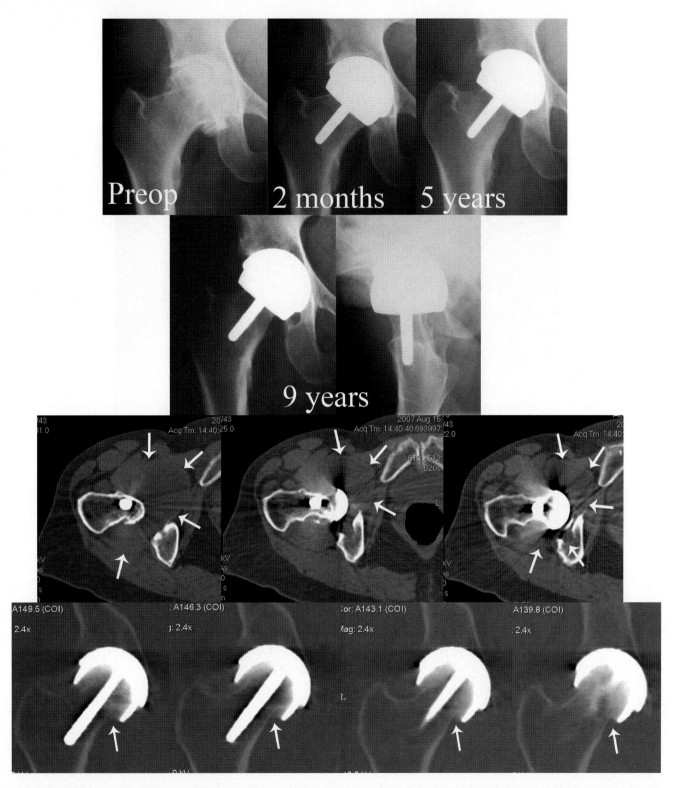

Fig. 27.11. Radiographic series of a woman who underwent a BHR at the age of 58 years. She is perfectly pleased with her 9-year results. Her 5-year radiograph showed medial neck thinning. Her 9-year radiographs showed the appearance of a small area of osteolysis in the ischium. Multislice CT scanning shows a large iliopsoas bursa (arrows) causing external pressure leading to medial neck thinning and the erosion in the ischium. No debris was detected in the fluid filling the bursa.

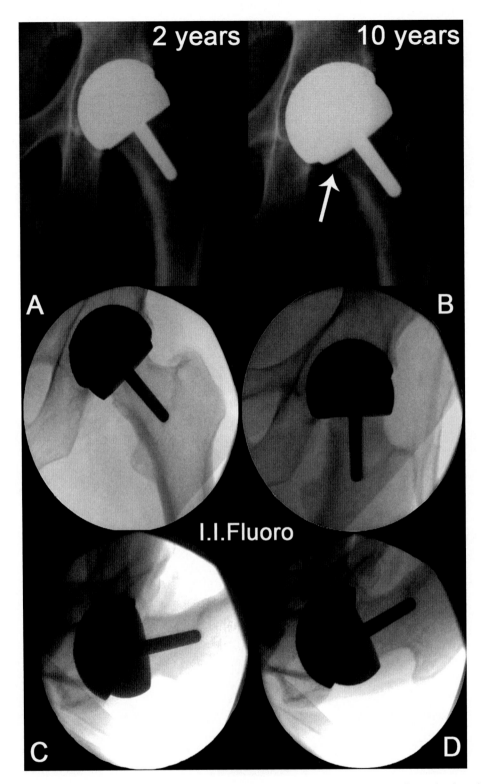

Fig. 27.12. Radiographs of a man who underwent a BHR 10 years ago at the age of 57 years. The 2-year radiographs show the presence of a tiny punched-out lesion at the medial head-neck junction that has persisted in the 10-year radiograph. Manipulation of the hip under image intensifier fluoroscopy (I.I.Fluoro) showed no impingement in the anteroposterior view (A) even in adducted position (B). However, the lateral view shows the femoral neck impinging on the cup in a position of flexion, adduction, and external rotation (C and D) at the site of the punched-out lesion.

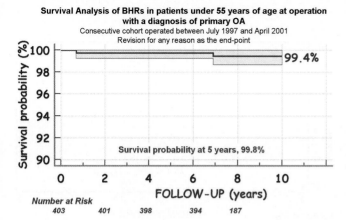

Survival Analysis of BHRs in patients under 55 years of age at operation
with a diagnosis of primary OA
Consecutive cohort operated between July 1997 and April 2001
Revision for any reason as the end-point

FIG. 27.13.

Four others failed due to infection at 3.8 years (1.7 to 9.7). The other two failures were due to femoral neck fracture 0.07 and 0.38 years after the operation. These are different from the typical pattern of bearing wear-related failures seen with conventional hip replacements in young patients. We published on a cohort of the first 403 consecutive BHRs in patients with OA under the age of 55 years earlier and continue to follow them up regularly. Their implant survival at 10 years is 99.4% (Fig. 27.13). An assessment of their workplace and leisure activities had revealed that 92% of the men with unilateral resurfacings play sport and 62% of them participate in impact sports.

Avascular Necrosis of the Femoral Head

BHR can work well in cases of femoral head avascular necrosis (AVN), and good results have been reported by Mr. Ronan Treacy in Birmingham, United Kingdom [3], and also from Chennai, India, and Seoul, South Korea. However, the results of AVN in any series are not as good as those in OA and other diagnoses. Caution must be exercised in the use of BHR in femoral head AVN.

Joint preserving surgery such as core decompression, bone grafting vascularized or nonvascularized, osteotomies, and so forth, have a role in the treatment of osteonecrosis before femoral head collapse occurs. However, in postcollapse patients (Ficat and Arlet grade III and IV), joint damage resulting from the incongruity and progressive cartilage loss inevitably lead to painful secondary arthritis necessitating an arthroplasty procedure. Because these patients are typically between the third and fifth decade, a conservative arthroplasty is desirable.

The results of hemiresurfacing and hemiarthroplasty are not predictable for several reasons. First, acetabular cartilage should be totally unaffected, and the patient should not have been symptomatic for long in order to expect success. Second, the slightest mismatch between the size of the femoral head compared with the inner diameter of the socket results in early failure. Success rates for hemiresurfacing vary from 84% at 3 years to 50% at 11 years. Persistent groin pain and acetabular erosion necessitating a revision are major causes for the poor results of a hemiresurfacing in AVN.

Furthermore, a later conversion to a regular resurfacing by adding a matching socket would result in greater acetabular bone loss. This is due to the fact that in order to exactly match the inner diameter of the acetabulum, the size of the component is slightly larger than the size of a regular primary total resurfacing femoral component for a given patient.

The results of total hip replacements are also generally worse in osteonecrosis compared with osteoarthritis [4] and vary from a failure rate of 0% at 18 months to more than 60% at 104 months. There are several reasons for this. Young age and absence of other restraining factors among idiopathic AVN patients put them in the high-expectation, high-activity group. Those on steroids and chemotherapy are more prone to infections. Dislocation rates after THR are reportedly higher in patients treated for AVN than for osteoarthritis. Posttraumatic patients who need complex reconstructions have a potentially higher failure rate.

There are 96 patients with a primary diagnosis of avascular necrosis of the femoral head treated with a BHR in our series (Fig. 27.14). Five (5.2%) of these failed at an average duration of 4 years (0.4 to 8.7 years) after the operation. Three (3.1%) of these were from further collapse of the femoral head and one each from femoral neck fracture and infection. We do not find the results of BHR in patients with femoral head AVN as good as those in either osteoarthritis or in the all-diagnoses combined group. The failure rate is higher compared with the failure rates seen in the all diagnoses series (1.65%) or the osteoarthritis series (1.4%).

The most disturbing feature is the 3.1% femoral head collapse rate, which is much higher than the 0.6% seen with the OA group. Survival probability with further collapse as the end point at 10 years for the two groups AVN and OA is 89.8% and 99.2%, respectively, and the difference between the two curves is statistically significant (Fig. 27.15). The probable explanation for the higher failure rate is that the pathologic factors that caused nontraumatic AVN (steroids, alcohol, etc.) continue to cause further femoral head collapse.

We therefore consider AVN a relative contraindication to resurfacing and tend to rely less and less on the BHR in cases with femoral head AVN. In young patients with AVN, we find the Birmingham Mid Head Resection (BMHR) prosthesis to be a reliable alternative. This device is explained in Chapter 23. It is a conservative arthroplasty device, too, and does not invade the medullary canal of the femoral shaft. Its stem offers the advantage of more physiologic proximal loading than do earlier designs of neck-conserving total hip replacement and therefore prevents stress shielding bone loss in the femoral neck.

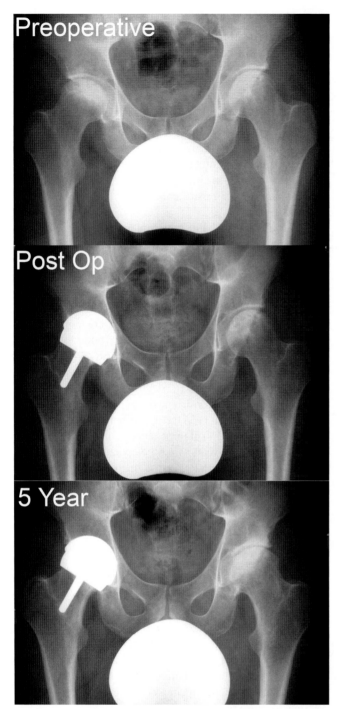

FIG. 27.14. A 28-year-old male engineer with three risk factors for AVN: steroids, high alcohol intake, and deep-sea diving. He had Ficat Arlet stage 3 AVN on his right hip and Ficat 2 on his left hip. He underwent a right-sided BHR and left-sided core decompression. He is pleased with his result, and there are no adverse features on his 5-year radiograph.

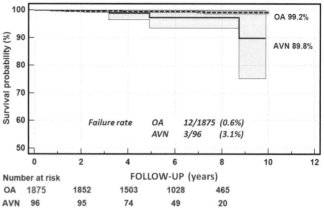

FIG. 27.15.

Post-traumatic and Early Destructive Arthritis

The results of BHR in arthritis secondary to previous trauma or in early destructive arthritis are also satisfactory (Fig 27.16). The more severe instances of trauma tend to develop avascular necrosis and therefore get filtered out into the AVN group. Cases of severe destructive arthritis often need a dysplasia socket or even a total hip replacement. Therefore, there could be a selection bias with regards to both these groups.

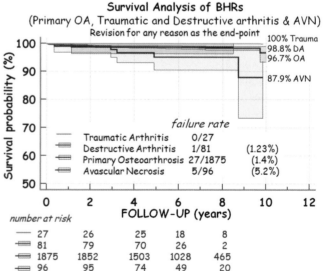

FIG. 27.16.

Inflammatory Arthritis and Post-Septic Arthritis

Total hip replacement (THR) arthroplasty has always been considered very effective in the treatment of painful end-stage inflammatory hip arthritis (IA) providing relief of pain and improvement in quality of life. The systemic nature of the disease and the inbuilt physical restraints ensure that patients do not wear out conventional hip replacements as quickly as someone with primary OA. However, recent developments in disease-modifying agents and cytokine inhibitors have made a quantum improvement in the quality of life and expectations of IA patients and have been indirectly and steadily dismantling these inbuilt restraints.

As opposed to 20 years ago, patients with IA and severe arthritic change who undergo a hip replacement today expect to go back to an active lifestyle. Being young, it is attractive to keep the procedure conservative. Furthermore, the incidence of dislocation is significantly higher in patients with IA compared with those with OA [5], which makes a large-diameter resurfacing more favorable than a conventional hip replacement.

However, the small stature and abnormal bony anatomy pose a challenge to a successful outcome with resurfacing. The thin cortices and poor bone stock increase the risk of a periprosthetic fracture after both resurfacings and replacements. With sound patient selection, we find that there are realistic chances of an excellent outcome with a resurfacing.

We reviewed our results of BHRs in patients with inflammatory arthritis and found 15 hips (12 patients) with ankylosing spondylitis (AS) operated at a mean age of 41.7 years and 45 hips (35 patients) with seronegative or rheumatoid arthritis (RA) treated with a BHR at a mean age of 40.6 years. In addition, there were five patients (five hips) who had secondary arthritis as a sequel to infective arthritis. In the entire cohort of 51 patients, one died 5 years later of an unrelated cause.

With revision for any reason as the end point, there were no failures among the AS patients. In the RA group, there was one failure from femoral neck fracture 2 months after operation giving a failure rate of 2.2%. The failure rate of BHRs

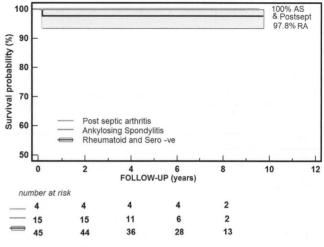

FIG. 27.18.

in this group of patients with inflammatory and post-infective arthritis is 1.56%, and the cumulative survivorship at 10 years is 98.4% (Fig. 27.17). None of the patients had a dislocation. Oxford hip scores and clinicoradiologic assessment did not reveal any significant adverse feature. Although the individual groups (Fig. 27.18) are small cohorts, the excellent survival rates in these young patients are no worse than the results obtained in many series with total hip replacements. The conservative nature of the procedure retains better revision options when the time comes for it.

Concerns have been raised regarding the effects of persistently elevated metal ion levels in patients with IA. The possibility of nephrotoxicity has also been a matter of concern as they happen to be receiving long-term potentially nephrotoxic medication as well. We have a few patients in our series who have had unilateral and bilateral MM resurfacings for IA in the past. They continue to be administered disease-modifying agents, and therefore their renal function is being periodically monitored by their physicians. We have reviewed these serial results and find that their renal function continues unaffected 10 years after resurfacing. Their metal levels also are no different from the levels obtained in patients with resurfacings performed for OA.

Childhood Hip Disorders

Childhood hip disorders not only lead to the development of early secondary arthritic change but also present with a range of anatomic abnormalities both on the femoral and acetabular sides. Congenital and developmental dysplasias result in a shallow socket and secondary changes in the femoral head and neck. As mentioned in Chapter 25, although traditionally dysplasia has been classified into congenital

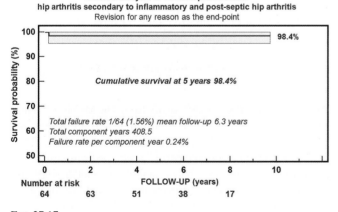

FIG. 27.17.

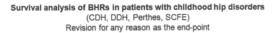

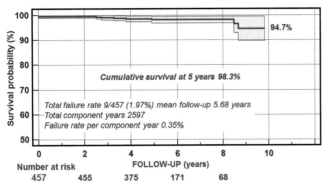

Fig. 27.19.

and developmental varieties, both these entities are, in reality, the same disease process. However, both these terms have been retained here, as they had been used as such in our database. Perthes disease and slipped upper femoral epiphysis (SCFE) lead to proximal femoral abnormalities and secondary socket changes. Post-Perthes arthritis is a particular challenge whereby the presence of a short, wide neck offers a poor foundation on which to seat the resurfacing femoral component. With a resurfacing procedure, very little can be done to improve femoral offset and leg length inequality. The hip in severe SCFE offers precious little peripheral support to the femoral component anterosuperiorly. Furthermore, the surgeon can be misled into seating the component in a poorly centered and aligned position. Both these situations are detrimental to a successful outcome with a resurfacing.

The BHR system has the option of a Dysplasia cup, which effectively addresses both primary acetabular dysplasia (CDH and DDH) and secondary dysplasia arising from a destructive arthritic change (Chapters 21 and 25). In this section, we look at the overall results of patients presenting with arthri-

tis secondary to childhood hip disorders as an etiology. The results of a regular BHR cup in mild to moderate dysplasia and a Dysplasia cup in severe acetabular insufficiency are also discussed.

The results of BHRs in this category are satisfactory with a survival probability of 98.3% between 5 and 8 years (Fig. 27.19). There have been no failures in patients with post-Perthes disease and SUFE. In both the congenital and developmental dysplasia groups, there has been one late failure each lowering their survival probability to 94.7% and 92.7%, respectively, at the tail end of the curve (Fig. 27.20).

Dysplasia

BHR in Mild to Moderate Dysplasia (Regular Cup)

The results we report here are from the Royal Orthopaedic Hospital, and one of us (C.M.) has compiled the data. Hip arthritis developing in patients with mild to moderate acetabular insufficiency can be managed with a regular BHR cup with a proximal and medial shift of the hip center of rotation. Sixty cases of hip arthritis secondary to Crowe grades I and II dysplasia treated with a regular cup BHR at a mean age of 47 years in a regional speciality orthopedic hospital in Birmingham by eight different surgeons over the past 10 years have been recently reviewed. At a median follow-up of 2.6 years, there have been two cup failures (failure rate, 3.2%; Kaplan-Meier survivorship at 8 years, 93%) (Fig. 27.21).

The primary stability in one cup was inadequate. It dislodged 3 days after the operation and was revised. Another failed with cup loosening at 3.2 years. There was a suspicion of hypersensitivity to metal and Aseptic lymphocytic vasculitis and associate lesions (ALVAL) in her, and she was revised to a non–MM bearing THR.

There have been no femoral failures in this group in contrast with another published series by Amstutz et al. [6] who reported metal on metal resurfacings with regular cups used in dysplastic hips (88% Crowe I and 12% Crowe II deficiencies). At an average follow-up of 6 years, 6 of 59 (10.2%) hips required conversion to a total hip arthroplasty, one due to repeated subluxations and five hips for femoral failures.

BHR in Severe Acetabular Insufficiency (Dysplasia Cup)

The data used in this subsection are from The McMinn Centre, and three of us (J.D., C.P., H.Z.) compiled the data. The socket in patients with severe acetabular insufficiency arising either from congenital/developmental dysplasia or from destructive or posttraumatic arthritis is too shallow. A regular BHR cup does not obtain adequate primary fixation stability in such a socket. Such patients need a Dysplasia BHR cup with supplementary screw fixation.

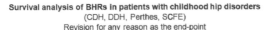

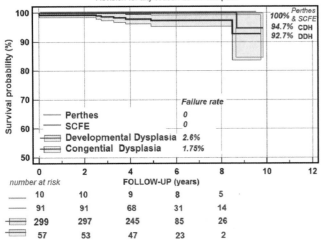

Fig. 27.20.

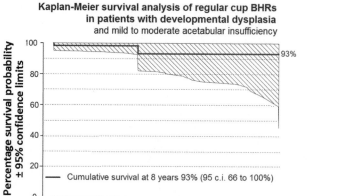

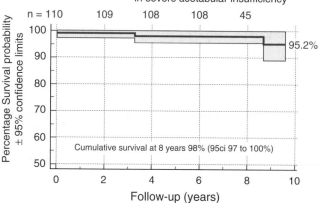

FIG. 27.21.

FIG. 27.23.

Earlier we reported on the results of a consecutive series of 110 hips (56 M, 54 F) in 103 patients with severe acetabular insufficiency treated with a dysplasia BHR between 1997 and 2000 [7]. The different primary pathologies leading to arthritis in this cohort are shown in Fig. 27.22. Mean age at operation was 47.2 years, and most women in the series were under the age of 55 years. One hundred three hips (94%) were Crowe grades II or III and 6 (6%) were Crowe grade I. One patient who underwent a simultaneous subtrochanteric derotation femoral osteotomy with AO plate fixation progressed to osteotomy union uneventfully. At a mean follow-up of 7.8 years (6 to 9.6 years), there are no cases of aseptic loosening of the cup. One patient died due to an unrelated cause 5 years after the operation. With reoperation or revision for any reason as the end point, there was a 2.7% conversion rate to a THR (one femoral neck fracture, one femoral head collapse, and one infection). The cumulative survivorship at 9 years is 95.2% (Fig. 27.23).

The absence of cup loosening in this series of patients with severe acetabular insufficiency is reassuring. Although a Dysplasia cup is more difficult to use than a regular cup, in situations where a regular cup is unlikely to be stable, the Dysplasia cup is proving to be a powerful tool in hip reconstruction. Should a revision become necessary in the future, the reconstituted socket provides a better foundation for stable cup fixation.

Conclusion

An overall failure rate of 1.65% with a 0.27% failure rate per component year and a 96.1% survival probability at 10 years indicate that the BHR device has lived up to its expectations and reached first base (i.e., a 10-year symptom-free run in young active patients). In what percentage of patients the device will continue on to the home run and outlive the user only time will tell, but as one young patient with an early resurfacing put it at his 10-year follow-up, "Even if the resurfacing fails at some stage in the future, the ten quality years that I have had are reason enough to justify my operation and I can still have a replacement if it fails."

Patient selection is important. In certain indications like extensive femoral head AVN in the young patient, the low survival probability with the BHR persuades us that it deserves to be better. A slightly more forgiving option such as the BMHR is preferable. In severe cases of Perthes disease, the chances of restoring anatomy are limited with the BHR. Using an intermediate option such as the BMHR in order to restore better hip function is preferable to accepting a suboptimal correction with the BHR. Finally, as the results from the Australian Register demonstrate, it must be stated that the results of one type of resurfacing cannot be extrapolated to others. Each resurfacing with its unique material, manufacture, and design is bound to behave differently in

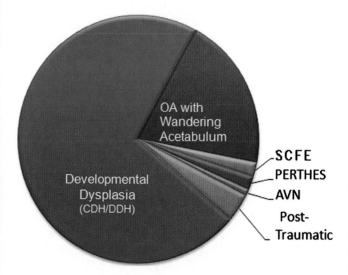

FIG. 27.22. Distribution of different etiologies in our study where the acetabular insufficiency necessitated a Dysplasia BHR.

real life, and the outcomes and longevity of each one will have to be demonstrated individually.

References

1. Hilmarsson S, Soderman P, Herbert P, Malchau H. An epidemiological analysis of a young total hip replacement population in Sweden. J Bone Joint Surg Br 88(Suppl 1):47–8.
2. Australian Orthopaedic Association National Joint Replacement Registry Annual Report 2006. Available at http://www.dmac.adelaide.edu.au/aoanjrr/documents/aoanjrrreport_2006.pdf. Accessed July 31, 2007.
3. Beaule PE, Lee JL, Le Duff MJ, Amstutz HC, Ebramzadeh E. Orientation of the femoral component in surface arthroplasty of the hip. A biomechanical and clinical analysis. J Bone Joint Surg Am 2004;86:2015–21.
4. DeLee JG, Charnley J. Radiological demarcation of cemented sockets in total hip replacement. Clin Orthop 1976;121:20–32.
5. Revell MP, McBryde CW, Bhatnagar S, Pynsent PB, Treacy RBC Metal-on-metal hip resurfacing in osteonecrosis of the femoral head. J Bone Joint Surg Am 2006;88:98–103.
6. Ortiguera CJ, Pulliam IT, Cabanela ME. Total hip arthroplasty for osteonecrosis: matched-pair analysis of 188 hips with long-term follow-up. J Arthroplasty 1999;14:21–8.
7. Zwartelé RE, Brand R, Doets HC. Increased risk of dislocation after primary total hip arthroplasty in inflammatory arthritis: a prospective observational study of 410 hips. Acta Orthop Scand 2004;75:684–90.
8. Amstutz HC, Beaule PE, Dorey FJ, Le Duff MJ, Campbell PA, Gruen TA. Metal-on-metal hybrid surface arthroplasty: two to six-year follow-up study. J Bone Joint Surg Am 2004;86:28–39.
9. Daniel J, Pradhan C, Ziaee H, Pynsent PB, McMinn DJW. Dysplasia Birmingham Hip Resurfacing arthroplasty for deficient acetabulae. Presented at: International Society for Technology in Arthroplasty, New York, 2006.

28
Complications and Revisions of the Birmingham Hip Resurfacing

Chandra Pradhan, Joseph Daniel, and Hena Ziaee

Introduction

Excellent early and medium-term survival rates with the Birmingham Hip Resurfacing (BHR) have been published from different centers around the world. The meticulous documentation maintained at the McMinn Centre allows us to critically analyze our failures and complications. In addition to our own follow-up, all our patients are independently followed up by the Outcomes Centres at either Oswestry or St Helier in the United Kingdom, and this leads us to believe that we have as far as humanly possible captured all our complications.

In this chapter, we present the complications and failures we experienced and the lessons we learned over the past 10 years with the BHR. It should be recognized that in the early years as we continued to develop our indications, techniques, protocols of rehabilitation, and so forth, we were pushing the boundaries in several cases (Figs. 28.1–28.3). Looking back at the preoperative radiographs of some of our successful follow-ups, we wonder whether we would take the risk of resurfacing those hips today. The patients in question have had amazingly good clinical outcomes, but we no longer undertake BHRs in cases with such poor bone quality or grossly distorted anatomy. Neither do we advise others to try hip resurfacing in such cases.

Several criteria including revision, reoperation, radiologic adverse features, and so forth, have been used in the past to calculate survival analysis. Survival is an ultimate test of device success, but even the Swedes now recognize that this has the disadvantage of being a slow methodology. Their Hip Arthroplasty Register from 2005 [1] therefore presents short-term complications as well (every form of reoperation within 2 years of the primary operation). Taking that into account and to allow the capture of every event in the short-term for each patient, we have used our BHR cohort with a minimum 2-year follow-up to calculate our failure rate. This includes all BHRs performed at our center between July 1997 and July 2005. In order to dispel any possible doubt, we point out that we have not had any revisions among the patients operated on since July 2005.

We also present the immediate complications encountered, both surgical and nonsurgical, during this period and the strategies we employed to reduce or prevent some of them. Prior to the final development of the BHR, we went through several models between 1991 and 1996 that were successive improvements in our quest toward an optimum bearing and fixation. The failure rates with those models are shown in Chapter 1.

General Complications

The 30-day mortality rates after primary hip arthroplasty in different regions of the United Kingdom have been reported as between 0.4% and 0.7% [2]. A study of more than 28,000 U.S. Medicare enrollees showed that, compared with controls, the mortality after a hip arthroplasty is increased in the early weeks after operation [3]. By 90 days, the mortality rate equals that in controls and in the next 5 years it is only two thirds that seen in controls. We have had no deaths during the first 90 days after a BHR. During the past 10 years, 40 patients who had a BHR procedure in our center died due to unrelated causes at an average of 4.3 years after the operation (range 9 months to 8 years). Mean age of these 40 patients at operation was 60.4 years and at death it was 64.7 years.

We have outlined the incidence of different categories of complications after surgical procedures in general, primary total hip replacements (THRs), and in our series of 2600 BHRs in Table 28.1. A more detailed list of early complications in our series of 2600 BHRs is presented in Table 28.2.

In addition to the revisions described later, six patients of the 2600 were readmitted during the first 2 years after their BHR operation, three of whom were admitted at our hospital and the rest elsewhere. A very obese lady (body mass index 45) had wound dehiscence and was admitted for debridement and resuturing of her wound. Another patient needed soft tissue repair for a recurrent hip dislocation and a third was admitted for hypoglycemia. The three who were admitted at other hospitals include two for suspected pulmonary embolism and one for septicemia of unknown cause.

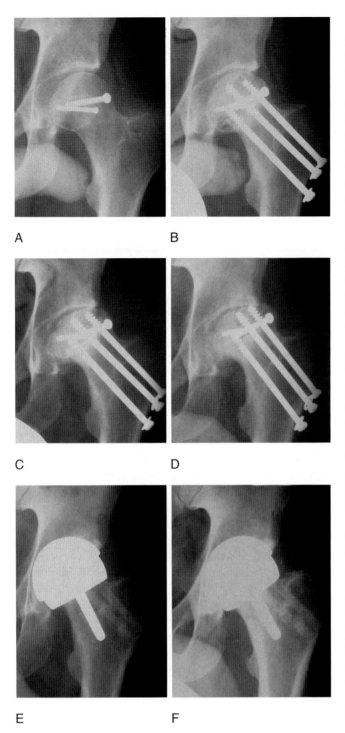

A

B

C

D

E

F

One patient who underwent a BHR in 1998 and a contralateral BHR in 2004 developed a cerebrovascular episode while in hospital, after the second procedure. She subsequently made a full recovery.

Short-term memory loss, confusion, acute renal failure, arrhythmias, and respiratory problems were transient and recovered fully with appropriate medical treatment. One patient had headache due to CSF leak after an epidural and was managed effectively with a blood patch. All cases of deep vein thrombosis (DVT) and two pulmonary emboli resolved fully without any sequelae. We do not use anticoagulants routinely although at the beginning of our BHR experience we used warfarin (Coumadin) (Bristol Myers Squibb, New York, USA) and later we used heparin. Our DVT prophylaxis is described in detail in Chapter 15. Since 2005, our practice has been to screen *all* postoperative patients with Doppler ultrasound to check for asymptomatic DVT. In the past 2.5 years, we have had no case of symptomatic DVT, and we find that even the asymptomatic below-knee DVT rate is very low without the use of anticoagulants.

We have had one case of air embolism. Acute cardiac collapse immediately followed insertion of the acetabular cup. We know of two other cases from elsewhere of air embolus immediately following insertion of the cup. One case was a BHR and one was a non-holed THR shell. The classic features of air embolus are acute cardiac collapse and the presence of a machinery murmur, heard with a stethoscope over the heart. In the context of hip arthroplasty, it follows immediately after the insertion of the cup, presumably from a bolus of air being injected with a particularly well-sealed cup-bone interface.

The emergency treatment is to tip the patient markedly head-down in an effort to displace air from the right heart chambers. External cardiac massage can sometimes be successful but if not, the air needs to be removed from the right heart either through a central venous line if already in place for central venous pressure (CVP) monitoring or by transthoracic needle aspiration of the right heart chambers. In our patient, we managed to reestablish a normal cardiac output eventually and his surgery was completed after re-prep and re-drape. He woke up with severe extensor spasm in his arms and legs and was unresponsive to commands. We feared a serious cerebral injury in this man, who was a 40-year old PhD scientist with a young family. Happily over the next 3 days, he made an apparently full recovery. He happened

FIG. 28.1. This 35-year-old man, an exhibition stand builder by trade, sustained a Pipkin fracture-dislocation of his left hip in a motorcycle accident. This was internally fixed with lag screws (A). Six months later, a femoral neck fracture through a stress-riser at a screw hole was treated with cancellous screw fixation (B). Over the next 2 years, he developed progressive collapse of his femoral head through AVN (C and D). At operation, it was found that nearly two thirds of the femoral head had collapsed and had to be reconstructed with a major cement build-up replacing the lost proximal femoral head. The screw holes were filled with autograft. Despite that cement build-up, the head-neck length has not been fully restored (E). The patient is

FIG. 28.1. (continued) extremely pleased with his result at the 5-year follow-up (F). Although he has had a good outcome, today we would not recommend hip resurfacing in the presence of such extensive bone loss. We feel that a cement build-up is unlikely to be durable in the long-term in a young active patient. We now regard the BMHR prosthesis as perfect for this type of pathology, where a proximally load transferring stem, osseo-integrated in viable bone, with full correction of the head-neck complex, gives us more hope for a good long-term result.

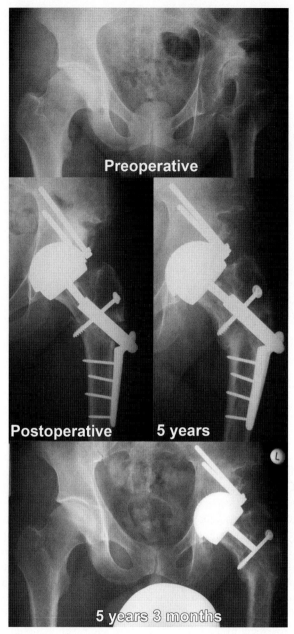

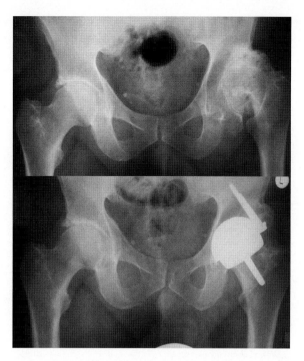

FIG. 28.3. This 47-year-old man presented with severe arthritis, a deformed femoral head, and wandering acetabulum. Regular nonsteroidal anti-inflammatory drug (NSAID) intake had also led to cystic change in the femoral head. The dysplastic acetabulum can easily be managed with the dysplasia cup and bone grafting as in this case. However, the superolateral femoral head is full of cysts, and although a successful outcome was achieved here, it is not recommended to risk femoral head collapse by resurfacing a hip with as poor bone quality as this. The BMHR or a THR would be considered safer options.

FIG. 28.2. A 37-year-old man with hip dysplasia and multiple previous operations including a Chiari pelvic osteotomy and extreme valgus femoral osteotomy. Reconstruction of this grossly deformed hip using a Dysplasia BHR and concomitant opening wedge subtrochanteric osteotomy with a custom hollow nail-plate device has given a reasonable postoperative anatomic restoration. The acceptable postoperative position has been lost, and the osteotomy has healed with a proximal femoral varus deformity. He has a normal gait, good hip function, and is pleased with his outcome. We are displeased with the result as a perfect anatomic restoration has not been achieved. This deformity in the femur will be troublesome if in the future he has to have a THR. Surgeons should be wary about performing hip resurfacing in the presence of such severe deformity. One of the goals of hip resurfacing is to leave the possibility of conversion to a future THR an easy procedure. A cementless THR stem in this man would have been a much easier technical exercise, with better fixation of the femoral osteotomy afforded by the stem in the femoral canal.

to have results from a bank of different tests of intelligence on file at his workplace. These were repeated before his 2-month outpatient review and were found unchanged from the previous tests. His hip is also fine 7 years after his BHR.

Local Complications

One patient who had wound dehiscence has been described earlier. Deep infections leading to a revision have been described later. There were no vascular injuries in our series of 2600 hip resurfacings. The most worrying local complication after any hip arthroplasty is partial or total nerve palsy, and we have described these in detail below.

Nerve Palsy

Sciatic and femoral nerve palsies are rare but disabling problems, with a reported incidence ranging between 2% to 8.5% after hip arthroplasty [4]. Risk factors include a diagnosis of posttraumatic arthritis or developmental dysplasia, severe limb lengthening, and previous operations.

Of the 2600 BHRs, there were 12 patients with transient partial sensory loss in different distributions who recovered fully. Total or partial motor loss developed in the sciatic nerve

TABLE 28.1. List of early complications after surgical procedures in general, primary hip replacements, and our series of 2600 BHRs.

Complications	Incidence of complications (%)		
	Surgery in general	Primary hip replacement	Birmingham Hip Resurfacing DM series
Mortality	2.7	(90-day) 0.97	0
Renal failure	5.4	0.5	0.03
General complications			
Septicemia	1.21	0.20	0.03
Acute gout/flare-up	2	0.69	0.35
Major cardiac events (MI, etc.)	13	0.23	0
Arrhythmias and other cardiac events	1.18	0.95	0.27
Respiratory complications excluding pulmonary embolism	0.79	1.7	0.27
Major cerebrovascular events	0.08	0.05	0.04
Transient and short-term memory loss/confusion, etc.	10.5	0.39	0.08
Pulmonary embolism	3	0.93	0.08
Paralytic ileus and other GI problems	1.12	0.32	0.19
Urinary infections	1.4	11.9	0.26
Readmission	1.59	(90-day) 4.6	0.23
Reoperation	7	0.53	0.15
Local complications			
Infection	1.89	0.5–3	0.42
Wound dehiscence	0.51		0.04
Vascular injuries	0.86	0.25	0
Neurologic injuries		2.13	0.65
Sensory events		0.15	0.38
Motor events		0.17	0.27
Symptomatic deep vein thrombosis	29	44	0.12
Revision		10-year, all diagnoses all ages ~5.8	1.63

TABLE 28.2. List of early complications in our series of 2600 BHRs.

Total number of hips	2600
90-day mortality	0
Readmission in the first 2 years (not including the revisions described later)	5
Cerebrovascular accident	1
Short-term memory loss/confusion	2
Foot drop (including one reoperation for exploration)	2
Sensory loss in sciatic/common peroneal nerve territory	2
Partial/total femoral palsy	5
Sensory loss in femoral nerve territory	8
Transient sensory loss in the hand/upper extremity	2
Unilateral loss of hearing	1
Hip dislocations that needed closed reduction	2
Revision of acetabular component for hip dislocation	1
Recurrent dislocations that needed soft tissue repair	2
Urinary catheterization	202
Urinary tract infection	7
TURP (Transurethral resection of prostate)	2
Transient acute renal failure	1
Chest pain	4
Myocardial infarction	0
Transient supraventricular tachycardia/atrial fibrillation	7
Chest infection	5
Pulmonary edema	2
Vascular injury	0
Symptomatic deep vein thrombosis	3
Symptomatic pulmonary emboli	2
Air embolism	1
Paralytic ileus	5
Flare-up of gout	9
Drug allergy	3
Wound dehiscence	1
Decubitus ulcer	4
CSF leak	1

distribution in two patients and in the femoral nerve territory in five patients, most of whom recovered fully as well.

One patient, who was able to move her foot and toes in the postoperative recovery room, developed ankle and toe dorsiflexor weakness later that evening and progressed to total foot drop the next morning. Her ankle and toe plantar flexors continued to function. In view of her progressive weakness, the possibility of pressure from a hematoma was considered, and surgical exploration was performed to rule out or to evacuate hematoma. At operation, there was no discontinuity in the sciatic nerve, nor did we find the presence of a hematoma. Although she had some improvement in the following months, she is still symptomatic and reports residual weakness in her ankle dorsiflexors. Another patient who developed complete femoral nerve palsy made a slow recovery and still had weakness at the end of 1 year.

A patient with a dysplastic hip and excess femoral anteversion dislocated her hip during the night after her operation and developed femoral nerve palsy. The acetabular component was revised to compensate for her excessive femoral anteversion. Her nerve function started recovering immediately and she had total recovery. All the other patients had transient partial nerve conduction blocks and recovered fully in weeks to a few months later.

Revisions

We had 43 revisions out of the 2600 BHRs (1.65%) over a period of 10 years. These can be broadly divided into six types (Fig. 28.4). It can be seen from the timeline of failures that 65% of all the revisions took place in the first 3 years after the operation (Fig. 28.5).

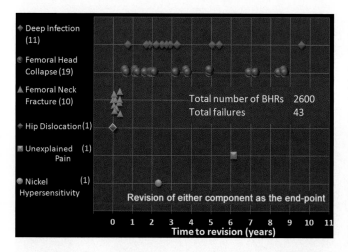

FIG. 28.4. Timeline of failures in the consecutive cohort of 2600 BHRs. Revisions of either component for any reason as the end point.

A breakdown of the incidence of the different reasons for failure shows that almost all the femoral neck fractures occur in the first few months. Femoral head collapse and infection continue to occur over a longer time span. There was one case of unexplained pain and one patient who tested positive for nickel allergy on lymphocyte transformation test. They were both revised to non–metal on metal (MM) bearing devices.

Femoral Neck Fracture

All the failure mechanisms that can affect a THR can affect a resurfacing as well. In addition, because the femoral head and neck are retained in a resurfacing, these patients carry the risk of two additional sites of possible failure, femoral neck fracture and femoral head collapse, leading to a failure of the femoral component. In the presence of a well-fixed socket, the femoral component can now be converted to a THR with a stem and a large-diameter modular head that matches the existing socket (Fig. 28.6).

There were 10 failures from femoral neck fracture in this series of 2600 resurfacings (0.38%). All of them occurred in the first 6 months after the BHR (Fig. 28.7). Mean age at operation among these 10 patients was 54.5 years. Three patients had a definite physical reason for a fracture. A 34-year-old woman underwent a bilateral BHR for rheumatoid arthritis and sustained a fracture after a fall at around 2 months after the operation. Another had a severe twisting injury at work 4 months after the operation, and a third went walking on a sandy beach at 3 weeks when he was supposed to be using his crutches. A 55-year-old man with an alcohol problem was the only one with this risk factor who fractured. Two patients were above the age of 65 years. One of them had severe coxa vara. This deformity makes it difficult not to lengthen the leg with a THR and therefore it is more tempting to do a resurfacing. However, her fracture shows us that age must be treated with respect when it comes to resurfacing, and it is better to err on the side of caution and perform a THR when in doubt.

The risk of fracture can be minimized by careful patient selection. Old age, osteopenia, the presence of large femoral head cysts, and alcohol abuse have been described as risk factors for these failures. We have not found any correlation between femoral neck fracture and a small femoral head size or high activity although these have been suggested as risk factors in the Beaule index. The Australian analysis of the incidence of femoral neck fractures in resurfacings also does not find such a correlation [5]. The femoral head sizes in our group of fractures ranged from 46 to 54 (mean, 48). We have not had any femoral neck fractures in the group that we found to be the most active (young patients with unilateral hip osteoarthritis in whom more than 60% participate in impact sports).

It has also been suggested that performing a bilateral resurfacing procedure puts the femur on the side operated first at risk of a fracture. This is attributed to the force used in implanting the second resurfacing while the patient lies in the lateral position on the just-resurfaced first hip. In our series of 2600 resurfacings for all diagnoses and in all age groups, 193

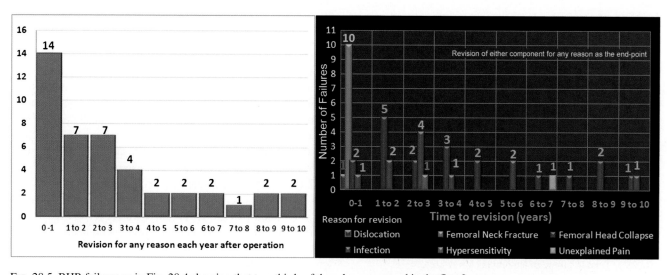

FIG. 28.5. BHR failures as in Fig. 28.4 showing that two thirds of them have occurred in the first 2 years.

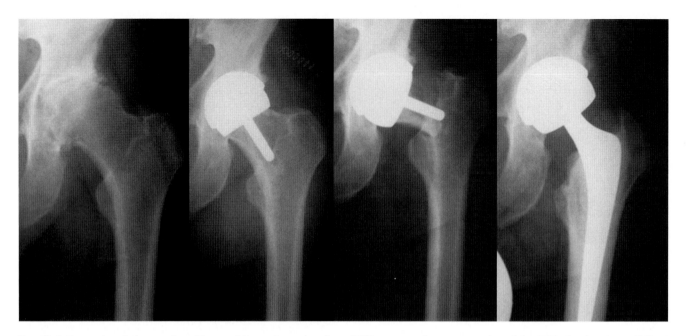

FIG. 28.6. Femoral neck fracture in a 56-year-old man 4 months after a BHR, converted to a stemmed modular THR, leaving the well-fixed cup *in situ*.

patients (386 hips) presented with bilateral end-stage arthritis and had both sides operated in the same hospital admission (14.8% hips of all resurfacings or 8% of all patients). One hundred thirty-three patients had the two operations a week apart, and 60 had them both together on the same day. All operations were carried out through either a traditional posterior or a mini posterior approach with the patient lying in the lateral position on the contralateral side. All patients had a check x-ray in hospital before discharge. Of the 193 bilateral resurfacing patients (386 resurfacings), only two hips failed from a femoral neck fracture. Both had the second operation a week after the first. One was the lady with rheumatoid arthritis referred to earlier. She made an uneventful recovery during the first 9 weeks and then sustained a significant fall and femoral neck fracture on the side operated first. The other was

a 56-year-old man with osteoarthritis who fractured his femoral neck at 3.5 months and he fractured on the side operated second. The low incidence of fractures (2 of 386, 0.5%) in this bilateral resurfacing series does not support the view that there is an increased risk of fracture from a bilateral procedure.

Young fit patients with bilateral hip arthritis prefer to undergo resurfacing of both hips during the same hospital admission in order to reduce the recovery and rehabilitation period. Even though the risk of fracture is not increased in bilateral procedures we hesitate to recommend a simultaneous bilateral resurfacing except for the most compelling reasons and that too only in patients who are in perfect medical fitness for anesthesia and surgery.

Femoral Head Collapse

Femoral head collapse is another complication that is unique to a resurfacing procedure. Unlike a femoral neck fracture, which is an acute event, a femoral head collapse is a slower process and can progress over several months before resulting in a failure or fracture. This may occur as a result of collapse of a previously avascular, osteopenic, or cystic segment. Femoral head collapse can also occur as a result of postoperative loss of blood supply to the femoral head. There have been conflicting reports on femoral head vascularity after a resurfacing that have been fully reviewed and summarized in chapters 9 and 10 by McMahon and Sugano and collaeagues.

The radiologic appearance of a collapsing femoral head in the early stages can often be mistaken for a stem loosening. During the treatment of a patient with femoral head cysts with resurfacing arthroplasty, very often the cyst is curetted and either bone grafted or filled with bone cement. If the grafting

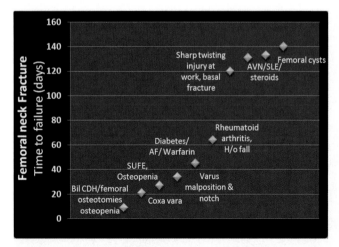

FIG. 28.7. Time to failure in femoral neck fractures.

is inadequate or does not incorporate, the resultant collapse leads first to a varus tilt of the femoral component. This results in displacement of the femoral stem leading to the appearance of a lucent line adjacent to the stem, with or without a sclerotic margin as a remnant of the original stem track. These lucent lines give rise to the appearance of a loose stem. The BHR stem, unlike that of a THR, is not intended for weight bearing and is designed to be loose from the outset (Fig. 27.10). The reason for the apparent stem loosening in this situation is *not* primarily due to wear-debris–induced bone loss around the stem as in a replacement. Displacement of the stem is secondary to displacement of the femoral head, and the femoral head collapse is the primary event that leads to failure in this situation. In a THR, the stem displacement is primary and is due to wear-debris–induced aseptic loosening, which leads to failure as the stem is the load-bearing and fixation structure in the construct.

In a varus position, the resurfacing component is rendered mechanically disadvantaged and leads to progressively increasing deformity, until at some point it fails with or without a precipitating factor such as a trivial injury. This can happen a few weeks after the initial collapse. In one instance, the patient carried on for a few years with a partial collapse and a femoral component that had slightly tilted into varus.

In our consecutive cohort of 2600 BHRs with a 2- to 10-year follow-up, there were 19 failures from femoral head collapse at a mean duration of 3.9 years (8 months to 8.7 years) after the index procedure (Fig. 28.8). They included 14 men and 5 women with an average age of 53 years (range, 34–70 years). In 12 cases, there were definite risk factors preoperatively, but in view of the patients' young ages, a resurfacing was preferred. A subluxing femoral head or a wandering acetabulum leads to severe stress-shielding of the lateral portion of the femoral head rendering it osteopenic leading to a postresurfacing

collapse. Several others with similar radiologic appearances have had good outcomes, and it is a difficult decision as to what level of osteopenia is compatible with long-term success. Patients with extensive AVN or cystic degeneration or early destructive arthritis are especially prone to late femoral head collapse, and we now prefer to use a Birmingham Mid-Head Resection (BMHR) prosthesis or a THR in such cases. These patients should be counseled regarding the possible need for an intraoperative conversion to a THR and assessed carefully at operation for the full extent of the damage and the quality of the rest of the femoral head bone. In 16 hips, only the femoral component was revised leaving the well-fixed acetabular component *in situ* (Figs. 28.9 and 28.10). Three others were converted to a polyethylene-containing THR.

Infection

The most serious complication with resurfacings as with any other form of arthroplasty is infection. The mechanisms, risk factors, and rates of infection with resurfacing are no different from those seen with THRs. In our consecutive series of 2600 BHRs, there were 11 cases of deep infection (0.4%) at a mean duration of 3.5 years (range, 0.8–9.6 years). Seven of these occurred in the first 3 years and four in subsequent years. There were 7 women and four men and their mean age at operation was 50.2 years (range, 39.6–57.7 years). These results compare well with rates of deep infection after primary total hip replacements, which vary between 0.5% and 3%.

The importance of controlling all the possible factors that contribute to infection, including patient factors, operating room environment, surgical technique factors, perioperative care, and prophylactic antibiotics, cannot be overemphasized and are as critical in resurfacing as in other forms of arthroplasty. Just as it is with THRs, late infection is very often hematogenous, and therefore adequate prophylaxis during high-risk procedures is needed (e.g., before potentially infective dental work).

Very often, deep infection may not present as a full-blown case of fulminant infection with local and systemic symptoms. Delayed deep infection can mimic any of the other modes of failure and can present in any of the following four clinicoradiologic patterns, in addition to the classic presentation of a full-blown infection. The development of these radiologic features can be attributed to infective endarteritis occurring in the femoral head and neck after persistent low grade infection.

(a) Progressively worsening hip pain leading on to a femoral neck fracture (Fig. 28.11)
(b) Femoral head collapse.
(c) Femoral neck thinning (Fig. 28.12)
(d) Cup loosening (Fig. 28.13)

In all these cases, the local symptoms may be generally vague and persistent and may or may not be related to activity or weight bearing. The radiologic signs are often atypical, and on investigation, inflammatory markers are raised. A high index

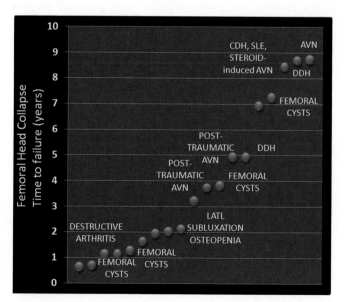

FIG. 28.8. Timeline of BHR failures from collapse of the femoral head.

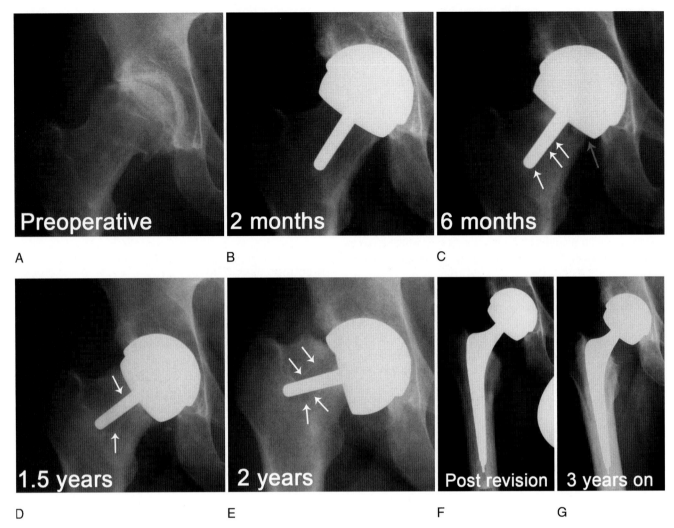

FIG. 28.9. The preoperative (A) and follow-up radiographs (B–G) of a 39-year-old man with severe hip arthritis with osteopenia and cystic change in the superolateral part of the femoral head. The early follow-up radiograph (B) does not reveal any adverse features. At 6 months (C), there are early changes in the femoral head neck junction (suggesting femoral head AVN, grey arrow) and a lucent line around the stem in zone 3 (white arrows). A further year later (D), the femoral head is clearly collapsing and the component tilting into varus with a clearly visible stem track lucency. He was able to carry on for a further 6 months before his femoral neck gave in and failed (E). Conversion to a THR using a cemented femoral stem and a modular component that matched the existing femoral head restored him (F, G). This is not aseptic stem loosening but femoral head collapse due to avascular necrosis.

of suspicion is needed to rule out infection in the presence of any suspicious atypism even in the absence of any systemic signs or symptoms.

When a patient with a resurfacing presents with one of the failure patterns described above and there is a suspicion of deep infection, a hematologic and biochemical profile including inflammatory markers, erythrocyte sedimentation rate (ESR), C-reactive protein (CRP), and white cell count are performed. Antibiotics should not be given in the interim until specimens from the joint have been obtained for analysis. In equivocal cases, a radioisotope bone scan and/or aspiration along with Harlow-Wood biopsy maybe needed. If the evidence points toward an infection, we prefer a two-stage revision, first a Girdlestone excision arthroplasty with gentamicin

beads implantation and systemic antibiotics according to the sensitivity of the organism. Nine of the 11 patients underwent this procedure. In a two-stage revision, we proceed to the second stage when inflammatory markers return to normal and confirmation regarding microbial clearance is obtained from image-guided aspiration/biopsy of the hip.

If the results are negative and the components have failed in one of the patterns described above, a one-stage procedure is performed. However, it is prudent to send the joint fluid and all the excised tissue for microbiological and histopathologic examination (HPE). If the results of either of these is positive for pathogenic infection, then treatment with appropriate antibiotics is instituted. In two patients, both clinical signs and symptoms and initial laboratory results did not suggest

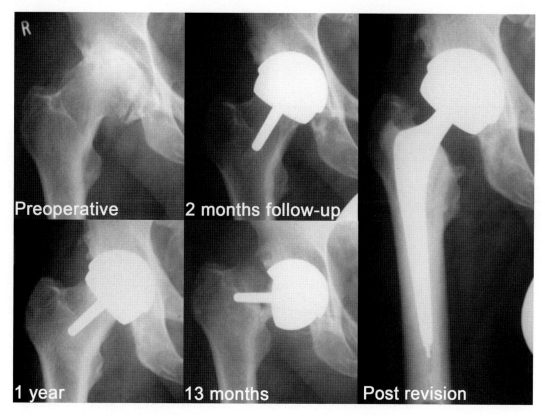

FIG. 28.10. A 58-year-old man underwent a BHR for destructive hip arthritis. He progressed well for a year after which he developed pain and stiffness. X-rays showed evidence of femoral head collapse, which within a month led to femoral neck fracture. He was converted to a THR leaving the socket *in situ.*

the presence of an infection. They were treated initially as a femoral head collapse with one-stage conversion to a THR. The diagnosis of infection was made only on the basis of unmistakable histopathologic evidence, and they were then treated with antibiotics with a good outcome.

During revision of a noninfected failed resurfacing, thick white pus-like sterile fluid is occasionally encountered at operation. A specimen should be sent for Gram staining. If sterile, one of the following two phenomena may be responsible for this fluid. Movement occurring between the ends of the collapsed or failed neck generate debris, which looks like thick white fluid. Thick whitish fluid has also been described in association with hypersensitivity. In the presence of this fluid, the intraoperative decision whether to treat the patient as established deep infection or as a noninfective failure is made all the more difficult. The final decision is based on an overall assessment of the patient, the inflammatory markers, Gram staining, and histopathology if immediately available.

Two female patients who had hip pain, systemic feeling of low-grade illness, and elevated inflammatory markers presented with a loose cup after a fall. At operation, there was purulent fluid, and it was obvious that they were infected. Both grew pathogenic organisms on culture. If the cup is not

loose, then it is dangerous to use force to take it out. The surgeon should use gouges and burrs to carefully detach the cup from its fixation surface first. Failure to do this can lead to a pelvic fracture, which is a dire situation.

Dislocation

There was one revision due to dislocation in our series of 2600 BHRs. This was in a woman with dysplasia and excess femoral anteversion as described earlier. The anterior dislocation occurred during the night after her operation. After relocation under general anesthesia, it was found that her hip was not stable. In order to stabilize her hip, the acetabular component had to be revised to a less anteverted position in order to compensate for the femoral anteversion. Her hip has been stable after that, and she has not dislocated in the past 5 years since the revision.

There were four other dislocations among our series that did not need a revision. In two of them, it followed a significantly violent fall tearing apart the posterior soft tissue structures of their hips. Both these dislocations were posterior. They both needed a soft tissue repair and are described in the "Reoperations" section of this chapter. In two others, the dislocation

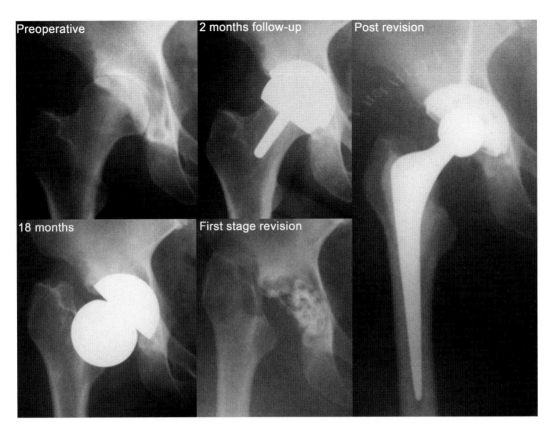

Fig. 28.11. A woman aged 53 years had an uneventful recovery after a BHR. She returned to an active lifestyle, and considered her hip as normal. She then developed hip discomfort, clunking in the hip, and a general feeling of being unwell. At 18 months, she experienced exacerbation of her pain and was x-rayed and found to have a femoral neck fracture. Her inflammatory markers were raised (pre-revision ESR was 36 and CRP 135). At operation, there was blood-stained pus in the hip joint that showed Gram-positive cocci on microscopy and later grew *Staphylococcus epidermidis*. Femoral neck looked white and dead. On histopathologic examination, all six specimens showed evidence of pyogenic infection. She underwent a two-stage revision to a THR.

occurred when they were being transferred from the operating table, and they were treated with closed reduction and have not dislocated since. Both these dislocations were anterior.

Large-diameter bearings have the benefit of having to translate a greater jump distance before a dislocation. One matched case series shows that metal on metal hips have lower dislocation rates than do hips containing polyethylene [6]. This is attributed to the suction-fit effect of metal on metal bearings. This dual advantage leads to a low dislocation rate in metal on metal resurfacings. However, the larger neck diameter in a resurfaced hip puts it at a higher risk of dislocation than that which is associated with a MM THR of the same bearing diameter. Therefore, dislocations are rare with well-implanted BHRs but they can happen. Careful attention to component placement is therefore very important.

Unexplained Pain

One 57-year-old woman made satisfactory progress for around 18 months after a BHR. She then developed hip pain after ice-skating while on holiday, which later continued as intermittent hip pain. Her radiographs showed neck thin-

ning. An ESR of 10 and a CRP level of 0.2 made an infection unlikely. A multislice computed tomography (CT) scan showed a moderately large iliopsoas bursa and medial neck thinning, possibly due to external pressure from the bursa. A lymphocyte transformation test showed that she was allergic to nickel. Her persistent symptoms and the proven presence of hypersensitivity warranted a revision, and we expected to find evidence of typical ALVAL in this our first confirmed case of hypersensitivity-related revision. Histopathologic examination of her tissues revealed only moderate lympho-plasmacytic infiltrate and no evidence of ALVAL. She has been revised to a titanium alloy stem Oxinium XLPE (cross-linked polyethylene) (Smith and Nephew Orthopaedics, Memphis, TN, USA) THR and has made satisfactory progress (Fig. 28.14).

Reoperations

Reoperation includes all those patients who needed a second operative procedure on the resurfaced hip to correct a complication during which neither component of the resurfacing had

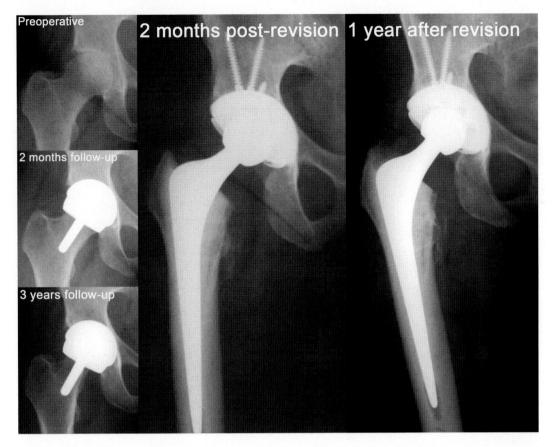

Fig. 28.12. A woman aged 55 years at operation who subsequently developed breast cancer and underwent a mastectomy and received chemotherapy. Three years after the resurfacing, she developed severe hip pain and neck thinning. Raised inflammatory markers (ESR 86 and CRP 76), frank pus on aspiration (*Staphylococcus aureus*), and histopathologic confirmation of pyogenic infection led to a two-stage revision to a THR.

to be revised. One overweight patient who had bilateral BHRs within 6 months of each other made good progress over the next 2 years. He then sustained a posterior dislocation of his left hip from a fall while trying to clean the guttering under the roof of his house. Recurrent dislocation ensued, which needed soft tissue repair. At operation, it was found that he had torn the posterior capsule and his hip had no posterior support at all. The capsule had to be reconstructed with flaps from the intact anterosuperior and inferior capsular segments, which were rotated and sutured on to the remnant of the posterior capsule. Perimysium from the vastus lateralis also was used as an additional flap to double breast the capsule. He recovered well from the reconstruction and has not had a dislocation in the 4 years since soft tissue repair. Another patient, a woman aged 55 years, developed recurrent dislocation after a fall in the shower early after her operation. She, too, recovered after a posterior capsular reconstruction and has not had a recurrence in the 3 years since her repair. There has been no problem with her contralateral hip on which a BHR had been performed around 7 years ago.

Conclusion

It has been said that there are three main causes of surgical complications: (1) the wrong operation done correctly, (2) the right operation done incorrectly, and (3) most frequently, the wrong operation done incorrectly. All three of these causes have the potential to lead to failures with resurfacings.

Constrained by the compulsions of patient age and activity, a surgeon might feel obliged to perform resurfacing in patients with doubtful-quality femoral head bone in some cases. In many instances, the benefit of the doubt may pay off and patients may have a good result, but that will not be universal. We find any case of failure a case too many, and having become wiser with the benefit of hindsight, we consider resurfacing a wrong operation in the presence of poor-quality femoral head bone by way of osteopenia, cystic change, and so forth. In addition, in conditions where severe proximal femoral abnormality exists such as severe cases of Perthes disease, slipped capital femoral epiphysis (SCFE), or femoral anteversion where the anatomy is so distorted that it leads to

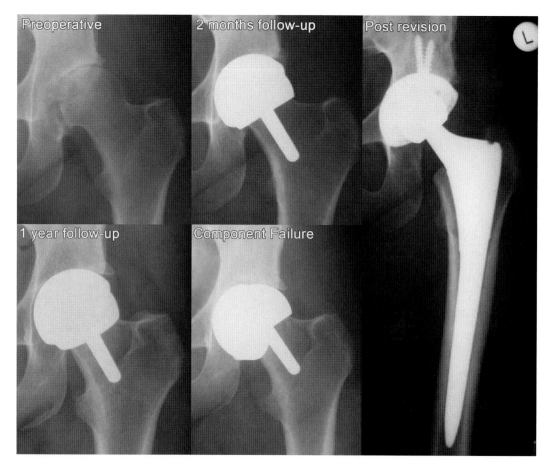

FIG. 28.13. A woman aged 45 years underwent a BHR for developmental dysplasia of the hip. Eighteen months later she developed intermittent pain in the hip. When pain became persistent, a bone scan was done followed by an aspiration and Harlow-Wood biopsy, which showed evidence of infection. In the interim, her cup became loose and dislodged. She underwent a two-stage revision to a total hip replacement.

suboptimal component positioning, we would rather perform a more invasive procedure such as a Birmingham Mid Head Resection or a THR.

Resurfacing can be the most appropriate procedure for a given patient and yet fail due to poor operative technique (right operation done wrongly). It is most vital to preserve femoral head viability for a successful long-term outcome with resurfacing, and every effort should be made to preserve it. Every attempt should be made to avoid notching or stripping soft tissue off the femoral neck. Femoral venting not only helps in reducing systemic embolization but also preserves blood supply to the femoral head and neck. Component malpositioning (in varus), reduced femoral head-neck offset, inappropriate

version of the femoral or acetabular components, and a high angle of cup inclination are all detrimental to a good outcome and long-term survival and should be avoided. One reassuring aspect about resurfacing, however, is that in a majority of these failures, the solution has been conversion to a total hip replacement, which would otherwise have been the treatment option for the original disease in the absence of hip resurfacing.

Acknowledgments. We gratefully acknowledge the expertise and help of Dr. John Wingate, FRCR, consultant radiologist, Birmingham, in the radiologic assessment presented in Chapters 27 and 28.

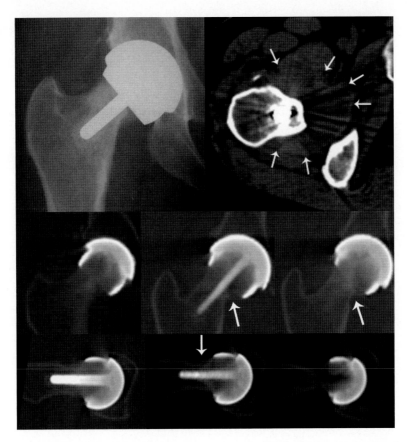

Fig. 28.14. Two-year radiographs and CT scanning images of a patient who was nickel-sensitive and developed neck thinning and persistent pain necessitating a revision. The CT showed a large iliopsoas bursa (arrows in top right picture) that, in the radiologist's opinion, had caused pressure on the femoral neck. The location and pattern of the medial neck thinning suggest that this is due to erosion of the neck as a result of external pressure from the bursa. Please note: A regular CT scan in the presence of a BHR is useless, with severe metal artifact degrading the images. Only some multislice CT scanners give good images in the presence of a BHR. Our radiologist uses a Siemens multislice CT, which provides us with excellent images around the hip and inside the femoral component. In addition to the hardware and software, a dedicated radiologist, prepared to achieve the perfect settings and reconstructions, is an essential ingredient.

References

1. Swedish National Hip Arthroplasty Register Annual Report 2005. Available at http://www.jru.orthop.gu.se/. Accessed August 24, 2007.
2. Williams O, Fitzpatrick R, Hajat S, Reeves BC, Stimpson A, Morris RW, Murray DW, Rigge M, Gregg PJ. National Total Hip Replacement Outcome Study Steering Committee. Mortality, morbidity, and 1-year outcomes of primary elective total hip arthroplasty. J Arthroplasty 2002;17:165–71.
3. Barrett J, Losina E, Baron JA, Mahomed NN, Wright J, Katz JN. Survival following total hip replacement. J Bone Joint Surg Am 2005;87:1965–71.
4. Oldenburg M, Müller RT. The frequency, prognosis and significance of nerve injuries in total hip arthroplasty. Int Orthop 1997;21:1–3.
5. Shimmin AJ, Back D. Femoral neck fractures following Birmingham hip resurfacing: a national review of 50 cases. J Bone Joint Surg Br 2005;87:463–4.
6. Clarke MT, Lee PT, Villar RN. Dislocation after total hip replacement in relation to metal-on-metal bearing surfaces. J Bone Joint Surg Br 2003;85:650–4.

29
Rehabilitation After the Birmingham Hip Resurfacing

Anne Hands, Hena Ziaee, and Chandra Pradhan

Rehabilitation starts at the immediate preoperative stage on admission to the ward. As well as physical rehabilitation, which comes after the operation, mental rehabilitation is also very important in reassuring and motivating the patient at the outset. All Birmingham Hip Resurfacing (BHR) patients choose their time of surgery as it is not a medical or surgical emergency. However, if their activity level has become very low at the time of surgery, then getting back to a high level of activity can be slow and prolonged. Maximum effort for maximum effect is key to a good outcome. We expect the patients to regain normal function on the operated hip and in the long-term to forget it has been operated on.

A care plan is constructed for each patient to take into account among other things the effect that comorbidities may have upon their postoperative rehabilitation.

Day of Operation (Day 0, Postoperative)

Stockings/Tyco Calf Compressor

Prior to the operation, the patient's legs are measured for a full-length Credalast (Credalast, Credenhill Surgical Hosiery Ltd., Ilkeston, UK) stocking for the to be operated leg and below knee T.E.D. (The Kendal Company, Mansfield, MA, USA), stocking for the other leg. The patient is taken in to the anesthetic room with a below-knee T.E.D. stocking applied to the nonoperative leg. The Tyco (Tyco Healthcare UK Ltd, Gosport, UK) intermittent calf compression appliance is applied to this leg after the patient is anesthetized. It is switched on during surgery. Immediately postoperatively, a Credalast stocking is put on to the operated leg to minimize swelling and help prevent thrombosis (Fig. 29.1).It should cover the wound dressing pads without any wrinkles otherwise it can cause local undue pressure. The second Tyco is put on the operated leg and a dough-nut ring (Fig. 29.2) is fitted just above the ankle to prevent heel pressure sores. These two stockings are worn throughout the hospital stay and continue to be worn for at least 6 weeks postoperatively. The Credalast can be removed after 6 weeks postoperatively and temporarily for washing, but if the swelling

in the leg reappears, it may be advisable to wear it again. The T.E.D. stockings are useful for long-haul flights in the future.

Drains

Our practice is to place the superficial drain proximally and the deep drain distally. A mixture of ropivacaine, ketorolac, and epinephrine is infiltrated particularly around the drains so that when the drains are removed at 10 hours postoperatively, minimum pain is experienced during their removal. Previous protocols had meant that the patients had experienced, some said, more pain on removal of the drains than from the operation. On rare occasions, where there is prolonged and heavy drainage, the drains are removed later, but usually within 24 hours postoperatively. Routine postoperative blood tests are done to check systemic functions and hemoglobin level. Herbal medicines such as Arnica and Rhus. Tox are started on the day of admission and are given during the in-patient stay plus for 1 week after discharge. This has been found by plastic surgeons to be very useful to keep bruising down, and we find herbal medicines quite useful in our patients, too. Pain relief may be given for a comfortable night's rest.

Patients sleep with a pillow between their legs or an abduction wedge but may sleep on the nonoperated side after the epidural has worn off (Fig. 29.3).

In the illustrations, the striped sock indicates the operated leg!

Recovery Ward

While the patient is in the recovery ward, an anteroposterior radiograph (mobile) of the pelvis is carried out routinely, as has been our practice for the past 5 years, first to ensure there is no dislocation and second to ascertain the component position. The quality of mobile x-rays is usually not very good, but our past experience of two dislocations while transferring the patient from operation table to bed taught us to do so. The patient under epidural anesthetic may not complain of pain, and a leg deformity may not be very obvious. The patients have both Tyco intermittent calf compression appliances switched on. Once the patient gains full consciousness and pulse, blood

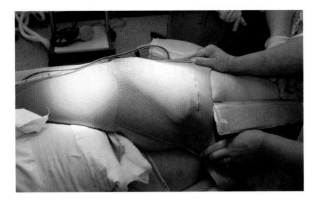

FIG. 29.1. A full-length Credalast stocking being put on.

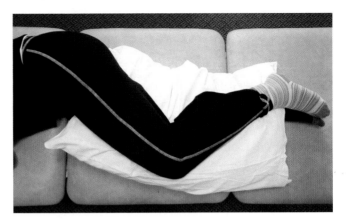

FIG. 29.3. Patient can sleep on the nonoperated side after the epidural anesthetic has worn off.

pressure, and oxygen saturations are satisfactory and stable, the patient is ready to go back to his or her room. Feet and quadriceps are checked to assess sciatic and femoral nerve functions by the recovery nurse before the patient is taken to the ward.

Dr. Lawrence Dorr [1] talks of a "healing-period" in his excellent book on hip arthroplasty. This is also the case with resurfacing patients. Postoperatively, the human body attempts to adjust and heal itself. The combination of an invasive operation, anesthesia, and a cocktail of drugs can throw bodily functions out of synchronization.

Day 1 Postoperative

Blood Test

The intravenous cannula is left *in situ* until postoperative blood results are back and 3 doses of prophylactic antibiotics have been given. Routine postoperative blood tests are done to check systemic functions and hemoglobin level. If a transfusion is required at this stage, the already saved serum is cross-matched. However, the need for a transfusion is now a rarity in our practice. Most of the patients do not require intravenous fluids, and they maintain good hydration and urine output with oral intake.

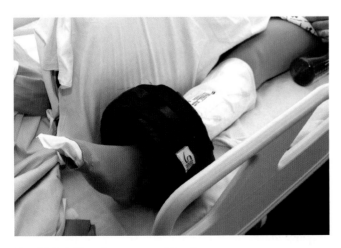

FIG. 29.2. A Tyco foot pump and doughnut.

Urine voiding can be difficult in some patients. If the usual nursing methods of encouraging passage of urine have not been successful, an indwelling catheter may be required until the patient is walking.

Physiotherapy

Physiotherapists usually attend the patient on day one after surgery. The physiotherapists need to be aware of postoperative instructions for each patient so that they can treat accordingly. If very soft bone is encountered during the procedure or if a Dysplasia cup is used with additional bone grafting of the acetabular roof, the patients may need to be taught partial weight bearing as advised, which may be for 2 to 3 months postoperatively. Encouragement and assistance in mobilization begins with a few simple exercises in bed and progresses to transferring from the bed to standing and taking their first few steps (Fig. 29.4).

Do's and Don'ts Prior to Mobilization

Prior to mobilization, the physiotherapist will have instructed "Do's and Don'ts," such as (1) no adduction past midline, (2) no internal rotation beyond midline, (3) no hip flexion beyond 90 degrees for a 6-week postoperative period, (4) to keep moving the feet to assist venous return, (5) deep breathing exercise to expand the lungs, (6) bending the unoperated knee and lift buttock off the bed using monkey pole to prevent pressure sore.

There is a series of bed exercises the patients are encouraged to do (Figs. 29.5).

The patient is stood with a nurse and physiotherapist and taught how to walk with a Zimmer frame. Some patient may feel dizzy because of postural hypotension.

Day 2 Postoperative

Walking is progressed and the patient is encouraged to use two elbow crutches (Figs. 29.6 and 29.7). Gait is monitored and corrected as necessary as many patients find it difficult to use the

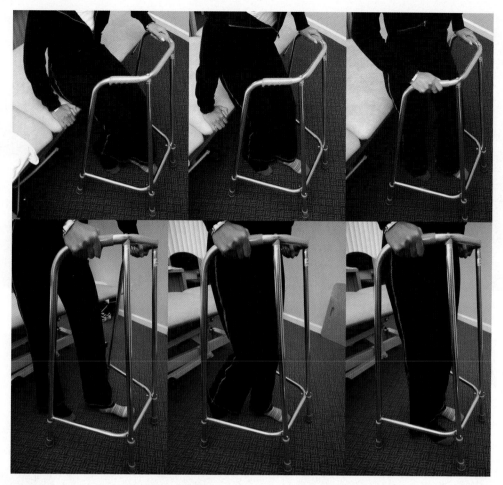

FIG. 29.4 One hand on bed, one hand on Zimmer frame. Move operated leg forward. Push onto hands and come into standing taking most of the weight onto the nonoperated leg. Draw operated leg back, level with other foot, and take weight evenly if possible. Move frame forwards. Move operated leg into frame taking weight as necessary on hands. Move nonoperated leg to join. Continue as able.

normal "heel-toe" pattern of walking at first. Sitting in a chair for short periods, no longer than 30 minutes is permitted (Fig. 29.8). Patients are advised how much walking to do independently. Further exercises are added to their routine, and they are encouraged to lie flat for half an hour twice daily to stretch the front of the hip. Nursing assistance is given in order to shower.

Patients are shown how to carry out simple tasks, such as putting on shoes and socks, without risking a dislocation (Fig. 29.9).

A shoehorn is used to help put shoes on, but remember to keep knees out and approach foot from inside the leg.

Do *not* rotate knees in when sitting in a chair, and do not try to pick up objects from the floor. *When In doubt, keep knees out!*

Patients gain a lot of confidence when they start walking along the corridors and see other patients also improving with their hip resurfacing.

The walks are taken either with the physiotherapist or the nurse, and as the patient gains more strength, the duration of the walk is increased. Initially, the patients are escorted by the physiotherapist changing to independent walking as they get more confident. Occasionally, patients may feel a click/

clunk on the operated side that disappears as muscle control is regained.

Day 3 Postoperative

By the third day, the patient should be able to independently transfer in and out of bed and be capable of showering and dressing with minimal help. Exercises again are progressed to include lateral rotation in some degree of hip flexion. By flexing the nonoperated leg toward the patient's chest and maintaining a straight position with the operated leg further, gentle stretching of the anterior hip structures is encouraged.

Care should be taken to encourage core stability (abdominal) so that the patient is using correct muscles at all times. Gait is progressed by introducing a 4-point pattern using elbow crutches (Fig. 29.10).

Patients do not need a raised toilet seat unless they are very tall.

These activities give the patients a real boost in their rehabilitation progress.

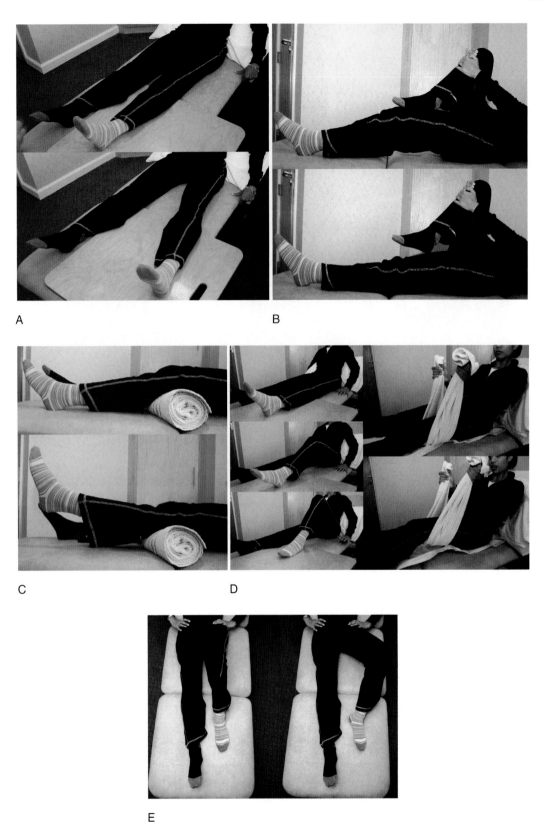

Fig. 29.5. (A) Place a sliding board under the operated leg. Slide leg out to side, as comfortable, and back to midposition. Ensure the pelvis is stable. This is easily done with the patients x-ray packet, which often comes to hand more easily than a board. (B) Bend nonoperated leg up toward chest as far as is comfortable and hold with both hands. Brace thigh on operated leg by pushing the knee into bed and hold for 5 seconds. (C) Place a rolled towel under the knee on the operated side, brace thigh, lift heel off bed and hold for 5 seconds. Lower slowly. (D) Bend the operated leg toward you, sliding the foot along the bed/board. Straighten leg back to starting position. A sling or towel may be used to assist the movement. The range of movement should gradually increase but to not more than 90 degrees hip flexion for at least 6 weeks. (E) Lie on back and bend operated knee to 50 degrees. Gently lower leg out. Ensure that the movement is from the hip and not pelvis.

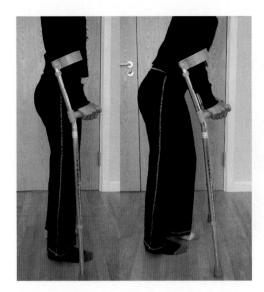

FIG. 29.6. When standing, ensure the back is straight and *not* bent.

If the patient is comfortable sitting for a short time, they are encouraged to do some gentle leg exercises to increase the strength in the legs (Figs. 29.11 and 29.12).

Standing exercises are also introduced (Figs. 29.13–29.17).

Days 4 to 5 Postoperative

Patients will be taught to ascend and descend stairs (Figs. 29.18 and 29.19).

They are encouraged to mobilize independently with periods of exercise and rest.

The patient is advised to continue with anti-deep-vein thrombosis (DVT) exercises when sitting.

They continue independent mobilization in corridor, shower, toileting, and dressing.

A good-quality pelvic radiograph is taken centered at the pubic symphysis, and a color Doppler scan is performed to assess possible deep venous thrombosis in the legs before patients are discharged.

Patients can be discharged after ultrasonography (USG) scan on or after the fourth postoperative day if they feel confident enough and are medically fit to do so.

Day 6 Postoperative

Nearly all patients are discharged by the sixth day, by which time they will have normally had considerable practice on stairs and walking along the corridors. Patients continue with home physiotherapy exercises as instructed on the ward. They are advised to think carefully about their home and stairs and ask their physiotherapist how to handle it. Patients are also shown how to bend and pick up small objects off the floor (Fig. 29.20). Our thromboprophylaxis regimen includes oral enteric-coated aspirin, which is started on the day of operation along with an H_2 receptor blocker. Patients who have

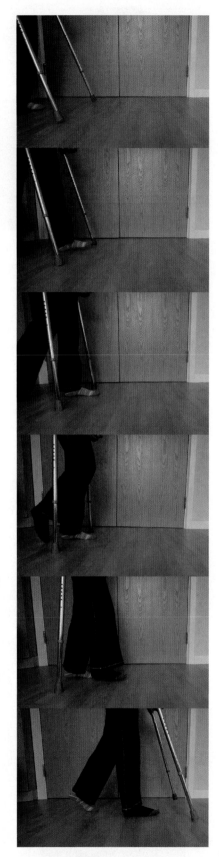

FIG. 29.7. Walking with crutches. Correct gait. Upright posture. Move both crutches forward. Move operated leg forward to join crutches, taking some weight on the operated leg and some on the crutches. Move the nonoperated leg forward. Continue with more steps.

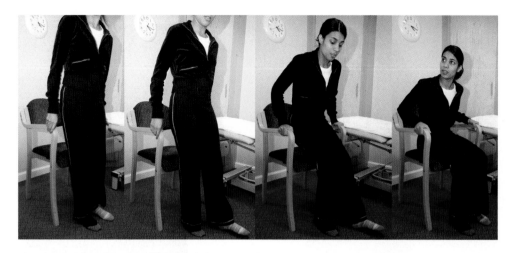

Fɪɢ. 29.8. How to sit and stand. Move back to feel chair behind legs. Chair height is important. Do not try and sit on a very low chair. Place hands onto arms of chair, move operated leg forward, but still on the ground, and sit down gently. Adjust position until comfortable. Reverse instructions for standing.

gastrointestinal intolerance to aspirin receive dipyridamole [Persantin (Persantin, Boehringer Ingelheim Ltd., Blackwell, Berks, UK)] or clopidogrel [Plavix (Plavix, Bristol-Myers Squibb Pharmaceuticals Ltd., Uxbridge, UK)]. These are continued for one month after discharge.

Before discharge, the patients will have done much ward corridor walking and plenty of stairs practice, and they may go out to the car park and gardens for a walk. Sometimes, we have found patients even going to the pub (bar) nearby. Generally, the patients feel better quickly and may do too much, which should be avoided because of the risk of femoral neck fracture.

Some patients prefer to take a train to return home; they can do so at this stage, but the problem is that they cannot carry heavy luggage. Such patients are advised to bring just a rucksack, which leaves the arms free for using crutches (Fig. 29.21).

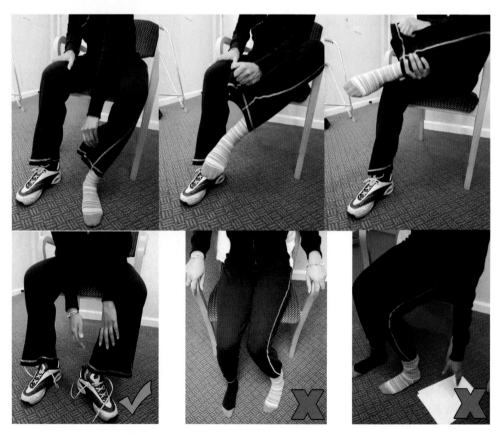

Fɪɢ. 29.9. How to put socks and shoes on.

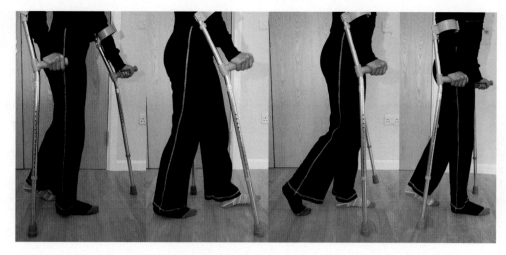

FIG. 29.10. Four-point gait walking with crutches: left crutch right leg; right crutch left leg.

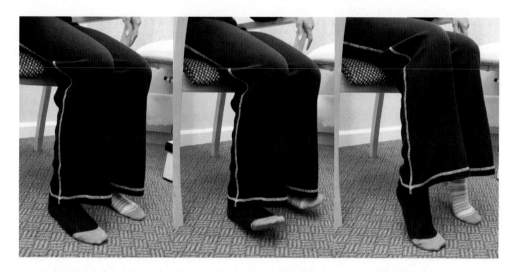

FIG. 29.11. Rock onto heels of both feet and then raise onto toes. Rocking motion.

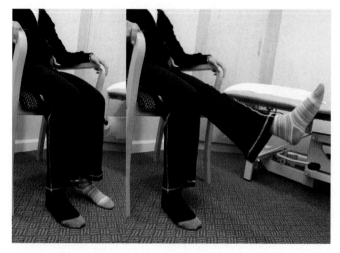

FIG.29.12. Sitting back in chair, straighten leg and hold for 3 seconds and then relax slowly.

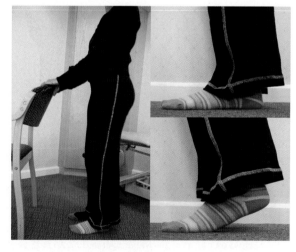

FIG. 29.13. Hold onto rail or chair. Place feet hip-width apart. Raise onto toes and lower, ensuring balance.

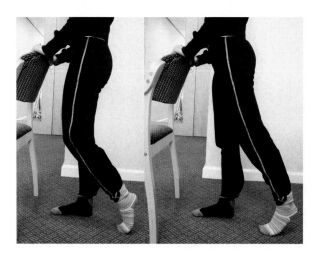

FIG. 29.14. Holding on to a railing or chair, move operated leg backwards and rest on toes. Nonoperated leg is taking most of the weight. Then straighten the operated leg by bracing the knee. Clench your buttocks together and keep your body straight. Hold this position for 5 seconds.

Patients are shown how to maneuver in and out of a car (Fig. 29.22).

Once the patients are home and in familiar surroundings, it is a good opportunity for them to work as much as they can on their hip but also take plenty of rest and not overdo it. Also, their appetite will recover.

Skin clips are removed by a district nurse or GP on the 12th postoperative day. Patients who would like to sleep on the operated side can do so at this stage with a pillow between the knees (this should be used until 6 weeks postoperatively). Usually, the area is sensitive, and massaging with some oil or cream will take away soreness arising from soft tissues.

Long-haul flights are not advised immediately postoperatively. Patients from the United States/Canada/Australia are advised to remain in the United Kingdom for a further

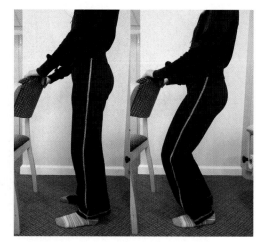

FIG. 29.16. Holding onto rail or chair, place feet hip width apart. Bend knees no further than 50 degrees and keep back straight.

week after discharge from hospital before undertaking flights home. They should take a walk during the flight every 30 to 40 minutes and take plenty of nonalcoholic drinks. They should do feet exercises and take aspirin. Patients are given a letter addressed to airlines requesting a seat with extra leg room. Patients should not go walking on sandy beaches in the early weeks after the BHR. Crutches are rendered ineffective in sand, and we have had one patient fracture his femoral neck with this activity. Patients from European countries can fly home directly after discharge from the hospital.

Four Weeks Postoperative

Before the patient is discharged, they will be shown how to walk with a stick (cane) as they usually transfer from crutches to a stick by 1 month postoperatively (Fig. 29.23). Patients are

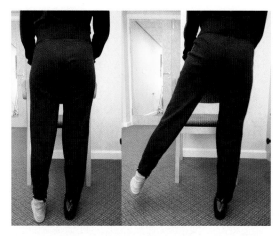

FIG. 29.15. Hold on rail or chair. Move operated leg to side as able. Hold for 5 seconds and lower back to starting position. Avoid moving trunk—only leg moves and not pelvis.

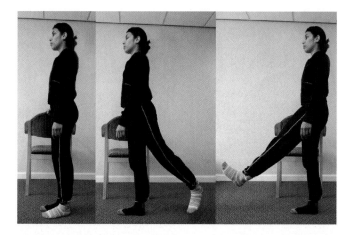

FIG. 29.17. Holding onto rail or chair, stand on the nonoperated leg. Keeping body still, from hips, slowly swing the operated leg backwards and forwards.

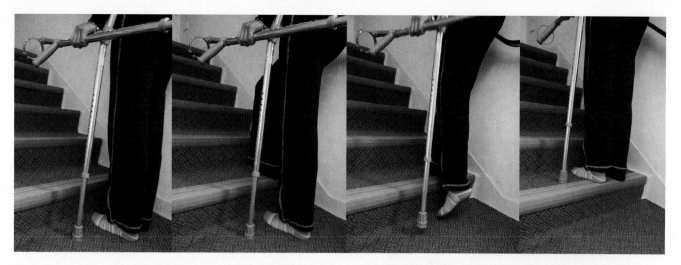

FIG. 29.18. Going *up*: Stand close to bottom step. Transfer crutches to hand furthest away from handrail, holding safely as illustrated. Hold rail with other hand. Put nonoperated leg onto first step. Push with hand on crutch and pull with hand on rail, raise operated leg and crutch onto first step. Progress up stairs. Stick to climbing one step at a time until able to walk without limp comfortably.

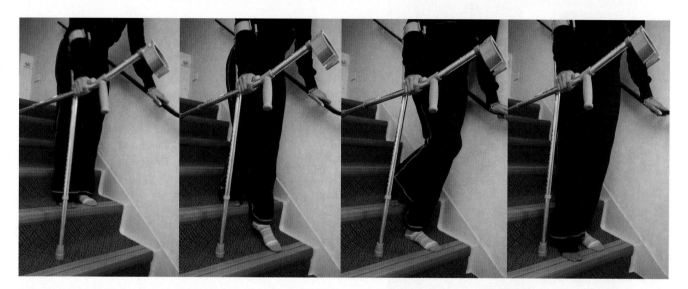

FIG. 29.19. Going *down*: Put elbow crutches into one hand, and hold hand rail with other hand, as illustrated. Move crutch onto stair below, move other hand down the rail. Operated leg moves down to join crutch on step. Then nonoperated leg moves to join on same stair. Proceed down slowly.

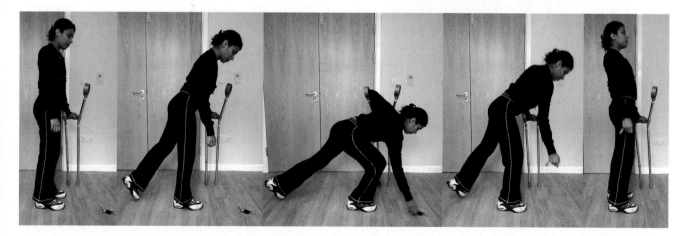

FIG. 29.20. Make an "H: with the crutches, holding both handles in the same hand. Keeping the operated leg straight, move it back and keep the toe on the floor. Slowly bend forward to pick up small objects (e.g., keys).

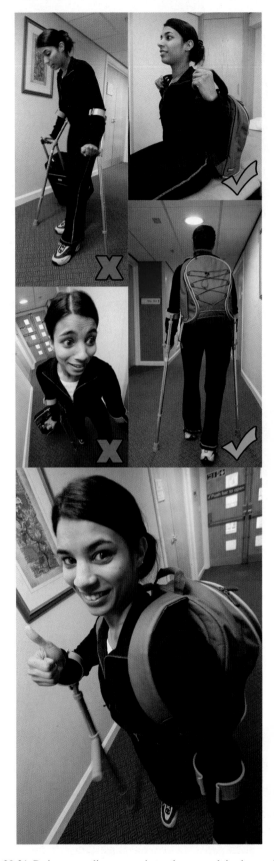

FIG. 29.21. Patients traveling on a train or plane are advised not to bring suitcases or trolleys because of the difficulty of carrying the case while using the crutches postoperatively. Use a rucksack instead. Ensure that the rucksack sits in the small of the back and straps are secure.

given a stick to take home, if they do not already have one, and use a stick for walking outdoors until outpatient review.

Driving

There is evidence that the reaction time on and off car foot pedals does not return to normal for 6 weeks. Depending on the side of operation, therefore, patients can drive an automatic car 3 weeks postoperatively but not a manual car until 6 weeks postoperatively.

Return to Work

Return to work depends on the nature of the job. We find most of the patients return to part-time work 4 to 6 weeks postoperatively and full-time work 6 to 8 weeks postoperatively. There are some patients who return to work early.

Six to 8 Weeks Postoperative

This is when the first postoperative review is done. Patients are requested to attend clinic where an up-to-date x-ray is taken, a postoperative questionnaire is completed by the patient, and a clinical examination is carried out. Assessment and improvements in patients mobility and flexibility are noted. At this stage, patients should have hip flexion of about 90 degrees. Now patients can attempt to flex the hip in excess of 90 degrees. They can also cross the operated leg to the midline.

Patients are shown and given an illustrated booklet of do it yourself (DIY) exercises to stretch the scar tissue around the operated hip to gain a good range of movement (Fig. 29.24). At this stage, most patients should be able to walk about 1 mile a day. Their common concern is they cannot put their socks on. They may have a slight limp because of their old walking habit. They also sometimes comment that they feel as though they are sitting on a wallet. This is due to scar tissue. Local massage with oil/cream should continue. The majority of patients will have stopped using a walking stick. It is important to use a stick in the opposite hand until one walks without a limp.

Hydrotherapy

Swimming in a pool is strongly recommended from 6 weeks postoperatively, in particular, breaststroke once daily for 20 minutes for a duration of 3 months. Circular movements in the water turn a good recovery to a great recovery much faster. Hence, patients who cannot swim are advised to hang on to the sides in the pool and perform the circular movements. Patients can use other swimming strokes, but breaststroke is the best one.

Patients are advised to gradually increase their level of activity, be it professional or social. The thought of returning to their "normal" life by doing the things they used to do (within moderation) is very good for boosting the patient's morale and speeding their recovery.

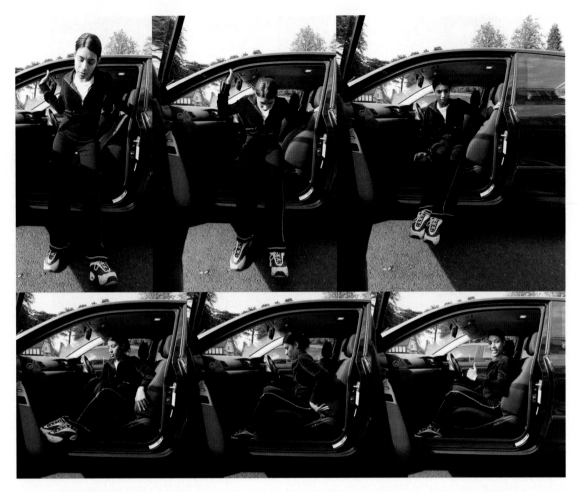

FIG. 29.22. How to get in and out of a car. Move car seat back as far as possible and recline slightly. Back up to the car and give elbow crutches to your companion. Hold onto back of seat with one hand and door frame or appropriate hand-hold position. Move operated leg forward, duck head and sit carefully down. Push bottom carefully back onto seat (if seat is fabric, use a plastic bin liner to slide on). With both feet together, move carefully round, lifting feet into car, and move into a comfortable position. Lift back of seat up for comfort. *Remove bin liner if used*. Travel home safely! No more than 40 minutes to 1 hour traveling is advised before getting out and walking around for 5 to 10 minutes. Follow the reverse instructions to get out of the car.

Gymnasium

Patients can attend a gym from 6 weeks postoperatively, doing static bike cycling, rowing, and other stretching exercises. They should concentrate on strengthening and stretching exercises but avoid impact loading. Gymnasium work and all sporting activity should be gradually built up.

Return to Activities

Sports and hobbies are banded into different groups depending on their level of impact loading through the hip (Table 29.1).

BHR patients have been found to continue to improve in bone strength in a dual-energy x-ray absorptiometry (DEXA) scan study [2] for 2 years postoperatively. Therefore, it is crucial that patients do not undergo high-impact loading activities until 1 year postoperatively. Patients who are keen to run

or jog are advised to start treadmill running with a good pair of shoes at 10 months postoperatively for 2 months. Then they can start road running 1 year postoperatively. Walkers can walk unlimited distance within comfort.

Golf/Tennis

These can be started gently 4 to 6 months after BHR surgery. During a strenuous golf swing, one can tear capsular soft tissues. This causes some bleeding and pain. The patients may get alarmed that they have dislocated or fractured the hip, and they need reassuring. In order to prevent this, golfers are asked to concentrate on getting back a full range of movement by means of hydrotherapy before returning to the golf course. Pitching and putting can start at 6 weeks postoperatively. In tennis, patients are told to play doubles initially and should be prepared to leave some balls if excessive stretching is required.

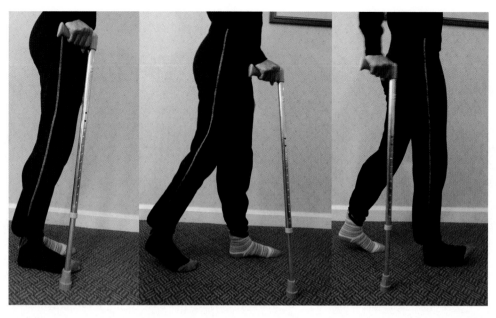

FIG. 29.23. How to walk with a stick. Hold stick on nonoperated side. Normal gait, stick moving forward with operated leg.

This pamphlet should be used as a reference following the demonstration of these exercises at your follow up consultation with Mr McMinn. If for any reason your post operative follow up consultation is delayed then these exercises should be started by you at 6 weeks from the date of your operation.

The following should be performed on a firm but comfortable surface to enable you to carry out the exercises without any discomfort.

It is recommended that you perform each exercise with 20 repetitions, morning and evening, and these exercises should be supplemented with 20 minutes of breast stroke swimming every day. Perform each exercise on both sides if you have had surgery to both hips.

The purpose of these exercises is to stretch the scar tissue around the hip and restore the range of hip movement.

Exercise 1
Lying flat on your back with your head on the bed or floor, grasp the knee of your un-operated side and pull towards your chest as far as you can. On your operated side your knee will naturally bend. Without relaxing your unoperated leg, tense your thigh and buttock muscles, to try and get the bottom of your knee flat. This will stretch the scar tissue in front of the hip. Maintain this stretched position for 5-10 seconds.

Repeat this movement 20 times.

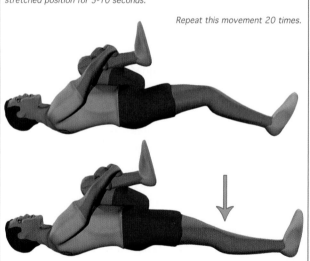

Exercise 2
Lie on your back, feet together and knees bent to around 45 degrees. Split your legs, moving your knees as far away from each other as possible, then return to the starting position. The object is that with gradual stretching the operated hip will come as far out as the unoperated hip.

Repeat this movement 20 times.

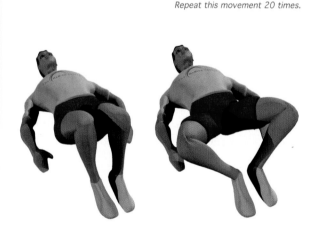

Please turn over...

FIG. 29.24. An example from the postoperative booklet showing exercises. These are also available on the Web site [3].

TABLE 29.1 Examples of severity of physical activity at work or home...

None.	Light work (Walking involved)
Needs Wheelchair/crutches for mobility. Needs help with sample household chores	Nursing. School teaching. Bench work. Assembly line work. Lifting/carrying less than 5kg. Washing clothes. Making beds. House cleaning. Care of small children. Weeding. Pruning. Professional sportspersons of low impact sports.
Sedentary work (Seated most of the time)	**Moderate work.**
Driving light vehicles, Reading, Writing, Office work, Working at computers.	Heavy service work. Heavy gardening work. Maintenance work. Truck driving. Loading/unloading goods less than 25kg. Care of physically disabled. Lifting and transferring patients. Professional sportspersons and coaches of moderate impact sports such as golf, bowling, ballet etc.
Semi-sedentary (Standing involved).	**Heavy work**
Feeding and distributing medicine in healthcare, Washing dishes. Fine mechanical service work. Bar tending.	Concreate founding/Felling trees. Digging ditches. Shovelling sand or chopping wood. Lifting or carrying more than 25kg. Policemen, Soldiers and Firemen on active duty, Professional sportspersons and coaches of high impact sports such as running, hockey, football, cricket etc.

Skiing

This can be started after 1 year postoperatively. Patients are told to miss a season before skiing after BHR surgery.

Future Long-Haul Flights

Patients should wear T.E.D. stockings and take one aspirin half an hour before a flight. In addition, they should walk around during the flight, avoid alcohol, and drink plenty of water and juices. Mr. McMinn advises patient to travel first class, British Airways, Thai Airlines, or Virgin upper-class, with a fully flat bed!

Dental Treatment

Antibiotic cover for dental treatment is required for the first 3 months after hip surgery. Thereafter, there is no need for antibiotic cover unless there is any evidence of infection/abscess being present. Under these circumstances, it is important to have antibiotic cover for dental treatment.

References

1. Dorr LD. Hip Arthroplasty. Philadelphia, Saunders Elsevier, 2006.
2. Kishida Y, Sugano N, Nishii T, et al. Preservation of the bone mineral density of the femur after surface replacement of the hip. J Bone Joint Surg Br 2004;86:185–9.
3. Available at: The McMinn Centre website, Rehabilitation section (www.mcminncentre.co.uk)

30
Recovery and Rehabilitation

Lawrence Kohan and Dennis R. Kerr

Ideally after any operation, recovery to full health and resumption of the normal activities of daily living should be immediate, and there should be no complications or side effects from any of the therapeutic interventions. In the real world, of course, it is unlikely that this ideal could ever be realized, but the focus of our efforts should be to approach this goal as closely as possible. Many patients who present for arthritis surgery on the hip are in good health, and often their only problem is arthritis. This is particularly the case for those presenting for hip resurfacing who tend to be younger (average age about 55 years) and fitter than the population presenting for total hip replacement (average age about 70 years). Additionally, both the Birmingham Hip Resurfacing procedure and the Birmingham Modular Head Total Hip Replacement are procedures that are compatible with immediate mobilization and present little risk of dislocation. Thus, we are presented with a unique opportunity to achieve rapid recovery and approach the ideal recovery more closely than previously possible.

There are several key tactics that must be considered that underpin the overall strategy directed at rapid recovery. They include:

• Appropriate anesthetic technique
• Active normalization of physiology after surgery
• Meticulous pain management
• Eliminating unnecessary interventions and medications
• Adequate preparation
• Immediate mobilization
• Reducing hospital stay

The process in summarized in the following sections (Fig. 30.1).

Adequate Preparation

Our experience has shown that a key element in achieving rapid recovery is extensive preoperative preparation. Because the patient may only be in hospital overnight, all the educative processes and discharge planning must be completed before coming to the hospital. Considerable effort must be invested in psychological and organizational preparation and in arranging support and assistance postoperatively. Setting the patient's expectations relating to pain management, and postoperative surveillance is best achieved by an extended preoperative consultation with the anesthetist and cannot be adequately dealt with on the day of surgery in a brief encounter. Important points relating to the preoperative anesthesia consultation include:

• Allow enough time for the consultation—typically about 30 minutes—preferably several days preoperatively.
• *Give the patient a written pain management plan, and discuss it in detail.*
• Tell the patient what to expect—pain levels, mobility, swelling, wound, temperature.
• Discuss time of discharge, home situation, and transport arrangements.
• Discuss how the medications will be supplied and how to take them.
• Discuss side effects and problems and how to get help.
• Arrange a contact procedure and ensure that the patient has all relevant phone numbers.

Appropriate Anesthetic Technique

The anesthetic technique chosen is very important in ensuring rapid recovery after hip surgery and if poorly handled can delay the whole process for hours. Goals include

• Preventing pain signals from ever reaching the spinal cord where central processing can amplify and extend the painful experience; and
• Ensuring rapid full recovery from anesthesia with minimal sedation, muscle weakness, or drug side effects such as nausea and vomiting.

We use a short-acting spinal anesthetic (3 mL bupivacaine 0.25%) designed to wear off, so that the patient can mobilize and

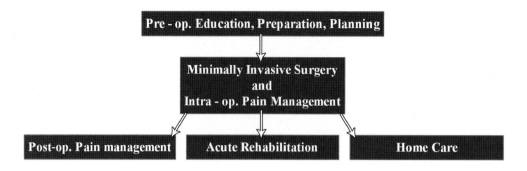

Fig. 30.1.

pass urine, rather than the more usual approach of trying to prolong the block to extend pain control. Leg movement is usually possible in the recovery room, and recovery of pain, autonomic, and bladder nerves is complete by about 3 hours postoperatively. This time frame also allows smooth transition to local infiltration analgesia for pain control as the local infiltration has time to spread and become established well before the spinal wears off. Opioids are not included in the spinal as they guarantee urinary retention and catheterization in a proportion of male patients and because pain is controlled without the use of opioids by the local infiltration analgesia technique. Because most of our patients expect to be asleep, we supplement the spinal with propofol and ketamine infusions to keep them lightly asleep.

Meticulous Postoperative Pain Management

Pain management should be a process rather than an event and must extend for the entire perioperative period. The process starts at the preoperative anesthesia consultation and well before the patient enters the hospital. The reaction to pain is conditioned by expectations especially if the patient has had an adverse experience with previous surgery. The combination of allaying their fears, setting their expectations, educating them about the process, and assuring them that you will be there for them whenever they need assistance is a powerful analgesic in its own right.

Our technique [1] for control of the acute postoperative pain is detailed in the section on that topic (Chapter 16). This approach to pain control aims to control pain at its source before central processing of the pain signals complicates matters and to do so in a way that avoids sedation, preserves muscle function, and enables rapid mobilization.

Eliminating Unnecessary Interventions and Medications

In order to mobilize patients, it is very important to dispense with anything that requires them to stay in bed. To this end, we do not routinely use urinary catheters, wound drains, invasive

monitoring, patient-controlled analgesia (PCA) machines, or epidurals for pain control; nor oxygen masks or nasal prongs or permanently connected ECG monitors or pulse oximeters. Routine postoperative monitoring is limited to intermittent routine nursing surveillance. Of course, exceptions are made for specific positive indications.

Active Normalization of Physiology After Surgery

Careful attention to detail and immediate action to correct any detectable pathophysiology promotes the recovery process. Most patients having hip surgery will lose some blood, and there will be some movement of fluid from the vascular compartment into the wound during the first 12 hours postoperatively. Although the need for blood transfusion is not frequent, it is important to maintain blood volume if hypotension is to be avoided. Two to 3 L of intravenous fluids are given over 18 to 24 hours postoperatively, and free oral fluids are encouraged. Hypotension is treated aggressively with plasma expanders such as 4% albumin or intravenous fluid boluses.

Hypoglycemia is also an impediment to rapid physiologic recovery, so all patients are presented with sandwiches and a sweet drink such as apple juice on arrival back in the ward, and they are served normal meals at the usual times.

Immediate Mobilization

Hip replacement or resurfacing procedures that use a large anatomic femoral component lend themselves to early mobilization. Once the prosthesis has been fixed in place, it is stable, and the patient can usually begin walking immediately. With adequate pain control and functioning musculature, it is possible for patients to walk within an hour or so after the procedure is completed provided physiologic disturbances (hypovolemia, hypoglycemia) are minimized and drug side effects eliminated.

Early and complete mobilization markedly reduces the incidence of postoperative thromboembolic complications [2] and improves early recovery of full joint movement. Also, if patients can stand and walk to the toilet within 4 hours of the surgery, urinary catheters are rarely necessary.

Getting people up and out of bed also improves cardiorespiratory function as expansion of the upright lung is assisted by gravity, and the chest and diaphragm operate at a mechanical advantage compared with their function in the recumbent position The effort involved also forces deep breathing and coughing.

Assuming the upright position also sets in train a series of cardiovascular reflexes that assist in restoring cardiovascular stability. Finally, mobilization boosts outlook and confidence.

Over the past 9 years, 8 of 700 Birmingham Hip Resurfacing (BHR) patients and 1 of 117 modular head BHR patients have had significant (>10 cm, axial vein) DVTs in the first 6 weeks after surgery, and we have had no pulmonary emboli recorded.

Perhaps the most important factor promoting early mobilization is the attendance of senior staff who have both the authority and experience to supervise and initiate the process. Left to themselves, patients will hardly move unless given permission and encouragement to do so. Our approach is to send specially trained staff, either our physiotherapist or nurse personal assistant, to the bedside 4 hours after the first intraoperative local anesthesia injection to get the patient up on a walking frame to walk out of the room and back and to walk to the toilet to pass urine. Often, this requires an intravenous fluid bolus of about 300 mL and on occasions a dose of atropine to prevent vasovagal fainting. Walking is compulsory provided the patient is deemed able, and if the patient objects, we argue with them especially as they have been well prepared to expect this initiative.

After successful completion of the first walk, patients are expected to take further walks every 2 to 3 hours until about 8 PM after which they may stay in bed if they wish. A walking frame is used on the first few occasions, but patients progress to using elbow crutches as soon as they are capable (often on the second walk). Toilet privileges are immediate on completion of the first walk, and sitting out of bed for short periods is encouraged and provides an opportunity to maintain general hygiene and refresh the bed linen, which may have become contaminated. The in-hospital mobilization schedule is completed early on the morning after surgery and is supervised usually (but not always) by a senior member of the medical team. The patient is required to demonstrate that they can transit from lying in bed to standing upright, climb a flight of stairs, walk about 30 meters, and manage the toilet all with minimal assistance before being certified as ready for discharge.

Physiotherapy assistance with early mobilization is important, especially as patients often need to be mobilized while the surgical team is still occupied in the operating room. The physiotherapist also has a role in preoperative education (including but not limited to the use of crutches and walking sticks and the provision of a mobilization program), teaching coping techniques such as managing stairs, toilet, and exiting bed, and providing a safety checkout for independent mobility.

In the first few days after leaving hospital, walking around the house every few hours and the normal activities of daily living are sufficient physiotherapy. The prime goal of this period is to recover from the operation and allow the wound to heal. Specific physiotherapy directed at developing problems can be arranged after a couple of weeks on the first or subsequent postoperative visits and can be accomplished on an outpatient basis.

Reducing Hospital Stay

Hospitals can be dangerous places. The risks patients are exposed to include:

• Infection with resistant organisms
• Medication errors
• Enforced bed rest
• Iatrogenic illness from overzealous interference

Nosocomial infection with multiresistant organisms has become a major problem in most hospitals. In many hospitals, inpatients are often sick, and cross-infection is inevitable under these circumstances. Over the past nine years, we have had only 4 deep infections recorded in over 700 BHR cases (0.6%) and no deep infections in 117 modular BHR patients. We attribute this result to our early discharge strategy. No patients were infected with multiresistant organisms, all four infected patients were successfully treated with antibiotics, and no prosthesis was removed on account of infection. If the patient has no pain and we are confident they will not develop pain, is independently mobile, is otherwise well, and has a suitable home environment, then the hospital can make little further positive contribution to his outcome and he should be discharged to the comfort of his own home. Early discharge also fosters an expectation of wellness, and placing patients in charge of their own management forces them to abandon the "sick role," both of which are positive contributors to full recovery. Finally, of course, early discharge significantly reduces the cost to the patient, often an important factor for them.

Our full discharge criteria are

• Adequate pain control (Numerical Rating Scale 0 to 3), top-up completed
• Physiologic stability

  ◦ No postural hypotension, no nausea
  ◦ Normal urine output, no urinary retention
  ◦ Clear head, minimal sedation

• Hemoglobin >80 g/L, no bleeding
• Oral intake of liquids and solids tolerated without nausea

- No uncontrolled comorbidities (e.g., diabetes, heart failure)
- Independent mobility

  ○ Transfer from bed to standing satisfactorily
  ○ Manage toilet
  ○ Walk approximately 30 m and manage one flight of stairs with minimal assistance

- Suitable attitude
- Suitable home with adequate assistance at home
- Suitable transport arrangements
- Adequate contact information and phone support

Over the past 9 years, 526 of 700 (75.1%) of our BHR patients and 41 of 117 (35%) modular head BHR patients were discharged directly home after a single overnight stay. The introduction of target controlled remifentanyl/propofol intravenous anesthesia and the use of Buprenorphine transdermal patches for residual pain control at the end of 2005 has enabled us to further improve these outcomes, such that between January 2006 and May 2008, 186/201 BHR patients (93%) and 20/32 (63%) modular head BHR patients were discharged home after a single overnight stay.

Postoperative Surveillance and Rescue

Readmission to hospital should be a rare event. Over the past 5 years, our readmission rate for all causes within the first 28 days after operation has been 2.6% for BHR and 1% for modular head Birmingham hip replacement patients. This rate is lower than our readmission rate when we routinely discharged patients 10 days after operation and reflects lower wound infection rates.

Nonetheless, it is not reasonable to send patients home immediately after surgery and expect them to fend for themselves entirely. They must believe they have support at all times and appreciate that if they strike trouble, help is immediately at hand by contacting the team. They will need some help at home, and we insist on having a responsible adult with them on the first postoperative night to comply with guidelines for day surgery.

TABLE 30.1. Postoperative surveillance

Period	Activity
Evening of surgery	Postoperative ward round by surgeon, anesthetist, and nurse
Morning after surgery	Pain catheter reinjected. Patient checked for adequacy of pain control and performance measured against discharge criteria
After discharge	Patients phone in on arrival at home
Postoperative day 2	Anesthetist phones to check on pain management before 10 AM
Days 4 to 6	Nurse assistant follows up with patient by phone, about day 4 or 5
Day 7	Office visit to nurse assistant
Day 10	Consultation with surgeon

Surveillance by the surgical team must not cease on discharge from the hospital. All the usual checks that used to happen in the hospital must now extend to the home. Our usual routine is described in the next section (Table 30.1).

A rescue plan must be in place if the patient gets into any difficulty such as uncontrolled pain, hemorrhage, or severe continuing nausea and vomiting. The vital link is communication—the patient must have a series of phone numbers to call if they need help so that they can be *sure* of contacting help at any time 24 hours per day. A well-oiled procedure for recovery to hospital needs to be in place should the need arise.

Notwithstanding the above considerations, not all patients can or should be discharged early. The most common reasons for discharge later than 24 hours are poor social support, no transport, remote location, no help, unsuitable house, cultural expectations, and third-party payers.

References

1. Kerr DR, Kohan L. Local infiltration analgesia: a technique for the control of acute postoperative pain following hip and knee surgery. A case study of 325 patients. Acta Ortho 2008;79.
2. Pearse EO, Caldwell BF, Lockwood RJ, Hollard J. Early mobilisation after conventional knee replacement may reduce the risk of postoperative venous thromboembolism. J Bone Joint Surg Br 2007;89:316–22.

31
Final Thoughts

Derek J.W. McMinn

The history of hip resurfacing is full of perplexing issues. The first puzzle relates to Charnley and his Teflon on Teflon double cup arthroplasty. It is recorded that there was absolute relief of pain in Charnley's earliest cases, and the range of hip movements under muscular control were impressive within the first 3 months after operation. As we know, these Teflon double cups failed and Charnley reported this [1]. However, he recorded the cause of failure in this operation as being due to ischemic necrosis of the femoral head. It can been seen on visiting the Wrightington museum that an outstanding failure mechanism from this procedure was marked wear of the implant material (Fig. 31.1).

It seems extraordinary that a man with such mechanical knowledge would ignore obvious wear-through of components and instead blame the failure on ischemic necrosis of the femoral head. It seems even more puzzling that Charnley would then move on to use Teflon cups against a metal total hip replacement component from 1958–1961, and, as we know, this experiment also ended in failure with many of these patients having to be revised because of severe pelvic osteolysis. Happily, much later, Charnley did explain the wear-through of the Teflon resurfacing components in a paper published in 1974 [2]. He explained that the Teflon surfaces stuck together in use, and he explained that the wear-through of the acetabular component was due to movement against bone. He described the presence of some unknown brown material at the Teflon-Teflon articulation that he believed was responsible for the two surfaces sticking together. There is no published histology from Charnley's resurfacing cases that I can find, but I wonder if the "ischemic necrosis" was really osteolytic destruction of the femoral head caused by a massive Teflon particle load. Charnley was focused on the issue of frictional torque, and Teflon, as part of the bearing couple, was obviously very attractive to him. He was not attracted to the idea of a metal on metal couple as I showed in Chapter 1. The pendulum comparator that Charnley constructed was complex, but he did have another demonstration in his laboratory that was a much more simple setup (Fig. 31.2). Here, metal on Teflon, metal on polyethylene, and metal on metal couples were tested with and without load.

The visitor was invited to rotate the bearing using a handle in the unloaded and loaded state and, of course, when load was applied, the metal on metal bearing was difficult to move. This convinced the visitor of the superiority of the metal on polyethylene articulation from a frictional torque viewpoint. The frictional torque offered by the metal on metal couple in this setup relates absolutely to the precise design of the metal on metal articulation. An equatorial or an annular bearing will tend to jam under load in this experiment, whereas a polar bearing metal on metal articulation will move freely under load (see attached DVD). I am amazed that McKee or Ring or Scales, all designers of metal on metal total hip replacement systems, did not attempt to show Charnley and other colleagues that if a polar bearing metal on metal articulation had been used in this experiment, then the observed frictional torque would be just as low as with a metal on polyethylene articulation. There seemed to have been an acceptance that Charnley had got it right and indeed McKee, Ring, and Scales all moved from metal on metal articulations to metal on polyethylene articulations for their own total hip replacements eventually. I am also surprised that the engineers, with whom Charnley associated at the time, did not point out to him that if he used a polar bearing metal on metal articulation, this would behave much better than the annular bearing couple he was favoring. It is also surprising to me that tribologists in the ensuing 40 years have not drawn this very obvious issue to the attention of orthopedic surgeons. Much of the bad press received by metal on metal bearings in the 1960s and 1970s would have been eliminated by this very simple experiment. This is all the more remarkable because Ring was obviously getting good results with his latest design of metal on metal implant and in 1989 reported 1085 patients treated between 1972 and 1979 with a 95.01% cumulative survival at 15 to 16 years [3]. As outlined in Chapter 1, there were considerable forces at work to stop metal on metal articulations in favor of metal on polyethylene articulations, but it does seem to me that a relatively poor defense of the metal on metal articulation was mounted. Certainly there were, and still are, issues relating to wear, metal ion production, and hypersensitivity with metal

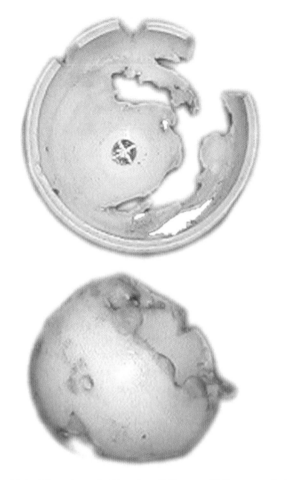

FIG. 31.1. Worn-through Charnley Teflon on Teflon resurfacing components.

on metal bearings. As Prof. Duncan Dowson pointed out, the wear of a metal on metal bearing needs to be kept in perspective. He taught us that the wear experienced by a metal on metal articulation over 15 years of use equates to the volume of one pin-head (Fig. 31.3).

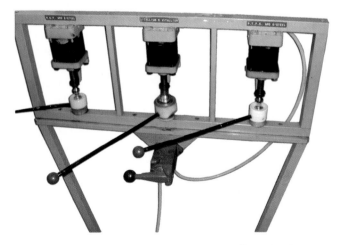

FIG. 31.2. Rig to feel the frictional torque of different bearing couples. (Image supplied courtesy of Mr. Martyn Porter, FRCS, and the Wrightington museum).

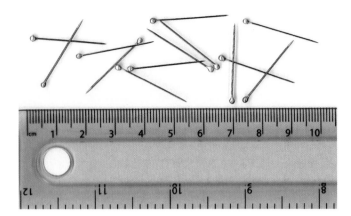

FIG. 31.3. From a lecture delivered by Prof. Duncan Dowson, "Joined at the Hip," London, 2002.

This pin-head volume of metal debris is broken down into many tiny particles that contribute to the metal ion exposure. However, surgeons know well that if wear-through of a polyethylene liner occurs with unintended articulation of the prosthetic femoral head against the acetabular cup shell, or, if impingement of a prosthetic femoral neck THR on an acetabular shell occurs, then the volume of metal debris shed rapidly exceeds the volume of one pin-head. No doubt improvement will be made in the coming years, reducing the wear from metal on metal articulations. However, we must all judge if it is sensible to take a risk with a new implant system to reduce the wear from one pin-head's worth over 15 years to half a pin-head's worth over 15 years. Is one pin-head's worth of metal wear definitely worse than half a pin-head's worth of metal wear occurring over 15 years?

I am sad that I was not able to include a chapter from my friend Dr. Hakan Borg in this book. He had his hip resurfaced by me 10 years ago and has kept up a phenomenal activity level since. When not skiing or swimming over the past few years, he has followed many patients on the Finnish registers who have had metal on metal THRs. Patients have been followed until death, and the metal on metal THR group has been matched with another group of normal Finnish citizens. The conclusion was that the metal on metal group live on average 1.5 years longer than the normal Finnish population [4]. Hart et al. have shown that increased metal ion levels in patients with metal on metal bearings cause a modest reduction in CD8 cells [5]. This is regarded as positive by Hart et al. as it may slow the ageing process. Perhaps these metal ions will turn out to be good for us. The health food industry certainly seems to think so, and a visit to such a store will show that many of these tonics and pills are laden with cobalt and/or chromium.

When I look at my efforts to make hip resurfacing work in the early years as outlined in Chapter 1, I am not proud of my performance. The reader will be forgiven for thinking that I was stumbling from crisis to crisis. As each new problem raised its ugly head, I took the advice of any surgeon who had enough experience of the subject to try and get out of the difficulty I was in. I singled out Mike Freeman earlier but actually that is unfair. In addition to his advice, at various times I took the advice of Furuya in Japan, Trentani in Italy, Wagner in Germany, Amstutz in the United States, and others. What happened? Trouble and then more trouble. I discovered early on that multiple cooks do not always make a good broth.

I often wonder what the landscape would be like if Zimmer had run with my first idea for a metal on metal resurfacing. As a new consultant, I had already looked around for what I considered to be the best acetabular component available and the best femoral component for my THRs. It made no difference to me if they weren't from the same company, all I wanted was the best. I decided on the uncemented Harris-Galante 1 cup and the cemented Exeter stem. This was my THR for many years in higher-demand patients (I still performed cemented cups in older patients), and time has shown that these implants were probably the best available then. Not everyone was happy. I remember Bill Harris not being too impressed that I was performing the Exeter collarless polished stem, and Robin Ling was aghast that I would ever want to do a cementless cup.

When I approached Ian Brown, PhD, the managing director of Zimmer UK in 1988, he knew exactly what I wanted and why. He knew about resurfacing designs and understood that they autodestructed because of polyethylene wear debris. He knew about metal on metal bearings and their manufacture as he had personally been involved in this. He was mad at himself because they had just thrown out a Thielenhaus machine that was thought to be redundant, but in its time was the "Rolls Royce" machine for metal on metal bearing manufacture. He was confident however that they could find a replacement. He knew about ingrowth surfaces, and Zimmer UK at the time applied fibermesh to various Zimmer products. I knew what I wanted. Just like my THR combination, I wanted a fibermesh coated, uncemented cup and a cemented femoral component, and Ian agreed. There we were, one surgeon and one very experienced engineer, agreeing the path ahead for a new implant. If the decision to proceed or not had been in the hands of Zimmer UK, there is no doubt in my mind that we would have done it. On the basis of everything I now know, this implant design would have been a winner and I, and more importantly many patients, would have been spared the early implant fixation problems that have been outlined. It would have been a clinical winner and, for Zimmer, it would have been a commercial winner. Just think of all the osteolysis caused in the 1990s by non–cross-linked polyethylene that could have been prevented by a good metal on metal resurfacing and a good metal on metal THR. The decision taken by the Zimmer organization not to proceed with this project will have cost them several hundred million dollars. And the reason? Marketing spin. "Surgeons are just not asking for that type of replacement." In 2003, Zimmer purchased Centerpulse, the developer of the Metasul metal on metal THR, for $3.2 billion. Did Centerpulse worry that they had no sales of metal on metal bearings when they started the Metasul development? Of course not! They were a genuine technology-driven company who were not interested in the immediately available fast buck. Too bad they were destroyed by oil contamination of products at a manufacturing plant in the United States. What lessons can we draw from this unfortunate train of events?

Will we ever see a Sir John Charnley or a Maurice Muller again? Probably not, unless there are big changes in the system. These men had clear ideas what they wanted from their implant designs and they had the power to make certain it happened. Did these men care what someone in sales or marketing thought about their designs? I doubt if they were ever subjected to contact from such people. What these men craved were top-quality engineers who could turn good ideas into quality products. Everything is different now, no one surgeon will ever design anything again unless there is radical change. The team approach is now the norm. It is rare to have two surgeons agree on a design; what happens when there are 10 surgeons on the design team? And then, of course, marketing have their say and regulatory departments have their say, not to mention a host of other hangers-on. What about the engineers? They will be told when the design is decided on! What I see are two things. Usually as an ill-considered response to a trailblazing new competitor product, I have seen designs emerge from these big teams that incorporate all the ideas of the team into the product. Everything is changed from products that went before, and if there are bad results from such a device, the question is, which of the 10 changes we made is causing the device to fail? This is not a hypothetical situation. One hip resurfacing device is performing badly on the Australian register. Multiple changes compared with predicate devices have been made, and now the question is, what should be changed? These types of experiments are only carried out in uncivilized countries, namely all countries outside the United States.

In the United States, there are also big design teams, only here the final product that emerges is very different. Regulatory affairs people decide what may be done. The design must not actually be different to predicate devices. The goal of the design team (apart from receiving a royalty payment) is to make the design appear to be different for marketing reasons. The end result is that nothing of any clinical importance is improved. The bizarre truth is that nearly all the implant companies are U.S. corporations, they have boring products for the United States for regulatory reasons, and, to a variable degree, have in addition experimental products for the rest of the world. This, I suggest, is not good for either the U.S. patients or patients elsewhere. Many of the top surgeons in the world work in the United States. Why are they considered such dimwits by the U.S. regulatory authorities? Surely, the U.S. surgeon is at least as well-equipped as surgeons elsewhere at deciding what is, and what is not, a good product for their patients?

Do the regulatory authorities always make the right decision? The Cormet 2000 resurfacing has just been given regulatory approval in the United States largely on the basis of 2-year clinical data, which is the normal U.S. IDE requirement. This implant started life as the McMinn 1996 resurfacing as outlined in Chapter 1. The big "improvement" made over the predicate device was the addition of plasma-sprayed titanium to the cup (see Chapter 6). The results of the McMinn 1996 started to dip at 5.5 years and produced an 86% survivorship at 10 years in addition to a 20% radiographic failure rate in unrevised patients. The regulatory authorities have made their decision on very short-term clinical data. Would a well-informed surgeon, free from the shackles of financial interest, view the evidence differently?

The trend over the past few years is that all small implant companies are bought by large U.S. corporations, who in turn amalgamate. Who is served well by this process? The shareholders of the corporations and employees with share options and bonuses are the beneficiaries. Distributors do well, often receiving commissions of 20% on sales. The corporations provide lubrication so the system works for them, with consultancy contracts for surgeons, royalty payments, and institutional financial support being commonplace to ensure brand loyalty. The costs associated with all this are enormous. It can only be afforded because of the fantastic profit margins available in the United States. As explained earlier, implant design is by committee, with little prospect of better implants resulting. Most of this process is intended to give the illusion of a "high tech" company with a major interest in design and development. That is why the spin doctors are involved in design teams. There is no intention of developing a "new" implant; that would be a regulatory and financial nightmare. In reality, surgeons have to cope with a smaller product range. When amalgamation of corporations happens, large numbers of lesser-known niche products are abandoned, and surgeons are forced to use the limited range of core products. Corporations ensure that their design teams have an international feel, but in effect the overseas surgeons are "political" appointees and are mere paid pawns in the process. How will the little-known surgeon working in some far-off land with a great idea for a new product get on in this system? He doesn't stand a chance. Ultimately, the losers will be patients, with potentially great ideas never tested. If for any reason the profit margins in the United States came down to the level of the rest of the world, there would be a serious meltdown of many corporations. A clampdown on lubrication would only increase company profits. The really serious problem would be third-party payers developing a taste for European-priced products, or worse still a cap on reimbursement for implants, like the system in France. I believe the system will melt down, and I predict chaos in large corporations with major "corrections" necessary. Small companies will come back into play, and this will be good for the "driven" designer surgeons irrespective of geographic location and ultimately good for genuine product development and patients.

The next puzzle relates to the history of metal on metal bearings, in particular, the history of metal on metal bearings in hip resurfacing. In Chapter 1, I outlined the history of hip resurfacing and metal on metal bearings from a very personal viewpoint and within my own experience. There have been two volumes of *Clinical Orthopaedics* that deserve attention. The first was in 1978, which attempted to review all the art at

the time. This volume concentrated on hip resurfacing. The second was in 1996, and this reviewed the reintroduction of metal on metal articulations and attempted to cover the history of metal on metal bearings. As I shall now show, both of these collector items have a very significant omission, and this omission has also been made in much of the history of this subject that has been written.

At an American Academy of orthopaedic surgeons' conference in 2001, I had a long meeting with Charles Townley (Fig. 31.4). What an interesting and innovative surgeon! He designed and implanted the first condylar total knee replacement. He had done much work on conservative hip arthroplasty, and it was on this subject that I wanted to get his views. At the time of our meeting, he was against metal on metal articulations, and he tried to encourage me away from metal on metal as a bearing material for my resurfacing. He was very focused (another one!) on frictional torque, and he believed that the frictional torque and wear of metal on metal articulations with the resultant ion exposure was not good. He was trying to encourage me down the route of using polyurethane because, as we all know, the theoretical advantages of a soft bearing with genuine fluid film lubrication are considerable. I found our conversation most stimulating, but he did reveal one fact at the time. He said he had done some metal on metal hip resurfacings but again he advised me against this. I pursued my quest for information on exactly what Townley had done, and now we know. Dr. Jim Pritchett has followed up a large cohort of Townley's and his own cases, and you will see that Townley's definition of "some" is understated. He performed 133 metal on metal resurfacings with a mean follow-up of 26 years and a zero failure rate.

If I get any credit for the introduction of modern metal on metal hip resurfacing, then Charles Townley deserves huge credit for having made this operation work many years ago.

Sadly, Charles Townley died recently, and I am going to give the last words in this book to Dr. Jim Pritchett so that the

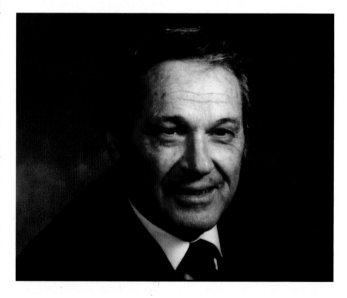

Fig. 31.4. Charles Townley at approximately 58 years (1916–2006).

history books can record correctly the tremendous work of a great innovator and show conclusively that metal on metal hip resurfacing is not new and can be remarkably successful.

References

1. Charnley J. Arthroplasty of the hip. A new operation. Lancet 1961;1:1129–1132.

2. Charnley J. Total hip replacement. JAMA 1974;230:1025–1028.

3. Ring P. Press-fit prostheses: clinical experience. In: Reynolds D, Freeman M, eds. Osteoarthritis in the Young Adult Hip. London: Churchill Livingstone, 1989:220–232.

4. Borg H. Personal communication, 2007.

5. Hart AJ, Hester T, Sinclair K, Powell JJ, Goodship AE, Pele L, Fersht NL, Skinner J. The association between metal ions from hip resurfacing and reduced T-cell counts. J Bone Joint Surg Br 2006;88:449–454.

Conservative total Articular Replacement Arthroplasty: Minimum 20-Year Follow-Up

James W. Pritchett

Abstract Hip joint resurfacing is an attractive concept because it preserves rather than removes the femoral head and neck and may provide better functioning. We report the first long-term follow-up on total hip resurfacing. A total of 445 patients (561 hips) were followed for a minimum of 20 years or until death; only 23 patients were lost to follow-up. Patients received a metal femoral prosthesis with a small curved stem. Three types of acetabular reconstruction were used: (i) cemented polyurethane, (ii) metal on metal, and (iii) polyethylene secured with cement or used as the liner of a two-piece porous-coated implant. Long-term results were favorable with the metal on metal combination only. None of the 121 patients (133 hips) who received a metal on metal articulation experienced failure. The failure rate with polyurethane was 100%, and the failure rate with cemented polyethylene was 41%. Thus, although hip resurfacing using a metal on metal articulation with a curved-stemmed femoral component is a technically demanding procedure, the prosthesis is durable, and the clinical outcome is generally favorable.

Introduction

Hip joint resurfacing offers several functional benefits over total hip replacement: the size of the femoral head and neck remains close to normal, and the resurfaced hip is stable and capable of an excellent range of motion, proprioceptive feedback from the remaining metaphyseal bone may be preserved, and the joint retains a greater degree of normal biomechanical function [1,2,9,18,28,30,31]. It also offers several procedural benefits: postoperative infection is usually resolved easily because only a limited amount of implanted material is used; it is less invasive than is conventional hip replacement because it does not involve decapitation of the femur; and it results in less blood loss, is more stable, and rehabilitates more easily [19,30,31]. The disadvantages of this procedure include the possibility of femoral neck fracture or collapse of the femoral head due to osteonecrosis. Additionally, it is a demanding procedure that requires both anterior and posterior dislocation of the joint.

The first total hip resurfacing arthroplasty was developed by Charnley in 1951 using a polytetrafluoroethylene on polytetrafluoroethylene (Teflon or Fluon) bearing [10]. The procedure failed due to osteonecrosis of the femoral head. In the 1970s, hip resurfacing was popular in several centers in Europe, Japan, England, and the United States. Initial promising results gave way to unacceptable failure rates, however, owing to acetabular loosening, wear, or both. Less commonly, femoral neck fracture, osteonecrosis, or loosening of the femoral component occurred [11,15,24]. Interestingly, none of the other resurfacing designs used a femoral stem.

Resurfacing was largely abandoned again until the 1990s when it was resurrected for the same reasons that made it attractive initially: patients want an active lifestyle, they want to keep their bone, and they don't want to worry about having a failed intramedullary, stem-supported hip prosthesis [2,9,28].

The purpose of this report is to evaluate long-term results of a hip joint resurfacing prosthesis and comment on what we are doing today.

Materials and Methods

Patient Population

We evaluated 561 total hip joint resurfacing procedures that were performed in 445 private practice patients from 1960 to 1987. None of the patients had undergone a prior implant arthroplasty procedure, although a few had been treated previously for a dislocated hip or fracture. The underlying diagnosis was osteoarthritis in 334 patients (75%); osteonecrosis in 44 (10%); posttraumatic arthritis in 31 (7%); inflammatory arthritis in 18 (4%); and developmental dysplasia in 18 (4%) patients.

The patient population consisted of 218 women and 227 men with a mean body weight of 71 and 82 kg, respectively (range, 50–107 kg). The mean age was 52 years (range, 30–74 years) with 97 patients aged 30 to 40 years, 118 aged 40 to 50 years, 109 patients aged 50 to 60 years, 100 aged 60 to 70 years, and 21 patients aged 70 to 74 years. Institutional review board approval was obtained for this study.

Surgical Procedure and Implants

Each surgical procedure was carried out through an antero-lateral approach without trochanteric osteotomy. The hip was dislocated anteriorly, and the femur was prepared. The femoral head was downsized when possible using great care not to notch the femoral neck. The zenith of the femoral head was removed at an approximate 140-degree angle to the femur, and all at-risk bone was removed. Cylinder and chamfer cutters were used to complete the preparation of the femoral head [26]. Whenever possible, the femoral stem was placed parallel to the medial trabecular system [6,11,23]. Prostheses were placed using an interference fit, cemented, or porous-coated technique.

The type of prosthesis varied with the time at which the procedure was done. In the earliest procedures, the acetabular surface used was polyurethane. This polymer was prepared by mixing the prepolymer with resin and the catalyst at the time of surgery and shaped to the femoral prosthesis. Polyurethane served as both the anchoring cement for the femoral side and as the articular replacement and cement for the acetabulum. Although it is a "plastic," it had a fairly rough finish. Metal on metal implants were made of cobalt chromium (Depuy Co., Warsaw, IN; Howmedica Co., Rutherford, NJ; Zimmer Co., Warsaw, IN) (Figs. 31.5 and 31.6).

They were placed without cement on the acetabular side and with or without cement on the femoral side. The length of the stem varied from 27 to 165 mm with longer stems used more commonly in the earlier cases.

Polyethylene, which became available in the 1970s, was initially used in a thickness of 4.5 mm, which was later

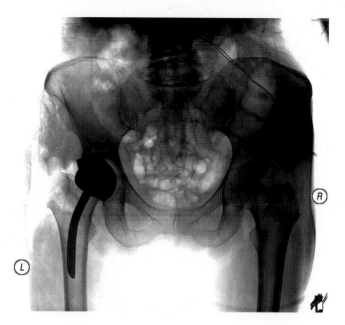

FIG. 31.6. Radiograph of cementless metal-on-metal prothesis.

increased to 6.0 mm and cemented in place using polymethyl-methacrylate. The two-piece metal-polyethylene component was porous-coated with a coxcomb fin for adjunctive fixation (Fig. 31.7).

Patient Follow-Up

Patients were followed prospectively and were asked to return at 1 year, 2 years, 5 years, and every 5 years thereafter. When

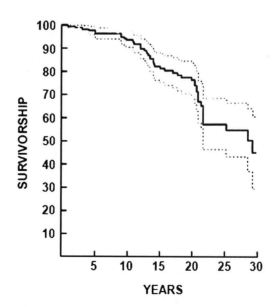

FIG. 31.7. Radiograph of cemented polyethylene cup on one side and a cementless acetabular prosthesis on the other.

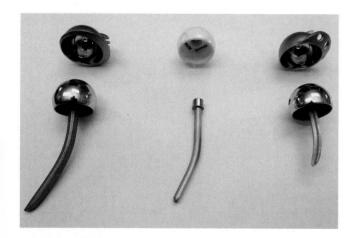

FIG. 31.5. Photograph of the curved stemmed metal on metal and ceramic surface replacements.

FEMORAL COMPONENT

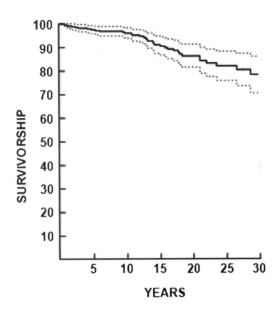

Fig. 31.8. Kaplan-Meier survivorship curve for the femoral component.

TABLE 31.1. Survivorship among patients treated with hip joint resurfacing.

	Number of patients (%)	Mean age of survivors (range) (years)
Overall survivorship		
Survivorship until death	374 (84)	80 (58–99)
<5 years	19 (5)	
5–9 years	24 (6)	
10–19 years	54 (14)	
20–30 years	166 (45)	
>30 years	111 (30)	
Patients alive at follow-up	71 (16)	75 (53–94)
Survival periods		
20–30 years	51 (72)	
30–40 years	18 (25)	
40 years	2 (3)	

this was not possible, they were asked to answer a written questionnaire or were contacted by telephone and interviewed using a standard telephone questionnaire. Patients were queried specifically about the need for additional surgery on their hip. If it had been required, they were asked to provide information about that procedure. The date of death was obtained by direct communication with the family. Information about the patient's hip function was obtained from the family for deceased patients.

Statistical Analysis

Patients were censored at death or at revision. End points consisted of revision or removal of either component for any reason. A 95% confidence interval (CI) was calculated for the Kaplan-Meier survivorship estimates [17]. Survivorship analyses were calculated for each type of acetabular reconstruction employed (Fig. 31.8). Failure was defined by removal or revision or the prosthesis or radiographic evidence of loosening. The Harris hip score was used to evaluate the surgical results [13].

Results

Clinical Results

Ninety-five percent of patients were followed until death or at least 20 years. By 2007, 374 (84%) of the 445 patients had died. The mean age at time of death was 80 years (range, 58–

99 years), and the mean survival time from surgery to the time of death was 22 years. The remaining 71 patients (16%) had been followed an average of 27 years (Table 31.1). The most common complications seen at any time during the follow-up period included deep infection, dislocation, and periprosthetic fracture. The periprosthetic fractures occurred sporadically anytime after the surgical procedure from 6 months to 36 years later. Less frequently, intraoperative fracture and nerve palsy occurred (Table 31.2).

Medical complications of various types occurred in approximately 5% of patients. In 21 procedures, technical difficulties—including poor exposure, change in intraoperative alignment and poor impaction of the cup or stem—were associated with obesity.

Patients were assessed for pain and function 2 years after the resurfacing procedure. Most patients experienced no pain, and only four (<1%) experienced severe pain. Of the 445 assessed for postsurgical activity, a third participated in athletics or strenuous work and only 22 (5%) did not work or participate in activities. Ninety percent were not limited in their activities (Table 31.3).

TABLE 31.2. Complications of hip joint resurfacing procedures.

Complications	Number of patients (%)	Comments
Deep infection	11 (2)	Over lifetime of prosthesis
Dislocation	5 (<1)	
Periprosthetic fracture (hips)	6 (>1)	Inter- and subtrochanteric
Femoral neck fractures	10 (1.7)	
Intraoperative femoral neck fracture	1	Converted to total hip replacement
Femoral nerve palsy	2	Both patients recovered
Sciatic palsy	5 (<1)	Recovery: 2 full; 2 partial; 1 limited due to peroneal and tibial involvement

TABLE 31.3. Functional results of hip joint resurfacing.

Pain	Number of patients (%)	Comments
Assessed 2 years after procedure		
No pain	459 (82)	
Slight pain	86 (15)	
Moderate pain	12 (2)	
Severe pain	4 (<1)	
Function: Postsurgical activity (Assessed 2 years after procedure in 445 patients)		
Highly active	147 (33)	Strenuous sports or job
Active and no limitations necessary	254 (57)	
Moderately active	22 (5)	
Inactive	22 (5)	
Patient satisfaction		
Satisfied with outcome	427 (96)	
Dissatisfied with outcome	18 (4)	Nine patients were dissatisfied because of a limp or weakness. Nine patients were dissatisfied because of pain.

Most patients reported satisfaction with their procedure (Table 31.3). However, 32 of 44 (73%) patients with osteonecrosis experienced prosthesis failure (mean time to failure 7 years). There were 27 (6%) patients who had undergone a resurfacing procedure on one side and a conventional total hip replacement on the other. All indicated that the hip that had undergone resurfacing was the "better hip." There was no difference in the outcomes in this series based on the gender of the patient.

The mean peak Harris Hip score improved from 57 (range, 8–79) to 92 (range, 63–100). Flexion improved from a mean of 83 degrees (range, 5–118 degrees) to a mean of 110 degrees (range, 65–140 degrees) between pre- and postoperative evaluations.

Radiographic Analysis

We attempted to place the femoral component in valgus. With the exception of patients with a preoperative diagnosis of osteonecrosis, there were no cases of femoral loosening or fracture when the femoral component was placed in valgus. Radiography revealed that in 28 hips (5%), the femoral component was in greater than 5 degrees more varus postoperatively than preoperatively compared with the medial trabecular system. It also revealed in some instances: malpositioned acetabular components; malpositioning of both the femoral and acetabular components; notched femoral necks; and incompletely seated femoral components (Table 31.4).

TABLE 31.4. Radiographic findings after hip joint resurfacing.

Radiographic finding	Number of hips (%)	Comments
Femoral component	28 (5)	>5 degrees more varus postoperatively measured vs. medical trabecular system
Acetabular component malpositioned	17 (4)	Includes 11 with hip resurfacing failure
Acetabular and femoral components malpositioned	6 (1)	Includes 3 with hip resurfacing failure
Notched femoral neck	11 (2)	Includes 3 with a femoral neck fracture
Femoral component incompletely seated	2 (<1)	Includes 1 with hip resurfacing failure

There was no difference in outcome based on the length the femoral stem.

Revision of the Resurfacing Prosthesis

All but two of the 141 revisions procedures involved a metal on polyethylene articulation; two involved a metal-on-polyurethane prosthesis. None of the metal-on-metal prostheses required revision (Table 31.5).

Both components were removed, and a new resurfacing prosthesis was inserted in two patients. The acetabular prosthesis alone was revised in 22 hips. The remaining 117 hips requiring revision were converted to a conventional total hip replacement.

Prosthesis Survival

The overall survivorship for the femoral prosthesis was 84% (Fig. 31.8). Failure was seen with every type of prosthesis except the metal on metal prosthesis (Table 31.5). The metal on metal patients had excellent results. Failure rates for the remaining prostheses ranged from 34% to 100%. The highest failure rate was seen with polyurethane. This bearing surface disappeared radiographically over time (Fig. 31.9); thereafter, this prosthesis seemed to function as a hemiarthroplasty.

Of the two patients requiring revision, one was converted to a metal on metal resurfacing, with a good outcome; the other underwent total hip replacement because of a femoral neck fracture. The cemented polyethylene acetabular prosthesis (Fig. 31.6) also resulted in notable failure and revision rates.

Fifteen patients received a two-piece cementless acetabular prosthesis in one hip and a cemented polyethylene in the other (Fig. 31.6). These patients also experienced notable failure rates (Table 31.5).

TABLE 31.5. Revisions of hip joint resurfacing prostheses.

	Type of prosthesis			
	Metal on polyurethane	Metal on metal	Metal on cemented polyethylene	Metal on two-piece cementless with polyethylene
Revision needed	2	0	105	34
Patients/hips	24/26	121/133	222/282	78/120
Mean follow-up, years (range)	24 (20–31)	26 (20–41)	25 (20–31)	21 (20–22)
Patients alive at follow-up	0	0	41	30
Patients lost to follow-up	0	2	15	6
Prosthesis failure rate	100%	0%	41%	34%
	Reason for failure			
More than one reason present in some patients	• Polyurethane wear (26) • Femoral neck fracture (1)	• N/A	• Loosening of acetabulum (76) • Polyethylene wear (30) • Loosening of femoral prosthesis (5) • Femoral neck fracture (6)	• Polyethylene wear (27) • Component loosening with migration (11) • Femoral neck fracture (3)

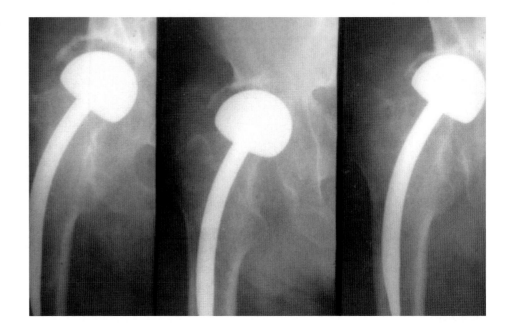

FIG. 31.9. Radiograph of a polyurethane acetabular resurfacing disappearing over time.

Discussion

To determine survivorship over a long period of time, we followed a large series of total hip resurfacing procedures. By following the patients for a minimum of 20 years or until death, we were able to determine their lifetime risk of failure. The high rate of follow-up and large number of patients followed until death suggests the survivorship estimates are valid.

Exposing and positioning the acetabular component with the femoral head in the way is technically difficult, and the preparation of the femoral head is demanding. The survivorship data in this series show more failures in the early years when compared with conventional hip replacement [34]. Failure resulted from unsatisfactory component positioning, loosening, and wear through of early acetabular resurfacing choices.

Complications that can occur with hip resurfacing include dislocation, postsurgical infection, nerve palsy, and fracture.

Dislocations are much less common with resurfacing than with conventional replacement, in part as a result of the larger head size with resurfacing, but also because of superior proprioception compared to total hip replacement. The anterior approach was used in this series and may also enhance stability, but we and others now use the posterior approach with very few dislocations [2,9,28]. The few infections that occurred were easily treated because of the minimal penetration of the prosthesis into the medullary space.

Femoral neck fracture is actually a rare complication after hip resurfacing [2,9,25,28]. Periprosthetic fractures including the femoral neck do occur after hip resurfacing but at a similar rate as periprosthetic fractures with conventional hip arthroplasty [3]. The rate of femoral fracture and loosening was low in all age groups in this series. This was in spite of the effort made to downsize the femoral head that resulted in femoral neck notching in some cases. The low fracture rate even in

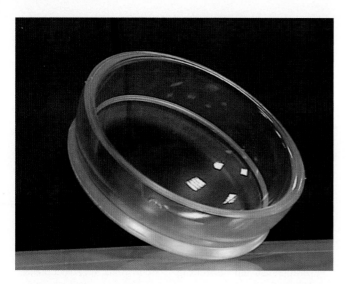

FIG. 31.10. Picture of flexible polyurethane acetabular component.

older individuals is attributed to valgus femoral component positioning. The loading forces on the femoral stem are optimal when they run parallel to the medial trabecular system with the femoral head perpendicular to it, and anatomic studies have shown that the medial trabecular system provides strength to the femoral neck. By contrast, varus positioning increases the tensile stress on the superior cortex, increases the medial compressive torque, and allows shear stress to develop at the prosthesis neck junction [16,24].

Most early resurfacing implants involved hemispherical preparation of the femoral head followed by placement of a hemispherical femoral implant; unfortunately, shear often resulted in loosening of these implants. These implants also did not have a femoral stem [11,15,24,32]. Several attempts have been made over the years to improve resurfacing implants: Gerard used a metal on metal prosthesis but did not fix the acetabular component to the pelvis; Mueller also performed metal on metal resurfacing procedures [12,21]. In this series, we used a prosthesis originally known as "cup-stem arthroplasty," in which the hemisphere was replaced by a flat-topped cylinder. The technique used to place this implant excised at-risk bone in the femoral head, and this may have contributed to the low failure rate. The head design provides compressive resistance stability, and a short, curved stem on the prosthesis adds varus stability without stress relieving the proximal femur [8,20,26,27]. A femoral stem is important in achieving satisfactory long-term results.

The difficulties with hip resurfacing in this series were primarily on the acetabular side. Well-performed femoral resurfacing rarely fails over time; this was true when an interference press-fit technique was used when neither cement nor porous coating was yet available. Early procedures involved the use of materials that did not provide an appropriate acetabular surface. Charnley used polytetrafluoroethylene in the first hip resurfacing procedure, and it failed [4,5]. In this series, polyurethane failed every time. However, polyurethane does not cause an osteolytic reaction; as a result, patients functioned generally well as it wore away. They had some pain, and radiographs of the hip joint looked as though a hemiarthroplasty had been performed (Fig. 31.9). Fortunately, the crude polyurethane used in the early days has now been reformulated. Our new polyurethane has very little wear, it is flexible, and the wear debris does not cause osteolysis. We are able to use our polyurethane cups with or without metal backing and with either a metal or ceramic femoral component (Fig. 31.10).

Another contributor to resurfacing arthroplasty failure in this series (and in others) was the use of cemented polyethylene acetabular components that loosened and wore through, often resulting in osteolysis [1,11,14,15,24]. Metal-backed cemented polyethylene sockets were not used in this series, but others have reported prosthesis failure when they were used in such procedures [22,29]. Our cross-linked polyethylene acetabular component worked better; particularly when used with a ceramic femoral prosthesis (Fig. 31.5).

Theoretically, avoiding a hard on hard joint surface should be advantageous. The strain distribution on the acetabular aspect is adversely affected by the stiffness of a metal component [16,33]. In this study, the use of polyethylene required removing an excessive amount of acetabular bone or insertion of a thin implant that would be prone to wear or loosening. Actually, more patients have the appropriate geometry for hip resurfacing with metal on metal implants than for other implants, because metal on metal devices make it is possible to couple thin heads of large diameter.

In our series, the metal on metal prosthesis was the second type of prosthesis tried. Metal on metal prostheses fell out of favor when polyethylene became available, until the drawbacks of polyethylene became apparent. Today, metal on metal is once again the most popular option. Patients who have received prostheses made of the newer metals do not yet have long-term follow-up. These devices, which require a porous-coated acetabulum and straight femoral stem, are similar to the metal on metal prostheses described in this report. The superior articulating characteristics of the metal surfaces available today suggest that excellent longevity can be expected [2,9,28]. Ions are released from the surface of these devices; the significance of this phenomenon remains unknown. However, no difficulties related to this issue were identified in this study [7].

Conclusion

Hip resurfacing is a technically demanding procedure, but it can be successful, and the results can be satisfying for the patient. Hip resurfacing requires good bone quality, and restitution of significant preoperative limb length inequality is not possible. Moreover, some acetabular deformities cannot be addressed. However, it is an attractive option for a young patient fearing a potentially difficult future revision.

References

1. Amstutz H. Surface replacement arthroplasty. In: Amstutz HC, ed. Hip Arthroplasty Edinburgh: Churchill Livingstone, 1991;295–332.
2. Amstutz H, Beaule P, Dorey F, LeDuff M, Campbell P, Gruen T. Metal-on-metal hybrid surface arthroplasty: two to six-year follow-up study. J Bone Joint Surg Am 2004;86:28–39.
3. Berry D. Epidemiology: hip and knee. Orthop Clin North Am 1979:30:183–190.
4. Charnley J. Arthroplasty of the hip-a new operation. Lancet 1961; 1:1129–1132.
5. Charnley J. Low Friction Arthroplasty of the Hip. Theory and Practice. New York: Springer 1979.
6. Clark J, Freeman M, Witham D. The relationship of neck orientation to the shape of the proximal femur. J Arthroplasty 1987;2:99–109.
7. Clark M, Lee P, Arora A, Villar R. Levels of metal ions after small and large diameter metal-on-metal hip arthroplasty. J Bone Joint Surg Am 2003;85:913–917.
8. Collier J, Kennedy F, Mayor M, Townley C. The importance of stem geometry, porous coating and collar angle of femoral hip prosthesis on the strain distribution in the normal femur. Trans Soc Biomater 1983;9:96.
9. Daniel J, Pynsent P, McMinn D. Metal-on-metal resurfacing arthroplasty of the hip in patients under 55 years with osteoarthritis. J Bone Joint Surg Br 2004;86:177–184.
10. Freeman M. Total surface replacement hip arthroplasty. Clin Orthop Relat Res 1978;134:2–4.
11. Freeman M, Cameron H, Brown G. Cemented double cup arthroplasty of the hip: a 5-year experience with the ICLH prosthesis. Clin Orthop Relat Res1978;134:45–52.
12. Gerard Y. Hip arthroplasty by matching cups. Clin Orthop Relat Res 1978;134:25–35.
13. Harris W. Traumatic arthritis of the hip after dislocation and acetabular fractures: Treatment by mold arthroplasty. J Bone Joint Surg Am 1969;51:737–755.
14. Head W. Total articular resufacing arthroplasty: analysis of failure in 67 hips. J Bone Joint Surg Am 1984;66:28–34.
15. Howie D, Campbell D, McGee M, Cornish B. Wagner resurfacing hip arthroplasty: the results of one hundred consecutive arthroplasties after eight to ten years. J Bone Joint Surg Am 1990;72:708–714.
16. Huiskes R, Streus P, Van Heck J. Interface stresses in the resurfaced hip: finite element analysis of load transmission in the femoral head. Acta Orthop Scand 1985;56:474–478.
17. Kaplan E, Meier P. Nonparametric estimation from incomplete observations. J Am Statist Assoc 1958;53:457–481.
18. Lilikaki A, Arora A, Villar R. Early rehabilitation comparing hip resurfacing and total hip replacement. Hip Int 2005:15:189–194.
19. Long J, Bartel D. Surgical variables affect mechanics of a hip resurfacing system. Clin Orthop Relat Res 2006;453:115–122.
20. Mesko J, Goodman F, Stanesco S. Total articular replacement arthroplasty: a three-to ten-year case-controlled study. Clin Orthop Relat Res 1994;300:168–177.
21. Mueller M. The benefits of metal-on-metal total hip replacement. Clin Orthop Relat Res 1995;311:54–59.
22. Pritchett J. Success rates of the TARA hip. Am J Orthop 1998;27:658.
23. Pritchett J, Perdue K. The neck shaft-plate shaft angle in slipped capital femoral epiphysis. Orthop Rev 1989;28:1187–1192.
24. Ritter M, Lutring J, Berend M, Pierson J. Failure mechanisms of total hip resurfacing. Clin Orthop Relat Res 2006;453:110–114.
25. Shimmin A, Back D. Femoral neck fractures following Birmingham hip resurfacing. J Bone Joint Surg Br 2005;87:463–464.
26. Townley C. Hemi and total articular replacement arthroplasty of the hip with a fixed femoral cup. Orthop Clin North Am 1982;13:869–893.
27. Townley C, Walker S. Intramedullary cup-stem arthroplasty of the hip. J Bone Joint Surg Am 1961;43:602.
28. Treacy R, McBryde C, Pynsent P. Birmingham hip resurfacing – A minimum follow-up of five years. J Bone Joint Surg Br 2005;87:167–170.
29. Treuting R, Waldman D, Hooten J, Schmalzried T, Barrack R. Prohibitive failure rate of the total articular replacement arthroplasty at five to ten years. Am J Orthop 1997;27:114–118.
30. Vail T, Mina C, Yergler J, Pietroban R. Metal-on-metal hip resurfacing compares favorably with THA at 2 years followup. Clin Orthop Relat Res 2006;123–131.
31. Vendiottoli P, Lavigne M, Roy A, Lusignan D. A prospective randomized clinical trial comparing metal-on-metal total hip replacement and metal-on-metal total hip resurfacing in patients less than 65 years old. Hip Int 2006:16:73–81.
32. Wagner H. Surface replacement arthroplasty of the hip. Clin Orthop Relat Res 1978;134:102–130.
33. Watanabe Y, Shiba N, Matsuo S, Biomechanical study of resurfacing arthroplasty: Finite element analysis of the femoral component. J Arthroplasty 2000;15:505–511.
34. Wroblewski B, Taylor G, Siney O. Charnley low-friction arthroplasty 19-25-year results. Orthopedics 1992;15:421–424.

Index

Printed in the United States of America

🐎 Springer